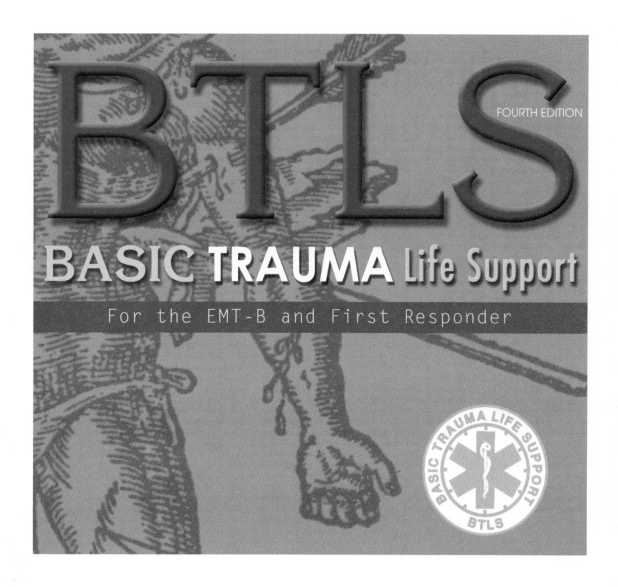

BTLS

FOURTH EDITION

BASIC TRAUMA Life Support

For the EMT-B and First Responder

Edited by
John Emory Campbell, MD, FACEP

Basic Trauma Life Support International, Inc.

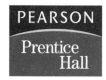

PEARSON

Prentice
Hall

Upper Saddle River, New Jersey 07458

Library of Congress Cataloging-in-Publication Data

BTLS : basic trauma life support for the EMT-B and the first responder /
edited by John Emory Campbell.—4th ed.

   p. ; cm.

  Includes index.

  ISBN 0-13-189378-5

  1. Emergency medicine.   2. Life support systems (Critical care)   3.
Emergency medical technicians.

  [DNLM: 1. Emergency Medical Services—United States.   2.
Emergencies—United States.   3. Life Support Care—methods—United
States.   4. Wounds and Injuries—United States.   WX 215 B916 2004   I.
Title: Basic trauma life support for the EMT-B and the first responder.
II. Campbell, John E.

RC86.7 .C342 2004

616.02′5—dc22

                                          2003024196

Publisher: *Julie Levin Alexander*
Publisher's assistant: *Regina Bruno*
Senior acquisitions editor: *Tiffany Price Salter*
Senior managing editor for development: *Lois Berlowitz*
Editorial assistant: *Joanna Rodzen-Hickey*
Senior marketing manager: *Katrin Beacom*
Channel marketing manager: *Rachele Strober*
Marketing coordinator: *Janet Ryerson*
Director of production and manufacturing: *Bruce Johnson*
Managing editor for production: *Patrick Walsh*
Production liaison: *Julie Li*
Production editor: *Bruce Hobart/Pine Tree Composition, Inc.*
Media editor: *John Jordan*
Media production manager: *Amy Peltier*
Media project manager: *Stephen Hartner*
Manufacturing manager: *Ilene Sanford*
Manufacturing buyer: *Pat Brown*
Creative director: *Cheryl Asherman*
Interior designer: *Mary Siener*
Cover designer: *Blair Brown*
Composition: *Pine Tree Composition, Inc.*
Printing and binding: *The Banta Company*
Cover printer: *Phoenix Color Corp.*

NOTICE ON CARE PROCEDURES

It is the intent of the authors and publisher that this textbook be used as part of an education program taught by qualified instructors and supervised by a licensed physician. The procedures described in this textbook are based upon consultation with paramedics, nurses, and physicians. The authors and publisher have taken care to make certain that these procedures reflect currently accepted clinical practice; however, they cannot be considered absolute recommendations.

The material in this textbook contains the most current information available at the time of publication. However, federal, state, and local guidelines concerning clinical practices, including, without limitation, those governing infection control and universal precautions, change rapidly. The reader should note, therefore, that new regulations may require changes in some procedures.

It is the responsibility of the reader to familiarize himself or herself with the policies and procedures set by federal, state, and local agencies as well as the institution or agency where the reader is employed. The authors and the publisher of this textbook and the supplements written to accompany it disclaim any liability, loss, or risk resulting directly or indirectly from the suggested procedures and theory, from any undetected errors, or from the reader's misunderstanding of the text. It is the reader's responsibility to stay informed of any new changes or recommendations made by any federal, state, and local agency as well as by his or her employing institution or agency.

NOTICE ON GENDER USAGE

The English language has historically given preference to the male gender. Among many words, the pronouns, "he" and "his" are commonly used to describe both genders. Society evolves faster than language, and the male pronouns still predominate our speech. The authors have made great effort to treat the two genders equally, recognizing that a significant percentage of EMS Providers are female. However, in some instances, male pronouns may be used to describe both males and females solely for the purpose of brevity. This is not intended to offend any readers of the female gender.

Pearson Prentice Hall™ is a trademark of Pearson Education, Inc.
Pearson® is a registered trademark of Pearson plc
Prentice Hall® is a registered trademark of Pearson Education, Inc.

Pearson Education LTD.
Pearson Education Singapore, Pte. Ltd
Pearson Education, Canada, Ltd
Pearson Education–Japan
Pearson Education Australia PTY, Limited
Pearson Education North Asia Ltd

Pearson Educaçion de Mexico, S.A. de C.V.
Pearson Education Malaysia, Pte. Ltd
Pearson Education, Upper Saddle River, New Jersey

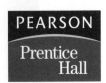

10 9 8 7 6 5 4 3 2 1
ISBN 0-13-189378-5

BTLS
25th Anniversary Edition

The 25th Anniversary Edition is dedicated in memory of Shirley M. Kimble, EMT-P. Shirley excelled at being a paramedic, a teacher, and a leader. During her term on the Board of Directors of BTLS her dedication, leadership, and infectious enthusiasm inspired us. Like a fragrant flower she blessed our lives for a little while and then all too soon she was gone. In an organization dedicated to saving lives it hurts that much more to lose someone you love. We miss you, Shirley.

From the BTLS Board of Directors and the whole BTLS family

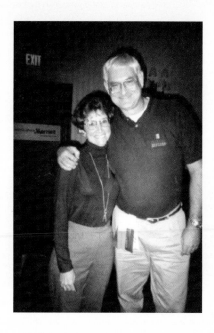

CONTENTS

AUTHORS

BTLS for the EMT-B and First Responder

Roy L. Alson, PhD, M.D., F.A.C.E.P., F.A.A.E.M.
Associate Professor of Emergency Medicine
Wake Forest University School of Medicine
Medical Director, NC Baptist Hospital AirCare
Assistant Medical Director, Forsyth County EMS

Gail V. Anderson Jr., M.D., F.A.C.E.P.
Medical Director
Harbor-UCLA Medical Center
Assistant Dean
UCLA School of Medicine
Los Angeles, California

James J. Augustine, M.D., F.A.C.E.P.

Jere F. Baldwin, M.D., F.A.C.E.P., F.A.A.F.P.
Chief, Department of Emergency
Medicine and Ambulatory Services
Mercy Hospital
Port Huron, Michigan

Russell Bieniek, M.D., F.A.C.E.P.
Medical Director of Emergency Services
Saint Vincent Health System
Erie, Pennsylvania

Walter J. Bradley, M.D., M.B.A., F.A.C.E.P.
Director, Trauma and Emergency Services
Trinity Medical Center
Rock Island, Illinois

John E. Campbell, M.D., F.A.C.E.P.

Leon Charpentier, EMT-P

James H. Creel Jr., M.D., F.A.C.E.P.

Ann M. Dietrich, M.D., F.A.A.P., F.A.C.E.P.
Attending Physician
Emergency Department
Columbus Children's Hospital
Clinical Assistant Professor
Ohio State University
State Medical Director
Ohio Chapter, BTLS

Raymond L. Fowler, M.D., F.A.C.E.P.

Jonathan I. Groner, M.D., F.A.C.S., F.A.A.P.
Trauma Medical Director
Children's Hospital
Columbus, Ohio

Donna Hastings, EMT-P
EMS Program Director
Grant MacEwan Community College
Edmonton, Alberta, Canada

Leah J. Heimbach, J.D., R.N., NREMT-P
General Counsel
WVU Hospitals, Inc.
Morgantown, West Virginia

Pam Kirkpatrick, R.N.
Program Director
AirMedTeam
Rocky Mountain Helicopters
Redding, California

Roger J. Lewis, M.D., Ph.D., F.A.C.E.P.
Associate Professor of Medicine
UCLA School of Medicine
Director of Research
Department of Emergency Medicine
Harbor-UCLA Medical Center

David Maatman, NREMT-P/IC
Educator
Cook Research & Education Institute
Spectrum Health
Grand Rapids, Michigan

Richard N. Nelson, M.D., F.A.C.E.P.
Associate Professor of Clinical Emergency Medicine
The Ohio State University
College of Medicine
Medical Director
Emergency Department
The Ohio State University Medical Center

Jonathan G. Newman, M.D., NREMT-P, F.A.C.E.P.
Emergency Physician
United Hospital Center, Inc.
Clarksburg, West Virginia
Clinical Faculty
West Virginia University
Morgantown, West Virginia

Paul M. Paris, M.D., F.A.C.E.P., L.L.D. (Hon.)
Andrew B. Peitzman, M.D., F.A.C.S.
Director, Trauma Services and
Surgical Critical Care
University of Pittsburgh Medical Center

Paul E. Pepe, M.D., M.P.H., F.A.C.E.P., F.C.C.M.

Jonathan M. Rubin, M.D., F.A.A.E.M.

Corey M. Slovis, M.D, F.A.C.P., F.A.C.E.P.
Professor of Emergency Medicine and Medicine
Chairman, Department of Emergency Medicine
Vanderbilt University Medical Center
Nashville, Tennessee
Associate EMS Medical Director
Nashville Fire/EMS

John T. Stevens, NREMT-P
Douglas County Fire/EMS
Paramedic Instructor
Carroll Technical Institute
Douglasville, Georgia

Ronald D. Stewart, O.C., M.D., F.R.C.P.C., F.A.C.E.P., D.S.C. (Hon.)
Professor of Emergency Medicine
Professor of Community Medicine and Epidemiology
Dalhousie University
Halifax, Nova Scotia
Canada

Arlo Weltge, M.D., F.A.C.E.P.
Assistant Professor
Emergency Medicine
UT-Houston Medical School
Medical Director
Houston Community College System
Program in EMS
Medical Director
P & S Ambulance Service

Howard Werman, M.D., F.A.C.E.P.
Associate Professor
Department of Emergency Medicine
The Ohio State University
College of Medicine and Public Health
Columbus, Ohio

Katherine H. West, B.S.N., M.S.Ed., C.I.C.

Janet M. Williams, M.D.
Associate Professor
Department of Emergency Medicine
Director
Center for Rural Emergency Medicine
West Virginia University
Arthur H. Yancy II, M.D., M.P.H., F.A.C.E.P.

INTRODUCTION

The first prehospital trauma course ever developed, Basic Trauma Life Support, was introduced in August of 1982. BTLS began as a local project of the Alabama Chapter of the American College of Emergency Physicians. Because of a similar need for trauma training for Basic EMTs, Basic Trauma Life Support for Basic EMTs and First Responders was first offered in 1988. After many years of dedicated work by volunteer instructors from every level of emergency medicine, BTLS has become internationally accepted as the training course for prehospital trauma care. The original BTLS course was modeled after the Advanced Trauma Life Support course (for physicians) so that the surgeon, emergency physician, trauma nurse, and EMT would think and act along similar lines. The courses differ in many respects because the prehospital situation differs markedly from the hospital.

The American College of Emergency Physicians and the National Association of EMS Physicians endorse Basic Trauma Life Support. The U.S. National Registry of Emergency Medical Technicians recognizes the course for 16 hours of credit for continuing education for all levels of EMTs. More than just a packaged course, BTLS has become an international organization of instructors of prehospital trauma care. Each local chapter is represented at the international meetings. The purpose of the organization is to foster trauma training worldwide and to maintain up-to-date high standards for the BTLS course.

Basic Trauma Life Support International, with the experience of training hundreds of thousands of students over the last 22 years, is responsible for the fourth edition of BTLS for Basic EMTs and First Responders. Authors include distinguished trauma surgeons, emergency physicians, emergency nurses, and paramedics. The authors are balanced between those in academics and "field providers." We have attempted to make changes that make the book more practical and thus more relevant to the real environment of the prehospital situation. Because EMS varies widely over the world, we have added some optional skill stations. There are several chapters that are not included in the course itself but that are pertinent to trauma care.

This course is designed for the EMT-B or First Responder, who must initially evaluate and stabilize the trauma patient. Since this is a critical time in the management of these patients, this course is intended to teach the skills necessary for rapid assessment, resuscitation, packaging, and transport. It also stresses those conditions that cannot be stabilized in the field and thus require immediate transport. It is recognized that there is more than one acceptable way to manage most situations, and your Medical Director may modify the procedures described here. You should have the physician who provides Medical Direction to your service go over the material and give you advice on how the procedures are done in your area. When teaching this course, the techniques taught here may be modified to correspond to local or regional standards.

The primary objectives of the course are to teach you the correct sequence of evaluation and the techniques of resuscitation and packaging of the patient. Thus Chapters 1 to 3 are key to this course. You will be given enough practical training to perform these drills rapidly and efficiently, thus giving your patient the greatest chance of arriving at the emergency department in time for definitive care to be lifesaving.

ACKNOWLEDGMENTS

Special thanks to these friends of BTLS who provided invaluable assistance with ideas, reviews, and corrections of the text. This was such a big job, and there were so many people who contributed, that I am sure I have left someone out. My apologies in advance. It is sad to be getting old and forgetful.

Ronald Audette, NREMT-P

Roy Alson, M.D., F.A.C.E.P.

Jere Baldwin, M.D., F.A.C.E.P.

David Barrick, B.S., NREMT-P

David Burkland, M.D., F.A.C.E.P.

Jackie Campbell, R.N.

Leon Charpentier, EMT-P

Dennis Cheek, Ph.D., R.N., C.C.R.N.

Jay Cloud

John Commander, EMT-P

Buddy Denson, EMT-P

David Effron, M.D., F.A.C.E.P.

Daniel Ferreira, M.D.

Cathy Gibson, B.S., EMT-P

K. H. Han, M.D., F.R.C.S., F.F.A.E.M.

Donna Hasting, EMT-P

Leah Heimbach, J.D., R.N., NREMT-P

Eduardo Romero Hicks, M.D.

David Maatman, NREMT-P/IC

Brian Mahoney, M.D., F.A.C.E.P.

Kevin D. Neilson, M.D.

Jonathan Newman, M.D., F.A.C.E.P.

Randy Orsborn, EMT-P

William Pheifer III, M.D., F.A.C.S.

John T. Stevens, EMT-P

Ron Stewart, M.D., F.A.C.E.P.

Robert Waddell II, EMT-P

Arlo Weltge, M.D., F.A.C.E.P.

Brian J. Wilson, NREMT-P

Another special thanks goes to the following photographers who donated their work to help illustrate the text.

Roy Alson, M.D., F.A.C.E.P.

Brant Burden, EMT-P

Leon Charpentier, EMT-P

Buddy Denson, EMT-P

Pamela Drexel, Brain Trauma Foundation

David Effron, M.D., F.A.C.E.P.

Kyee Han, M.D.

Eduardo Romero Hicks, M.D.

Bonnie Meneely, EMT-P

Nonin Medical, Inc.

Bob Page, NREMT-P

William Pheifer III, M.D., F.A.C.S.

Don Resch

Sam Splints

Thanks to Southern Union State Community College EMS Department and Opelika Fire Department for their help in photographing spinal immobilization scenes.

F.F. Kenny Allen

A.O. Keith Burnett, EMT-P

Lt. Lynn Callahan Jr.

Herbie Clark, EMT-P

Buddy Denson, EMT-P

F.F. Steve Miller

Capt. James C. Morgan Jr., EMT-P

Josh Stevens, EMT-P

BTLS COURSE

ABOUT THE COURSE

Basic Trauma Life Support for the EMT-B and First Responder is a 16-hour comprehensive course covering the skills necessary for rapid assessment, resuscitation, stabilization, and transportation of trauma patients. Created for the EMT-B and First Responder, the primary objectives of the course are to teach the correct sequence of evaluation and the techniques of resuscitation and packaging a patient.

NOTES FOR TEACHERS

Though suitable as a reference text about prehospital trauma care, this book is designed to be part of an organized hands-on course. An Instructor's Guide and slides are available to be used in teaching the BTLS course, which is monitored and certified in each area by the local chapter of Basic Trauma Life Support International, Inc. If you wish to arrange a certified course in your area but do not know the address of your local chapter coordinator, you may write or call:

Basic Trauma Life Support International, Inc.
1 South 280 Summit Avenue
Court B
Oakbrook Terrace, Illinois 60181
Phone: 1-800-495-BTLS

NOTES FOR STUDENTS

The BTLS course is an intensive, demanding experience that requires preparation in advance of the actual course. You should begin studying the book no less than 2 weeks before the course. The actual course is designed not to tell you, but rather to show you and allow you to practice managing trauma patients. If properly prepared, you will find this course to be the most enjoyable you have ever taken.

The first 19 chapters are essential and should be studied thoroughly in the weeks preceding the course. You will be tested on this material. The appendices contain important chapters, but due to time constraints they are not included in the course. You will not be tested on the appendices.

Appendix A contains some optional skills. If any optional skills are to be taught in the course, you will be notified in advance so that you may study them.

For information about BTLS or if you would like to place an order for textbooks, call 1-800-495-BTLS.

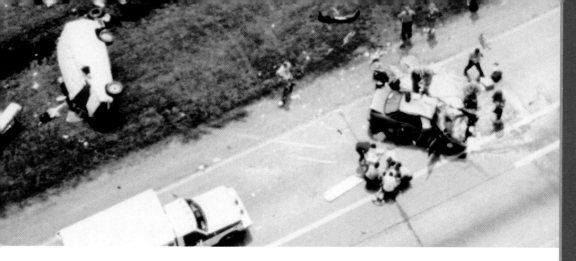

Scene Size-Up

James H. Creel, Jr., M.D., F.A.C.E.P.

Objectives

Upon completion of this chapter, you should be able to:

1. Explain the relationship of time to patient survival and explain how this affects your actions at the scene.

2. Discuss the steps of the Scene Size-up.

3. List the two basic mechanisms of motion injury.

4. Discuss mechanisms and settings for blunt versus penetrating trauma.

5. Identify the three collisions associated with a motor vehicle crash (MVC) and relate potential patient injuries to deformity of the vehicle, interior structures, and body structures.

6. Name the five common forms of MVCs.

7. Describe potential injuries associated with proper and improper use of seat restraints, head rests, and air bags in a head-on collision.

8. Differentiate lateral-impact collision from head-on collision based on the three collisions associated with a MVC.

9. Describe potential injuries from rear-end collisions.

10. Explain why the mortality rate is higher for victims ejected from vehicles in MVCs.

11. Describe the three assessment criteria for falls and relate them to anticipated injuries.

12. Identify the two most common forms of penetration injuries and discuss associated mechanisms and extent of injury.

13. Relate three factors involved in blast injuries to patient assessment.

(Photo courtesy of Bonnie Meneely, EMT-P)

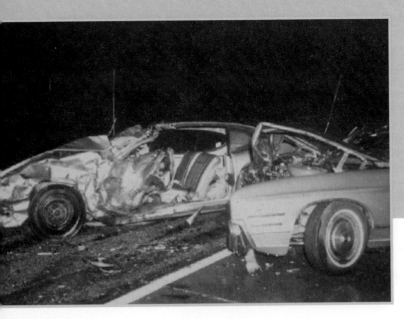

CASE STUDY

Dan, Joyce, and Buddy of the Emergency Transport Service have been dispatched to a two-car collision in which one auto ran into the side of the other. They are informed that a rescue truck is on-scene and attempting to extricate one of the drivers. How do they go about sizing up the scene when they arrive? What should they do before they approach the patients? What equipment should they carry with them when they approach the patient(s)? What injuries should they expect in a collision of this type? Keep these questions in mind as you read the chapter. The case study will continue at the end of the chapter.

INTRODUCTION

Trauma, the medical term for injury, continues to be our most expensive health problem. The fourth leading cause of death for all ages, trauma is the leading cause of death for children and adults under the age of 45 years. For every fatality, there are 10 more patients admitted to hospitals and hundreds more treated in emergency departments. The cost of injury is estimated to be over $210 billion annually. This represents a cost twice that of cardiovascular disease and cancer combined. The price of trauma, in both physical and fiscal resources, mandates that we learn more about this disease to treat its effects and decrease its incidence (see Appendix H, Injury Prevention and the Role of the EMS Provider).

PHILOSOPHY OF ASSESSMENT AND MANAGEMENT OF THE TRAUMA PATIENT

For the severely injured patient, survival is time-dependent. The direct relationship between the timing of definitive (surgical) treatment and the survival of trauma patients was first described by Dr. R. Adams Cowley of the famous Shock-Trauma Unit in Baltimore, Maryland. He discovered that when seriously injured patients were able to gain access to the operating room within an hour of the time of injury, the highest survival rate was achieved (approximately 85%). He referred to this as the "golden hour."

The golden hour begins at the moment the patient is injured, not at the time you arrive at the scene. Rarely is there much of the hour left when you begin your assessment, so you must be very well organized in what you do. In the prehospital setting you do not have a golden hour but rather a "platinum ten minutes" in which to identify live patients, make treatment decisions, and begin to move patients to the appropriate medical facility. This means that every action must have a lifesaving purpose. Any action that increases scene time but is not potentially lifesaving must be deleted. Not only must you reduce evaluation and resuscitation to the most efficient and critical steps, you must also develop the habit of assessing and treating every trauma patient in a planned logical and sequential manner so you don't forget critical actions. We have found it best to proceed in a "head-to-toes" manner so that nothing is missed. If you jump around during your assessment, you will inevitably forget to evaluate something important. Teamwork is very important since many actions must be done at the same time.

It has been said that medicine is a profession that was created for obsessive-compulsive people. Nowhere is this more true than in the care of the trauma patient. Often the patient's life depends on how well you manage the details. Not all of the details occur at the scene of the injury. You or a member of your team must:

1. Maintain your ambulance or rescue vehicle so that it is serviced and ready to respond when needed.
2. Know the quickest way to the scene of an injury.
3. Know how to size up a scene in order to recognize dangers and mechanisms of injury.
4. Know which scenes are safe and if not safe, what to do about it.
5. Know when you can handle a situation and when to call for help.
6. Know when to approach the patient and when to leave with the patient.
7. Know your equipment and maintain it in working order.
8. Know the most appropriate hospital and the fastest way to get there.

As if this were not enough, you also have to know:

1. Where to put your hands.
2. Which questions to ask.
3. What interventions to perform.
4. When to perform the interventions.
5. How to perform critical procedures quickly and correctly.

If you think the details are not important, then leave the profession now. Our job is saving lives, a most honorable profession. If we have a bad day, someone will pay for our mistakes with suffering or even death. Since the early beginnings of Emergency Medical Services (EMS), lives have been lost by patients and, unfortunately, even rescuers, for mistakes in every one of the details listed above. Many of us can recall patients that we might have saved if we had been a little smarter, a little faster, or a little better organized. Make no mistake, there is no "high" like saving a life, but you will carry the scars of your failures all of your life. Your mind-set and attitude are very important. You must be concerned but not emotional, alert but not excited, quick but not hasty. Above all, you must continuously strive for what is best for your patient. When your training has not prepared you for a situation, always fall back on the question: What is best for my patient? When you no longer care, burnout has set in and your effectiveness is severely limited. When this happens it is best to seek help (yes, all of us need help when stress overcomes us) or seek an alternative profession.

Since 1982 the Basic Trauma Life Support (BTLS) organization has been identifying the best methods to get the most out of those few minutes that we have to save the patient's life. We know that not all patients can be saved, but our goal is never to lose a life that could have been saved. The knowledge in this book can help you make a difference. Learn it well.

SCENE SIZE-UP

On-scene trauma assessment begins with certain actions before you approach the patient. Failure to perform these preliminary actions may jeopardize your life as well as the life of your patient. Sizing up the scene is a critical part of trauma assessment. This assessment includes body substance isolation (BSI) review, evaluating the scene for dangers, determining the total number of patients, determining essential equipment needed for this particular scene, and identifying the mechanisms of injuries. Scene Size-up actually begins at dispatch, when you begin to anticipate what you will find at the scene. You should begin to think about what equipment you will need and whether other resources (more units, special extrication equipment, multicasualty incident [MCI] protocols) may be needed. While information from dispatch is useful to begin to think about a plan, don't rely on this information too much. Information given to the dispatcher is often exaggerated or even completely wrong. Be prepared to change your plan depending on your own survey of the scene.

STEPS OF THE SCENE SIZE-UP

1. Body substance isolation review
2. Scene safety
3. Initial triage (total number of patients)
4. Essential equipment/additional resources needed on-scene
5. Mechanism of injury

BODY SUBSTANCE ISOLATION REVIEW

Trauma scenes are among the most likely to subject the rescuer to contamination by blood or other potentially infectious material (OPIM). Not only are trauma patients often bloody; they frequently require airway management under adverse conditions. Personal protective equipment (PPE) is always needed at trauma scenes. Protective gloves are always needed, and many situations will require eye protection. It is wise for the rescuer in charge of airway management to have a face shield or eye protection and mask. In highly contaminated situations impervious gowns with mask or face shield may also be needed. Remember to protect your patient from body fluids by changing gloves between patients.

SCENE SAFETY

Begin assessing the scene for hazards as you approach. Your first decision is to determine the nearest safe place to park the ambulance or rescue vehicle. You would like the vehicle as close as possible, and yet it must be far enough away from the scene for you to be safe while you are performing the scene assessment. Next, determine if it is safe to approach the patient(s). Things to consider are:

1. *Crash/rescue scenes:* Is there danger from fire or toxic substances? Is there danger of electrocution? Are there unstable surfaces or structures present such as ice, water, slope, or buildings in danger of collapse? Areas with potential for low oxygen levels or toxic chemical levels (sewers, ships' holds, silos, etc.) should never be entered until you have the proper protective equipment and breathing apparatus. You should never enter a dangerous area without a partner and a safety line attached.

2. *Crime scenes:* There may be danger here even after the crime has been committed. You should have law enforcement personnel at the scene, not only for the safety of you and the victims, but also to help preserve evidence.

3. *Bystanders:* You and the victim(s) may be in danger from bystanders. Are bystanders talking in loud, angry voices? Are people fighting? Are weapons present? Is there evidence of the use of alcohol or illegal drugs? Is this a domestic violence scene? You may not be recognized as a rescuer but rather as a symbol of authority and thus attacked. Are there dangerous animals present? Request law enforcement personnel if there is any sign of danger from violence.

Consider whether the scene poses a continued threat to the patient. If there is danger of fire, water, structure collapse, toxic exposure, etc., the patient may have to be moved immediately. This does not mean that you should expose yourself or your partners to unnecessary danger. You may need to call for special equipment and proper backup from the police, fire department, or power company. If the scene is unsafe you should make it safe or try to remove the patients from the scene without putting yourself in danger. Sometimes there is no clearly good way to do this. Use good judgment. You are there to save lives, not give up your own.

TOTAL NUMBER OF PATIENTS

Determine the total number of patients now. If there are more patients than your team can effectively handle, call for backup. Remember that you usually need one ambulance for each seriously injured patient. If there are many patients, establish medical command and initiate multicasualty incident (MCI) protocols. Are all patients accounted for? If the patient(s) is unconscious, and there are no witnesses of the incident, look for clues (schoolbooks or diaper bag, passenger list in a commercial vehicle) that other patients might be present. Carefully evaluate the scene for other patients. This is especially important at night or if there is poor visibility.

ESSENTIAL EQUIPMENT/ADDITIONAL RESOURCES NEEDED

If possible, carry all essential medical equipment to the scene. This prevents loss of time returning to the vehicle. Remember to change gloves between patients. The following equipment is always needed for trauma patients:

1. Personal protection equipment (see previous discussion)
2. Long backboard with effective strapping and head motion-restriction device
3. Appropriately sized rigid cervical extrication collar
4. Oxygen and airway equipment (suction and bag-valve mask [BVM] should be included)
5. Trauma box (bandage material, blood pressure cuff, stethoscope)

If special extrication equipment, more ambulances, or backup personnel are needed, call now! You are less likely to call for help when involved in patient care.

MECHANISM OF INJURY

Once you determine that it is safe to approach the patient, begin to assess for the mechanism of injury. This may be apparent from the scene itself but may require questioning the patient or bystanders. Energy transmission follows the laws of physics; therefore, injuries present in predictable patterns. Knowledge and appreciation of the mechanism of injury allow you to maintain a high index of suspicion to aid in the search for injuries. Missed or overlooked injuries may be catastrophic, especially when they become known only when the compensatory mechanisms are exhausted. Remember that patients who are involved in a high-energy event are at risk for severe injury. *Five to 15 percent of these patients, despite normal vital signs and no apparent anatomic injury on the initial exam, will later exhibit severe injuries that are discovered on repeat examinations.* Therefore, a high-energy event signifies a large release of uncontrolled energy, and you should consider the patient injured until you have proven otherwise. It is important to be aware of whether the mechanism is generalized (MVC, fall from a height, etc.) or focused (stab wound of abdomen, hit in head by hammer). Generalized mechanisms require a rapid trauma survey while focused mechanisms may only require a more limited exam of the affected areas or systems.

Factors to be considered are direction and speed of impact, patient kinetics and physical size, and the signs of energy release (e.g., major vehicle damage). There is a strong correlation between injury severity and automobile velocity changes as measured by the amount of vehicle damage. It is important that you consider these two questions:

1. What happened?
2. How was the patient injured?

Mechanism of injury is also an important triage tool and is information that must always be reported to the emergency physician or trauma surgeon. Severity of vehicle damage has also been suggested as a nonphysiologic triage tool.

Motion (mechanical) injuries are by and large responsible for the majority of the mortality from trauma in the United States. This chapter will review the most common mechanisms of motion injuries and will stress the injuries that may be associated with these mechanisms. It is essential to develop an awareness of mechanisms of injury and thus have a high index of suspicion for occult injuries. Always consider the potential injury to be present until it is ruled out in a hospital setting.

There are two basic mechanisms of motion injury, blunt and penetrating. Patients may have injuries from both at the same time.

 BASIC MECHANISMS OF MOTION INJURY

1. Blunt injuries
   a. Rapid forward deceleration (collisions)
   b. Rapid vertical deceleration (falls)
   c. Energy transfer from blunt instruments (baseball bat, blackjack)
2. Penetrating injuries
   a. Projectiles
   b. Knives
   c. Falls upon fixed objects

MOTOR VEHICLE COLLISIONS

Various injury patterns will be discussed in the following examples, which include automobiles, motorcycles, all-terrain vehicles (ATVs), personal watercraft, and tractors. The important concept to appreciate is that the kinetic energy of motion must be absorbed, and this absorption of energy is the basic component in producing injury. Motion injury may be blunt or penetrating. Generally, blunt trauma is more common in the rural setting, and penetrating trauma is more common in the urban setting. Rapid forward deceleration is usually blunt but may be penetrating. The most common example of rapid forward deceleration is the MVC. You should consider all MVCs to occur as three separate events (see Figure 1-1):

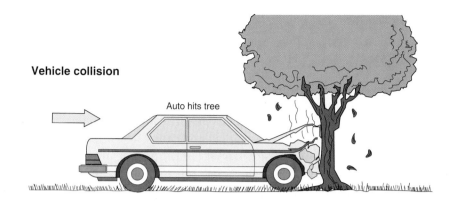

Vehicle collision

Auto hits tree

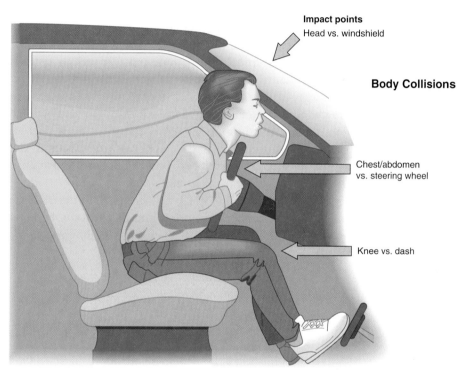

Impact points
Head vs. windshield

Body Collisions

Chest/abdomen
vs. steering wheel

Knee vs. dash

Organ collision

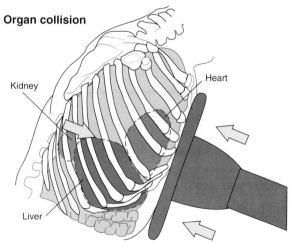

Kidney

Heart

Liver

The energy of body
collision is transmitted
to the interior.

Figure 1-1 The three collisions of a motor vehicle
collision.

1. The machine collision
2. The body collision
3. The organ collision

Consider approaching an MVC in which an automobile has hit a tree head-on at 40 miles per hour. The tree brings the auto to an immediate stop by transferring the energy into damage to the tree and the automobile. The person inside the auto is still traveling at 40 miles per hour until he strikes something that stops him (steering wheel, windshield, dashboard, etc.) by transferring energy into damage of the person and the surface struck. The organs inside the person are also traveling at 40 miles per hour until they are stopped by striking a stationary object (inside of skull, sternum, steering wheel, dashboard, etc.) or by their ligamentous attachments (aorta by ligamentum arteriosum, etc.). In this auto versus tree example, appreciation of the rapid forward decelerating mechanism (high-energy event) coupled with a high index of suspicion should make you concerned that the victim may have possible head injury, cervical spine injury, myocardial contusion, any of the "deadly dozen" chest injuries, intra-abdominal injuries, and musculoskeletal injuries (especially fracture or dislocation of the hip). To explain the forces involved here, you must consider Sir Isaac Newton's first law of motion: "a body in motion remains in motion in a straight line unless acted upon by an outside force." Motion is created by force (energy exchange), and therefore force will stop motion. If this energy exchange occurs within the body, damage of the tissues is produced. This law is well exemplified in the automobile crash. The kinetic energy of the vehicle's forward motion is absorbed as each part of the vehicle is brought to a sudden halt by the impact. Remember that the body of the occupant is also traveling at 40 miles per hour until impacted by some structure within the car such as the windshield, steering wheel, or dashboard. With awareness of this mechanism, one can see the multitude of injuries that may occur. The following are clues you should be aware of:

1. Deformity of the vehicle (indication of forces involved—energy exchange)
2. Deformity of interior structures (indication of where the patient impacted—energy exchange)
3. Deformity (injury patterns) of the patient (indication of what parts of the body may have been impacted)

You also must be aware that there can be other collisions other than the three mentioned above. Objects inside the automobile (books, bags, luggage, and other persons) will become missiles traveling at the original speed of the auto and may strike persons in front of them (see Figure 1-2). These are called *secondary collisions*. A good example of this is when a parent is holding a child in her lap and crushes the child between her and the dashboard in a deceleration collision.

In many auto collisions there are also additional impacts when the auto strikes another auto and is then in turn struck by an auto following. Also vehicles frequently deflect from hitting one object and then collide with a second or even third vehicle or stationary object. These are much like a rollover collision in that the persons inside the vehicle are subjected to energy transfer from multiple directions. It is often more difficult to predict injuries in these cases and you must quickly but carefully look for clues inside the vehicle.

MVCs occur in several forms, and each form is associated with certain patterns of injury. The five common forms of MVCs are the following:

1. The head-on collision (frontal)
2. The T-bone or lateral-impact collision (lateral)
3. The rear-impact collision (rear)

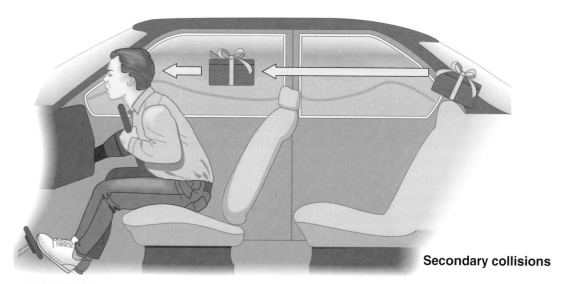

Figure 1-2 Secondary collisions in a deceleration MVC.

4. The rollover collision
5. The rotational collision

Head-On Collision

In this type of MVC, an unrestrained body is brought to a sudden halt, and the energy transfer is capable of producing multiple injuries.

Windshield injuries occur in the rapid forward decelerating type of event, in which the unrestrained occupant impacts forcefully with the windshield (see Figure 1-3). The possibility for injuries is great under these conditions. Of utmost concern is the potential for serious airway and cervical spine injury. Remembering the three separate collision events, note the following:

Machine collision: deformed front end

Body collision: spider web pattern of windshield

Organ collision: coup/contracoup brain, soft tissue injury (scalp, face, neck), hyperextension/flexion of cervical spine

From the spider web appearance of the windshield and an appreciation of mechanism of injury, you should maintain a high index of suspicion for possible occult injuries of the cervical spine. The head usually strikes the windshield, resulting in direct trauma to the face and head. External signs of trauma include cuts, abrasions, and contusions. These may be quite dramatic in appearance; however, the key concern is airway maintenance with motion restriction of the cervical spine and evaluation of level of consciousness.

Steering wheel injuries most often occur to an unrestrained driver of a vehicle in a head-on collision. The driver may subsequently also impact with the windshield. The steering wheel is the vehicle's most lethal weapon for the unrestrained driver, and any degree of steering wheel deformity (check under collapsed

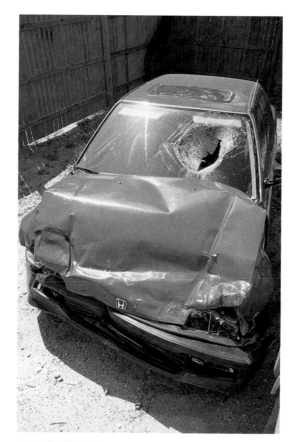

Figure 1-3 In a head-on collision, most injuries are inflicted by the windshield, steering wheel, and the dashboard.

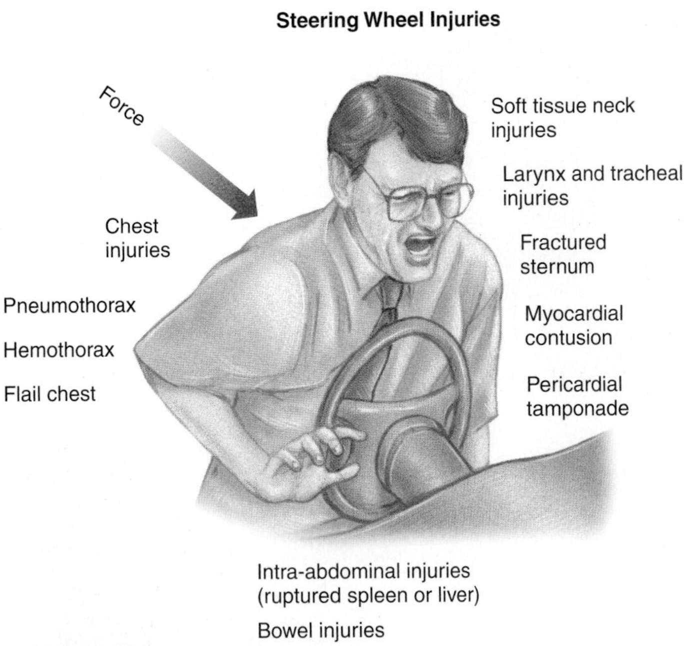

Steering Wheel Injuries

Force

Chest injuries

Pneumothorax

Hemothorax

Flail chest

Soft tissue neck injuries

Larynx and tracheal injuries

Fractured sternum

Myocardial contusion

Pericardial tamponade

Intra-abdominal injuries (ruptured spleen or liver)

Bowel injuries

Figure 1-4 Steering wheel injuries.

airbags) must be treated with a high index of suspicion for face, neck, thoracic, or abdominal injury. The two components of this weapon are the ring and column (see Figure 1-4). The ring is a semirigid plastic-covered metal ring attached to a fixed inflexible post—a battering ram. Utilizing the three-collision concept, check for the presence of the following:

Machine collision: front-end deformity

Body collision: ring fracture/deformity, column normal/displaced

Organ collision: traumatic tattooing of skin

The head-on collision is entirely dependent upon the area of the body that impacts with the steering wheel. Signs may be readily visible, with direct trauma such as lacerations of mouth and chin, contusion/bruises of the anterior neck, traumatic tattoos of the chest wall, and bruising of the abdomen. These external signs may be subtle or dramatic in appearance, but more important, they may represent the tip of the iceberg. Deeper structures and organs may harbor occult injuries due to shearing forces, compression forces, and displacement of kinetic energy. Organs that are susceptible to shearing injuries due to their ligamentous attachments are the aortic arch, liver, spleen, kidneys, and bowel. With the exception of small-bowel tears, these injuries are sources for occult bleeds and hemorrhagic shock. Compression injuries are common with the lung, heart, diaphragm, and urinary bladder. An important sign is respiratory distress, which may be due to pulmonary contusions, pneumothorax, diaphragmatic hernia (bowel sounds in chest), or flail chest. Consider a bruised chest wall as a myocardial contusion that requires electrocardiogram monitoring.

In short, the steering wheel is a very lethal weapon that is capable of producing devastating injuries, many of which are occult. Steering wheel deformity is a cause for alarm and must heighten your index of suspicion. You must also relay this information to the receiving physician.

Dashboard injuries occur most often to an unrestrained passenger. The dashboard has the capability of producing a variety of injuries, depending upon the area of the body that strikes the dashboard. Most frequently, injuries involve the face and knees; however, many types of injuries have been described (see Figure 1-5).

Applying the three-event concept of collision, you will note:

Machine collision: deformity of the car

Body collision: fracture/deformity of the dash

Organ collision: facial trauma, coup/contracoup brain, hyperextension/flexion of the cervical spine, and knee trauma

Facial, brain, and cervical spine injuries have already been discussed. Like chest contusion, knee trauma may represent only the tip of the iceberg. Knees commonly impact with the dashboard. This may range from the simple contusion noted about the patella to the severe compound fracture of the patella. Frank dislocation of the knees can occur. In addition, this kinetic energy may be transmitted proximally and may result in fracture of the femur or fractured/dislocated hip. On occasion the pelvis can impact with the dash, resulting in acetabulum fractures as well as pelvic fractures. These injuries are associated with hemorrhage that may lead to shock. Maintain a high index of suspicion and always palpate the femurs as well as gently squeeze the pelvis and palpate the symphysis pubis.

Deceleration collisions are the most common to have secondary collisions from people or objects in the back of the vehicle. These secondary missiles can cause deadly injuries.

T-Bone or Lateral-Impact Collision

The mechanism of the T-bone collision is similar to that of the head-on collision, with the addition of lateral energy displacement (see Figure 1-6).

Applying the three-collision concept, look for the presence of the following:

Machine collision: primary deformity of the car—check the impact side (driver/passenger)

Body collision: degree of door deformity (e.g., arm rest bent, outward or inward bowing of door)

Organ collision: cannot be predicted by external exam alone; consider organs underneath areas of external injury

The most common injuries to look for are the following:

Head: coup/contracoup due to lateral displacement

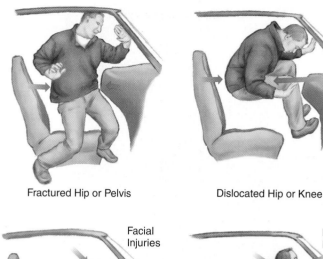

Fractured Hip or Pelvis   Dislocated Hip or Knee

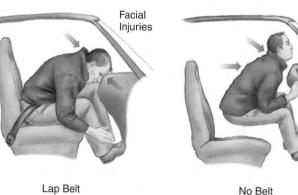

Lap Belt   No Belt

Figure 1-5 Dashboard injuries.

Neck: lateral displacement injuries range from cervical muscle strain to subluxation with neurological deficit

Upper arm and shoulder: injuries on the side of the impact

Thorax/abdomen: injury due to direct force either from inward bowing of door on the side of the impact or from unrestrained passenger being propelled across seat

Pelvis/legs: occupants on the side of the impact are likely to have pelvic, hip, or femur fractures

Injuries of the thorax vary from soft tissue injuries to flail chest, lung contusion, pneumothorax, or hemothorax. Abdominal injuries include those of solid or hollow organs. Pelvic injuries may include fracture/dislocation, bladder rupture, and urethral injuries. Shoulder girdle or lower-extremity injuries are common, depending on the level of the impacting force.

Rear-Impact Collision

In the most common form of rear-impact collision, a stationary car is struck from the rear by another moving vehicle (see Figure 1-7). Or a slower-moving car may be impacted from the rear by a faster-moving car. The sudden increase in acceleration produces posterior displacement of the occupants and possible hyperextension of the cervical spine if the headrest is not properly adjusted. If the seat back breaks and falls back into the rear seat, there is greater chance of lumbar spine injury. There also may be rapid forward deceleration if the car suddenly strikes something in the front or if the driver applies the brakes suddenly. You should note deformity of the auto anterior and posterior as well as interior

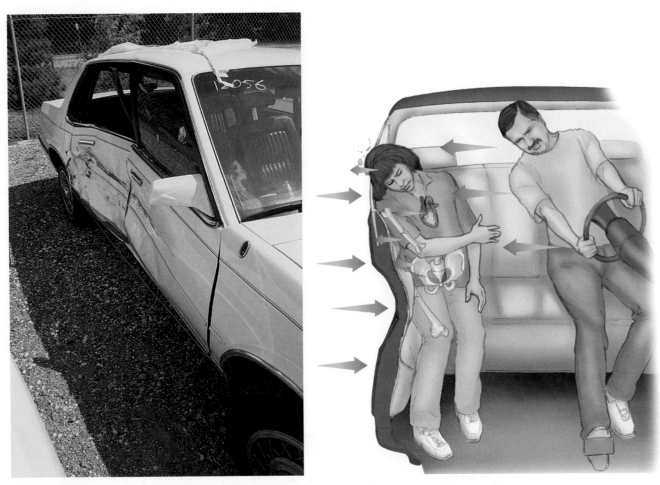

Figure 1-6 In a lateral impact collision, most injuries are inflicted by intrusion of the door, armrest, side window, or door post.

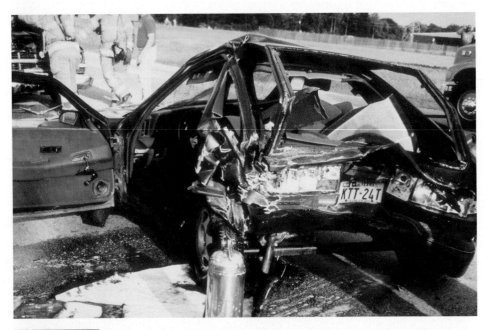

Figure 1-7 In a rear impact collision, there is a potential for neck and back injury. *(Photo courtesy of Bonnie Meneely, EMT-P)*

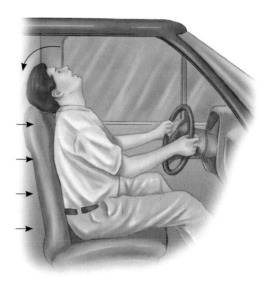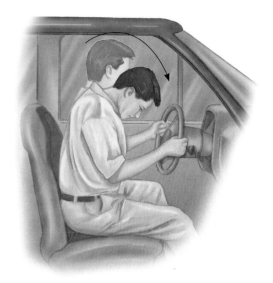

a. Victim moves ahead while head remains stationary. Head rotates backward. Neck extends.

b. Head snaps forward. Head rotates forward. Neck flexes.

Figure 1-8 Mechanism of cervical spine injury in rear-impact collision.

deformity and headrest position. The potential for cervical spine injuries is great (see Figure 1-8). Also be alert for associated deceleration injuries.

Rollover Collision

During a vehicle rollover, the body may be impacted from any direction; thus the potential for injuries is great (see Figure 1-9). The chance for axial loading injuries of the spine is increased in this form of MVC. Rescuers must be alert for clues that imply that the car turned over (e.g., roof dents, scratches, debris, and deformity of roof posts). There are

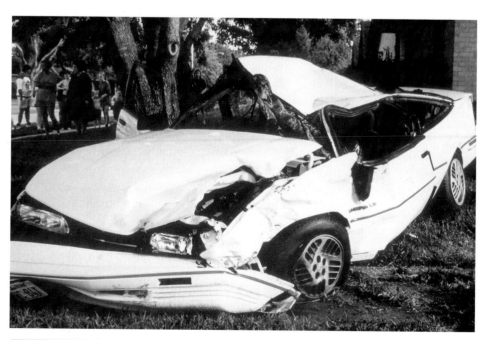

Figure 1-9 In a rollover collision, there is a high potential for injury. Many mechanisms are involved, and unrestrained victims are frequently ejected. *(Photo courtesy of Bonnie Meneely, EMT-P)*

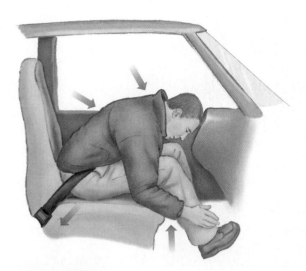

Figure 1-10

Clasp-knife effect.

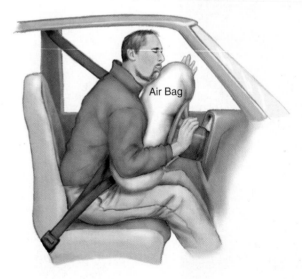

Air Bag

Air Bag and 3-Point Restraint
Prevents Collisions 2 and 3

Figure 1-11 Air bag and three-point restraint.

more lethal injuries in this form of accident because there is a greater likelihood of occupants being ejected. Occupants ejected from the car are 25 times as likely to be killed.

Rotational Collision

A rotational mechanism is best described as what occurs when one part of the vehicle stops and the rest of the vehicle remains in motion. A rotational collision usually occurs when a vehicle is struck in the front or rear lateral area. This converts forward motion to a spinning motion. The results are a combination of the frontal-impact and the lateral-impact mechanisms with the same possibilities of injuries of both mechanisms.

Occupant Restraint Systems

Restrained occupants are much more likely to survive because they are protected from much of the impact inside the auto and are restrained from being ejected from the auto. These occupants are, however, still susceptible to certain injuries. The lap belt is intended to go across the pelvis (iliac crests), not the abdomen. If the belt is in place and the victim is subjected to a frontal deceleration crash, his body tends to fold together like a clasp knife (see Figure 1-10). The head may be thrown forward into the steering wheel or dashboard. Facial, head, or neck injuries are common. Abdominal injuries occur if the lap belt is positioned improperly. The compression forces that are produced when a body is suddenly folded about the waist may injure the abdomen or the lumbar spine.

The three-point restraint or cross-chest lap belt (see Figure 1-11) secures the body much better than does a lap belt alone. The chest and pelvis are restrained, so life-threatening injuries are much less common. The head is not restrained, and therefore the neck is still subjected to stresses that may cause fractures, dislocations, or spinal cord injuries. Clavicular fractures (at the point where the chest strap crosses) are common. Internal organ damage may still occur due to organ movement inside the body.

Like belt restraints, airbags (passive restraints) will reduce injuries in victims of MVCs in *most* but not all situations. Airbags are designed to inflate from the center of the steering wheel and the dashboard to protect the front-seat occupants in case of a frontal deceleration accident. If these function properly, they cushion the head and chest at the instant of impact. This is very effective in decreasing injury to the face, neck, and chest. You should still stabilize the neck until it has been adequately examined. Airbags deflate immediately, so they protect against only one impact. The driver whose car hits more than one object is unprotected after the initial collision. Airbags also do not prevent "down and under" movement, so drivers who are extended (tall drivers and drivers of small low-slung autos) may still impact with their legs and suffer leg, pelvis, or abdominal injuries. It is important for occupants to wear chest and lap belts even when the car is equipped with airbags. Research has recently shown that some drivers who appear uninjured after deceleration accidents have been found to have serious internal injuries. A clue to which driver may have internal injuries is the condition of the steering wheel. A deformed steering wheel is just as important a clue in an auto equipped with an airbag as in those that are not. This clue may

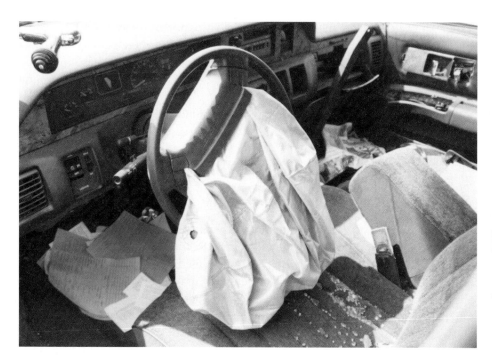

Figure 1-12

Lift the collapsed airbag to note whether there is a deformity of the steering wheel. *(Photo courtesy of Robert S. Porter)*

be missed because the deflated airbag covers the steering wheel. Thus a quick "lift and look" under the airbag should be a part of the routine examination of the steering wheel (see Figure 1-12). Many autos are now equipped with side airbags in the doors; some have airbags that come down from the roof to protect the head; and at least one make of auto has airbags under the dash to protect the legs. These obviously give much needed extra protection. There are dangers associated with airbags. Small drivers who bring the seat up close to the steering wheel may sustain serious injuries as the bag inflates. Infants in car seats placed in the front seat may be seriously injured by the airbag.

In summary, when at the scene of an MVC, you must note the type of collision and the clues that imply that high kinetic energy has been spent (e.g., deformities of the vehicle). Maintain a high index of suspicion for occult injuries and thus keep scene time to a minimum. These observations and clues are essential to quality patient care and must be relayed to Medical Direction and the receiving physician.

Tractor Accidents

Another large motorized vehicle with which you must be familiar is the tractor. The U.S. National Safety Council reports that one-third of all farm accident fatalities involve tractors. There are basically two types of tractors: the two-wheel drive and the four-wheel drive. In both, the center of gravity is high, and thus the tractors are easily turned over (see Figure 1-13). The majority of fatal accidents are due to the tractor turning over and crushing the driver. Most overturns (85%) are to the side; these are less likely to pin the driver because he or she has a chance to jump or be thrown clear. Rear overturns, although less frequent, are more likely to entrap

REAR OVERTURNS   SIDE OVERTURNS

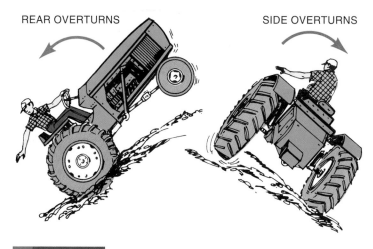

Figure 1-13 Tractor accidents.

and crush the driver because there is almost no opportunity to jump free. The primary mechanism is the crush injury, and the severity depends on the part of the anatomy that is involved. Additional mechanisms are chemical burns from gasoline, diesel fuel, hydraulic fluid, or even battery acid. Thermal burns from hot engine parts or ignited fuel are also common.

Management consists of scene stabilization followed quickly by the primary survey and resuscitation. The following checklist is used in scene stabilization:

1. Engine off?
2. Rear wheels locked?
3. Fuel situation and fire hazard addressed?

While you are surveying the patient, other rescuers must stabilize the tractor. The center of gravity must be identified before any attempt is made to lift the tractor. The center of gravity of the two-wheel-drive tractor is located approximately 10 inches above and 24 inches in front of the rear axle. The center of gravity of a four-wheel-drive tractor is closer to the midline of the machine. Because tractors usually overturn on soft ground and their centers of gravity are tricky to determine, great care must be taken during lifting to avoid a second crush injury. Because of the weight of the tractor and the length of time (usually prolonged) the driver is pinned, anticipate serious injuries. Often, the patient will go into profound shock as the compressing weight of the tractor is removed—similar to what happens when antishock trousers are suddenly deflated. Rapid, safe management of tractor accidents requires special exercises in lifting heavy machinery as well as good trauma management.

Small-Vehicle Crashes

Other small vehicles that fall into the motion injury category include the motorcycle, the ATV, the personal watercraft (PWC), and the snowmobile. The operators of these machines are not encased within them, and, of course, there are no restraining devices. When the operator is subjected to the classic head-on, lateral-impact, rear-end, or rollover collision, the only forms of protection are the following:

1. Evasive maneuvering
2. Helmet usage
3. Protective clothing (e.g., leather clothes, helmet, boots)
4. Use of the vehicle to absorb kinetic energy (e.g., bike slide)

Motorcycles: It is extremely important for motorcycle riders to wear helmets. Helmets help prevent head injury (which causes 75% of motorcycle deaths). However, helmets give no protection to the spine. The operator of a motorcycle involved in a crash is much like an ejected automobile occupant. Injuries depend on the part of the anatomy subjected to kinetic energy. Because of the lack of protective encasement, there is a higher frequency of head, neck, and extremity injuries. Important clues include deformity of the motorcycle, distance of skid, and deformity of stationary objects or cars. Again, a high degree of suspicion, appreciation of environmental clues (skid marks, vehicle deformity), identification of load-and-go, and strict BTLS protocols constitute the optimal standard of prehospital care.

All-Terrain Vehicles: The ATV was designed as a vehicle to traverse rough terrain. They were used initially by ranchers, hunters, and farmers. Unfortunately, some people view the ATV as a fast toy. Careless misuse has resulted in an ever-increasing morbidity and mortality from accidents—sadly—frequently among the very young. The two basic designs are either three wheeled (no longer made and, so, rare) or four wheeled. The four-wheel design affords reasonable stability and handling, but the three-wheeled ATV has a high center of gravity and is very prone to rollover when turned sharply. Listed below are the four most common mechanisms:

1. Vehicle rollover
2. Fall-off of rider or passenger
3. Forward deceleration of rider from vehicle impact with stationary object
4. Impact of rider or passenger's head or extremities when passing too close to stationary objects (trees)

The injuries produced depend upon the mechanism and the part of the anatomy that is impacted. The most frequent injuries are fractures, about half of which are above and half below the diaphragm. The major bony injuries involve the clavicles, sternum, and ribs. Be very suspicious for head or spinal injury.

Personal Watercraft: The use of PWC, such as wave runners, has become very popular in water recreational activities. In 1995 there were approximately 750,000 PWC in operation in the United States. Between 1990 and 1997 there was a 400% increase in the number of injuries from PWC (2,860–12,000). The rate of emergency department-treated injuries related to PWC is about 8.5 times higher than the rate of that of motorboats. These watercraft are designed to be operated by the driver in a sitting, standing, or kneeling position, with one or more passengers located behind the driver in tandem. PWC are able to obtain high speeds very quickly. Mechanism for injury potential is very similar to the ATV. Rollovers impacting with the water at high speeds result in the same potential injury patterns. Collisions with other watercraft produce injury patterns similar to those encountered with motorcycle–auto collisions. Rectal and vaginal trauma may occur when rear-seat passengers or the driver fall off backwards, impacting the water (buttocks first) at high speeds. The likelihood of drowning (even with the use of personal flotation devices) is always a danger. Remember, water is not soft when a body impacts with it at high speeds; therefore you must assess and practice the same index of suspicion as with any high-energy event.

Snowmobiles: Snowmobiles are used both as recreational and utility vehicles. The snowmobile has a low clearance and a low center of gravity. The injuries common to this vehicle are very similar to those that occur with the ATV. Turnovers are somewhat more common, and since the vehicle is usually heavier than the ATV, crush injuries are seen more frequently. Again, the injury pattern depends on the part of the anatomy that is directly involved. Be alert for possible coexisting hypothermia. A common injury with the snowmobile is the "hangman" or "clothes line" injury that results from running under wire fences. Be alert for occult cervical spine injuries and potential airway compromise.

Pedestrian Injuries

The pedestrian struck by a car almost always suffers severe internal injuries as well as fractures. This is true even if the vehicle is traveling at low speed. The mass of the auto is so large that high speed is not necessary to impart high-energy transfer. When high speed is involved the results are disastrous. There are two mechanisms of injury. The first is when the bumper of the auto strikes the body, and the second is when the body, accelerated by the transfer of forces, strikes the ground or some other object. An adult usually has bilateral lower leg or knee fractures plus whatever secondary injuries occur when the body strikes the hood of the car and then later the ground. Children are shorter so the bumper is more likely to hit them in the pelvis or torso. They usually land on their heads in the secondary impact. When answering a call to an auto–pedestrian accident, be prepared for broken bones, internal injuries, and head injuries.

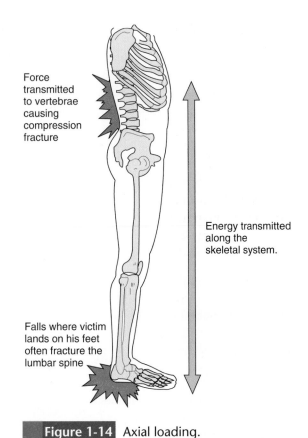

Figure 1-14 Axial loading.

Force transmitted to vertebrae causing compression fracture

Energy transmitted along the skeletal system.

Falls where victim lands on his feet often fracture the lumbar spine

FALLS

The mechanism for falls is vertical deceleration. The types of injuries sustained depend upon three factors, listed below, that you must identify and relay to Medical Direction:

1. Distance of fall

2. Anatomic area impacted

3. Surface struck

The primary groups involved in vertical falls are adults and children under the age of five. In children, the falls most commonly involve males and occur mostly in the summer months in urban high-rise multiple-occupant dwellings. Predisposing factors include poor supervision, defective railings, and the curiosity associated with that age group. Head injuries are common in falls by children because the head is the heaviest part of the body and thus impacts first. Adult falls are generally occupational or due to the influence of alcohol or drugs. It is not uncommon for falls to occur during attempts to escape from fire or criminal activity. Generally, adults attempt to land on their feet; thus their falls are more controlled. In this landing form, the victim usually impacts initially on the feet and then falls backwards landing on the buttocks and outstretched hands. Classically, this "lover's leap" fall may result in the following injuries (see Figure 1-14):

1. Fractures of the feet or legs

2. Hip and/or pelvic injuries

3. Axial loading to the lumbar and cervical spine

4. Vertical deceleration forces to the organs

5. Colles' fracture of the wrists

The greater the height, the greater the potential for injury. However, do not be deceived into believing that there is little risk for serious injury in a short-distance fall. Surface density (concrete versus sawdust) and irregularity (gym floor versus staircase) also influence the severity of injury. Relay information about distance fallen and surface struck to Medical Direction with other pertinent information.

PENETRATING INJURIES

Numerous objects are capable of producing penetrating injuries. These range from the industrial saw blade that breaks off at an extremely high rate of speed to the foreign body hurled by a lawn mower. Most high-velocity objects are capable of penetrating the thorax or abdomen. However, the more common forms of penetrating wounds come from the knife and gun.

Knife-wound severity depends on the anatomic area penetrated, the length of the blade, and the angle of penetration (see Figure 1-15). Remember, an upper abdominal stab wound may cause intrathoracic organ injury, and stab wounds below the fourth intercostal space may have penetrated the abdomen. The golden rule with knife wounds that still have the blade inside—do not remove the knife.

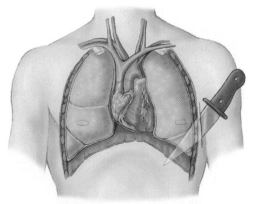

Stab wounds at nipple level or below frequently penetrate the abdomen.

Figure 1-15 Stab wounds.

Most penetrating wounds inflicted by firearms are due to handguns, rifles, and shot-guns. Important factors to obtain, if possible, are the type of weapon and its caliber and the distance from which the weapon was fired. However, remember that you treat the patient and the wound, not the weapon.

Wound Ballistics

Because the kinetic energy (kinetic energy = 1/2 mass × velocity^2) produced by a projec-tile is mostly dependent upon velocity, weapons are classified as high or low velocity. Weapons with velocities less than 2,000 ft/sec are considered low velocity and include essentially all handguns and some rifles. Injuries from these weapons are much less destructive than those sustained from high-velocity weapons, such as a military rifle. Low-velocity weapons are certainly capable of lethal injuries, depending on the body area struck. More civilians are killed by low-velocity bullets because they are more often shot by low-velocity weapons. All wounds inflicted by high-velocity weapons carry the addi-tional factor of hydrostatic pressure. This factor alone can increase the injury.

Factors that contribute to tissue damage include:

1. *Missile size:* The larger the bullet, the more resistance and the larger the permanent tract.
2. *Missile deformity:* Hollow point and soft nose flatten out on impact, resulting in a larger surface area involved.
3. *Semijacket:* The jacket expands and adds to surface area.
4. *Tumbling:* Tumbling of the missile causes a wider path of destruction.
5. *Yaw:* The missile can oscillate vertically and horizontally (wobble) about its axis, resulting in a larger surface area presenting to the tissue.

The wounds consist of three parts:

1. *Entry wound:* Usually smaller than the exit wound; may have darkened, burned edges if bullet is fired from very close range (see Figure 1-16).
2. *Exit wound:* Not all entry wounds will have exit wounds, and on occasion there may be multiple exits due to fragmentation of bone and missile; generally, the exit wound is larger and has ragged edges (see Figure 1-16).
3. *Internal wound:* Low-velocity projectiles inflict damage primarily by damaging tissue that the missile contacts; high-velocity projectiles inflict damage by tissue contact and transfer of kinetic energy to surrounding tissues (see Figure 1-17a and b).

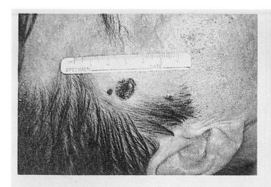
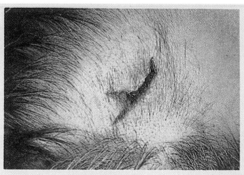

ENTRANCE WOUND (Bullet — Close Range)

EXIT WOUND (Bullet)

Figure 1-16 Comparison of entrance and exit wounds.

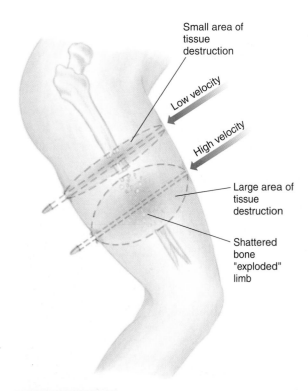

Small area of
tissue
destruction

Low velocity

High velocity

Large area of
tissue
destruction

Shattered
bone
"exploded"
limb

Figure 1-17 a High-velocity versus low-velocity injury.

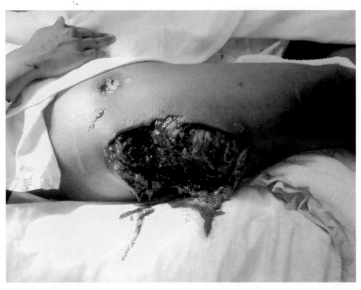

Figure 1-17 b Example of high-velocity wound of leg.
(Photo courtesy of Roy Alson, M.D.)

Damage is related to the following:

a. Shock waves

b. Temporary cavity, which is 30 to 40 times the bullet's diameter and creates immense tissue pressures

c. Pulsation of the temporary cavity, which creates pressure changes in the adjacent tissue

Generally damage done is proportional to tissue density. Highly dense organs such as bone, muscle, and liver sustain more damage than less-dense organs such as lungs. A key factor to remember is that once a bullet enters a body; its trajectory will not always be in a straight line. Any patient with a missile penetration of the head, thorax, or abdomen should be transported immediately. Personnel who have been shot while wearing a flak vest should be managed with caution; be alert for possible cardiac and other organ contusion.

In shotgun wounds, injury is determined by kinetic energy at impact that is influenced by:

1. Powder

2. Size of pellets

3. Choke of muzzle

4. Distance to target

Velocity and kinetic energy dissipate rapidly as distance is traveled. At 40 yards the velocity is one-half the initial muzzle velocity.

PEARLS: BASIC BALLISTIC INFORMATION

Caliber:
the internal diameter of the barrel; this corresponds to the ammunition used for the particular weapon

Rifling:
a series of spiral grooves in the interior surface of the barrel of some weapons

Ammunition:
case, primer, powder, and bullet

Bullet Construction:
usually solid lead alloy; may have a full or partial copper or steel jacket. The shape of the nose of the bullet may be rounded, flat, conical, or pointed. The bullet nose may also be soft or hollow (for expansion or fragmentation)

Treat the patient and not the weapon.

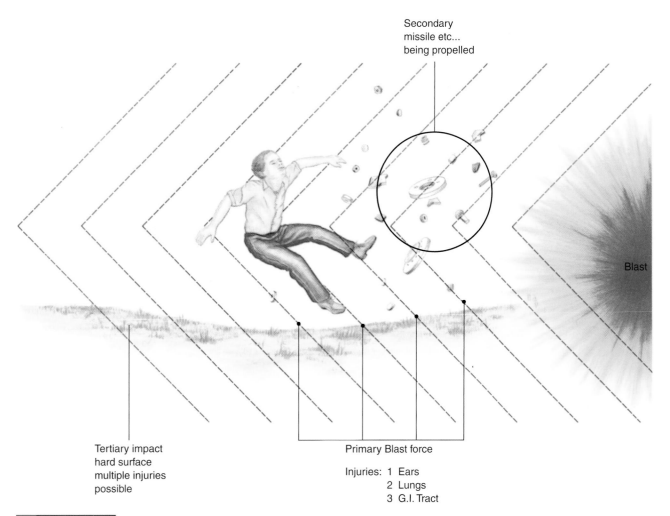

Secondary
missile etc...
being propelled

Blast

Tertiary impact
hard surface
multiple injuries
possible

Primary Blast force

Injuries: 1 Ears
2 Lungs
3 G.I. Tract

Figure 1-18a Explosions can cause injury with the initial blast, when the victim is struck by debris, or by the victim being thrown against the ground or other fixed objects by the blast.

BLAST INJURIES

Blast injuries in this country occur primarily in industrial settings such as grain elevator and gas fume explosions. However, as threat of terrorist activity is now both common and world-wide, blast injury management must be added to BTLS training and knowledge.

The mechanism of injury by blast/explosion is due to three factors:

1. *Primary:* initial air blast
2. *Secondary:* patient being struck by material propelled by the blast force
3. *Tertiary:* body being thrown and impacting on ground or other object

Injuries due to the primary air blast are almost exclusive to the air-containing organs. The auditory system usually

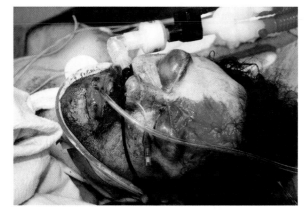

Figure 1-18b Tertiary injury from being thrown into a wall by the blast. *(Photo courtesy of Roy Alson, M.D.)*

involves ruptured tympanic membranes. Lung injuries may include pneumothorax, parenchymal hemorrhage, and, especially, alveolar rupture. Alveolar rupture may cause air embolus that may be manifested by bizarre central nervous system symptoms. Gastrointestinal tract injuries may vary from mild intestinal and stomach contusions to frank rupture. Always suspect lung injuries in a blast victim.

Injuries caused by the secondary factors may be penetrating or blunt and tertiary injuries are much the same as when as person is ejected from an automobile (see Figure 1-18a and b).

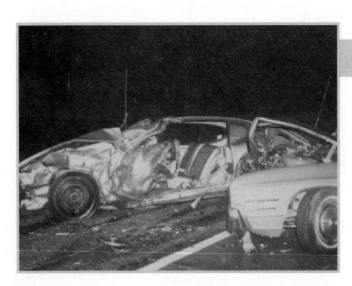

(Photo courtesy of William Pfeifer, M.D.)

CASE STUDY

Dan, Joyce, and Buddy of the Emergency Transport Service have been dispatched to a two-car collision in which one auto ran into the side of the other. They are informed that a rescue truck is on-scene and attempting to extricate one of the drivers. While driving to the scene they decide that Joyce will act as team leader on this case. On arrival, Joyce gets the trauma box and cervical collars and begins the Scene Size-up. Dan gets the oxygen and airway equipment and Buddy gets the backboard. Joyce notes that the police are on-scene and the scene is safe. The team dons personal protective equipment; each carries his part of the essential equipment to the scene as they approach. Neither vehicle had any passengers other than the driver. The first car has front-end damage, the airbag deployed, and the driver is walking around with no complaints. The second car was struck in the driver's door with major intrusion into the passenger compartment. The driver is pinned in the vehicle and extrication requires removing the door in order to free him. He is alert and oriented but complains of chest and abdominal pain. After extrication, Dan stabilizes the cervical spine and applies the non-rebreather oxygen mask while Joyce performs the assessment. Joyce's Rapid Trauma Assessment reveals crepitation of the lower ribs on the left with a tender, distended abdomen and an unstable pelvis. Breath sounds are decreased on the left and the chest is dull to percussion. The patient is in shock. They quickly package the patient and immediately load-and-go. Vital signs: BP 70/40, pulse 140, respiration 28. The patient states he has no allergies, takes no medications, has always been healthy, and last food was about four hours ago. Joyce calls her On-Line Medical Direction (OLMD) and reports that she is transporting a patient who is in shock. She suspects that the patient has rib fractures, a hemothorax, intra-abdominal injuries, and a fractured pelvis. OLMD tells them to transport the patient to the local level-one trauma center. The trauma team is mobilized and waiting when they arrive. The patient is found to have a fractured pelvis, ruptured spleen, fractured left ribs, and a hemothorax. He requires surgery and multiple blood transfusions but eventually recovers and returns to work. The emergency physician credits prompt prehospital management with helping save the patient's life.

CASE STUDY WRAP-UP

The mechanism of injury of a T-bone or lateral-impact collision is straight deceleration for the auto hitting the side of the other auto. For the auto that sustains the lateral-impact, the mechanism depends on the height of the blow. A sports utility vehicle or large truck would strike the auto higher than a passenger car and so would more likely cause upper chest, shoulder, neck, and head injuries. A passenger car would strike lower and, depending on how low, would be more likely to cause pelvis fractures, intra-abdominal injuries, rib, and lower chest injuries. With major intrusion into the passenger compartment you expect these to be serious injuries. All patients in shock are load-and-go. The pneumatic antishock garment could not be used in this case because of the chest and abdominal injuries.

SUMMARY

Trauma is the most serious disease affecting young people. Being a rescuer is among the most important professions but requires great dedication and continuous training. Saving patients who have sustained severe trauma requires attention to detail and careful management of time. Teamwork is essential, as many actions must occur at the same time.

At the scene of an injury, there are certain important steps to perform before you begin care of the patient. Failure to perform a Scene Size-up will subject you and your patient to danger and may cause you to fail to anticipate serious injuries that your patient may have sustained. You must take proper BSI precautions, assess the scene for dangers, and determine the need for (and call for) special backup or special equipment. Then assess the total number of patients and initiate proper protocols if there are more patients than your team can manage.

You must identify the mechanism of injury and consider it as part of the overall management of the trauma patient. What happened? What type of energy was applied? How much energy was transmitted? What part of the body was affected? If there is an MVC, you must consider the form of the crash as well as survey the vehicle's interior and exterior for damage. Tractor accidents require careful stabilization of the machine to prevent a second injury to the patient. Falls require identification of distance fallen, surface struck and position of the patient upon impact. Stab wounds require knowledge of the length of the instrument as well as the angle at which it entered the body. When evaluating a shooting victim you need to know the weapon, caliber, and distance from which it fired.

Information about the high-energy event (e.g., falls, vehicle damage) is also important to the emergency physician. Be sure not only to record your findings but to give a verbal report to the emergency department physician or trauma surgeon when you arrive. With this knowledge and a high index of suspicion, you can give your patient the greatest chance of survival.

BIBLIOGRAPHY

1. Branche, C. M., J. M. Conn, and J. L. Annest. "Personal Watercraft-Related Injuries." *JAMA,* Vol. 278, No. 8 (August 1997), pp. 663–665.

2. Greenberg, M. I. "Falls from Heights." *Journal of the American College of Emergency Physicians Emergency Procedures,* Vol. 7 (August 1978), pp. 300–301.

3. Huekle, D. F., and J. W. Melvin. "Anatomy, Injury, Frequency, Bio-mechanical Human Tolerance." Society of Automotive Engineers, Technical Paper No. 80098, February 1980.

4. McSwain, N. E. Jr. "Kinematics of Penetrating Trauma." *Journal of Pre-Hospital Care,* Vol. 1 (October 1984), pp. 10–13.

6. National Highway Traffic Safety Administration. *Occupant Protection Facts.* Washington, DC: National Center for Statistics and Analysis, U.S. Department of Transportation, June 1989.

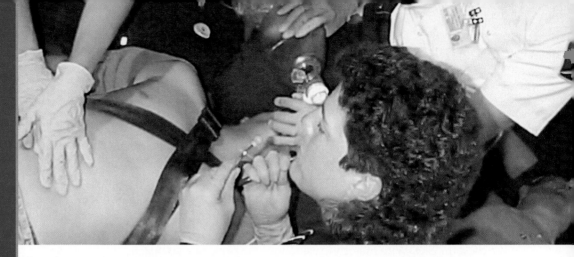

Chapter 2

Assessment and Initial Management of the Trauma Patient

John E. Campbell, M.D., F.A.C.E.P.

John T. Stevens, EMT-P

Leon Charpentier, EMT-P

Objectives

Upon completion of this chapter, you should be able to:

1. Describe the steps in trauma assessment and management.

2. Describe the Initial Assessment and explain how it relates to the BTLS Rapid Trauma Survey and the Focused Exam.

3. Describe when the Initial Assessment can be interrupted.

4. Describe when critical interventions should be made and where to make them.

5. Identify which patients have critical conditions and how they should be managed.

6. Describe the Detailed Exam.

7. Describe the Ongoing Exam.

(Photo courtesy of BTLS Ontario, Steve McNenly, Jennifer Lundgren, and Sheryl Jackson).

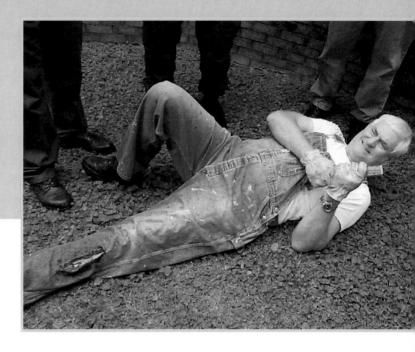

Dan, Joyce, and Buddy of the
Emergency Transport System have
been called to the scene of a construction accident where a man fell from a scaffold onto a pile of lumber. Their Scene Size-up
reveals that the scene is safe and there is only one victim. He has been pulled from the
lumber pile but appears to be pale and diaphoretic and has an obvious open fracture of
his left lower leg. He is clutching a piece of wood that is sticking out of his chest. How
would you approach this patient? What is the mechanism of injury? What type of assessment would you perform? What would you do first? Is this a load-and-go situation?
Keep these questions in mind as you read the chapter. The case study will continue at the
end of the chapter.

TRAUMA ASSESSMENT

The BTLS patient assessment surveys are consistent with U.S. Department of
Transportation patient assessment guidelines. The old BTLS Primary Survey has been
slightly modified to make it more flexible and to focus on life-threatening injuries.
Patients with trauma to a focused area (limited to a certain area of the body) or with
insignificant mechanisms of injury don't require an exam as comprehensive as the old
BTLS Primary Survey. The new *BTLS Primary Survey* is a combination of the **Scene Size-
up,** the **Initial Assessment** (which is the same for all patients), and the **Rapid Trauma
Survey** or the **Focused Exam** (depending on the situation). The **Detailed Exam** is the
same as the old BTLS Secondary Survey and the **Ongoing Exam** is the same as the old
BTLS Reassessment Survey. The Initial Assessment is a very brief exam of level of consciousness (LOC) and the ABCs to prioritize the patient and to determine if *immediately
life-threatening conditions* exist. The purpose of the BTLS Rapid Trauma Survey is to find
all life-threatening injuries and determine if the patient should have immediate transport.
The BTLS Rapid Trauma Survey differs from the Detailed Exam (Secondary Survey) in
that the Detailed Exam is an evaluation for *all* injuries, not just life-threatening ones.

The patient with the most minor-appearing injury will get a brief Initial Assessment
before you concentrate on the minor injury. Critical patients will get a much more comprehensive exam, but in each case the exam will begin in the same way (Initial
Assessment). The Scene Size-up will set the stage for how you will perform the rest of the
BTLS Primary Survey.

If there is a dangerous *generalized* mechanism of injury (auto crash, fall from a height,
etc.) or if the patient is unconscious, you should go from Initial Assessment directly to the

BTLS Rapid Trauma Survey. You would then perform interventions, transport, and possibly do a Detailed Exam en route.

If there is a dangerous *focused* mechanism of injury suggesting an *isolated* injury (bullet wound of thigh, stab wound to the chest, etc.), you would perform the Initial Assessment but the Focused Exam would be limited to the area of injury. The full BTLS Rapid Trauma Survey is not required. You would then perform interventions, transport, and possibly do a Detailed or Ongoing Exam.

If there is no significant life threat in the mechanism of injury (shot off big toe) you would do the Initial Assessment and *if normal,* go directly to a Focused Exam based on the patient's chief complaint. *The Detailed Exam would not be necessary.*

To make the most efficient use of time, prehospital assessment and management of the trauma patient is divided into five steps, and each step contains certain priorities (see Figure 2-1). These priorities are the foundation on which trauma care is built.

PATIENT ASSESSMENT USING THE PRIORITY PLAN
Evaluation of the Scene and Preparation for Patient Assessment and Management

Scene Size-Up: On-scene trauma assessment begins with certain actions before you approach the patient. It cannot be stressed too much that failure to perform preliminary actions may jeopardize your life as well as the patient's. Perform the Scene Size-up as described in Chapter 1.

Carry essential medical equipment to the scene. The critical patient may not have time for you to return to the vehicle for needed equipment. Remember to change gloves between patients. The following equipment is always needed for trauma patients:

1. Personal protection equipment (See chapters 1 and 22)
2. Long backboard with effective strapping and head motion-restriction device
3. Appropriately sized rigid cervical extrication collar
4. Airway kit (separate kits or separate sections for adult or pediatric patients)
   a. Oxygen
   b. Airway equipment
   c. Bag-valve mask (BVM)
   d. Suction
5. Trauma box (should be separate boxes for adult or pediatric patients)
   a. Dressings and bandages to aid in controlling bleeding
   b. Blood pressure cuff
   c. Stethoscope

Evaluation and Management of the Patient

As the team leader, you must focus on the rapid assessment of your patient. All decisions on treatment require that you have identified life-threatening conditions. Experience has shown that most mistakes occur because the team leader stops to make an intervention and forgets to perform part of the assessment. If interventions must be made, you should delegate these to your team members while you continue the assessment. Remember, *once you begin the BTLS Primary Survey, nothing interrupts the completion of the assessment except treatment of airway obstruction or cardiac arrest* (respiratory arrest or dyspnea can be addressed by Rescuer 2 while you continue the Initial Assessment). For critical patients, the goal should be to have on-scene times of five minutes or less.

Patient Assessment Using Priority Plan

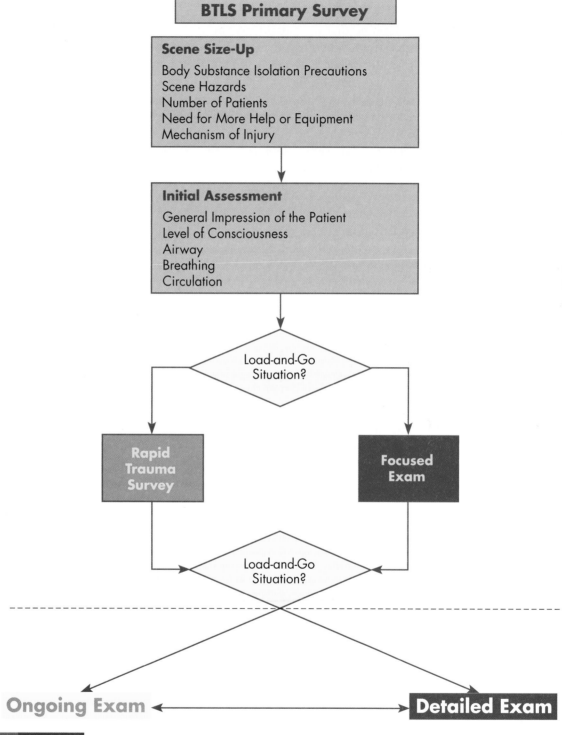

Figure 2-1 Steps in the assessment and management of the trauma patient.

Initial Assessment

The purpose of the Initial Assessment is to prioritize the patient and to determine the existence of immediately life-threatening conditions. The information gathered here is used to make decisions about critical interventions and time of transport. Once you determine that the patient may be safely approached, the assessment should proceed quickly and smoothly (the Initial Assessment and Rapid Trauma Survey should take less than two minutes). As you begin this assessment you should direct Rescuer 2 (who should have the cervical collar and airway equipment) to stabilize the patient's neck (if needed) and to assume responsibility for the airway. Rescuer 3 will place the backboard and the trauma box beside the patient while you are proceeding with your exam. This team approach makes the most efficient use of time and allows you to rapidly perform the Initial Assessment without performing airway interventions yourself, which can interrupt your thought process.

General Impression of the Patient on Approach: You have already assessed the scene, determined the total number of patients, and initiated MCI protocols if there are more patients than your team can effectively handle (see Chapter 1). Based on initial triage, begin evaluation of the most seriously injured patient first. As you approach, note the patient's approximate age, sex, weight, and general appearance. *The old and the very young are at increased risk.* Female patients may be pregnant. Observe the position of the patient, both her body position and her position in relation to her surroundings. Note her activity (is she aware of her surroundings, anxious, obviously in distress, etc.?). Does she have any obvious major injuries or major bleeding? Your observation of the patient in relation to the scene and the mechanism of injury will help you prioritize the patient.

Evaluate Initial Level of Consciousness while Obtaining Cervical Spine Stabilization: Assessment begins immediately, even if the patient is being extricated. The team leader should try to approach the patient from the front (face to face, so the patient does not turn her head to see you). If there is a mechanism of injury that suggests spinal injury, the second rescuer immediately, and gently, but firmly, stabilizes the neck in a neutral position. The team leader may need to initially stabilize the neck if there is not a second rescuer immediately available. If the head or neck is held in an angulated position and the patient complains of pain on any attempt to straighten it, you should stabilize it in the position found. The same is true of the unconscious patient whose neck is held to one side and does not move when you gently attempt to straighten it The rescuer stabilizing the neck must not release the neck until he or she is relieved or a suitable motion-restriction device is applied. The team leader should say to the patient, "My name is _____. We are here to help you. Can you tell me what happened?" The patient's reply gives immediate information about both the airway and the level of consciousness. If the patient responds *appropriately* to questioning, you can assume that the airway is open and the LOC is normal. If the response is not appropriate (unconscious, or awake but confused), make a mental note of the LOC by the AVPU scale (see Table 2-1). Anything below "A" triggers a systematic search for the causes during the Rapid Trauma Survey.

Assess the Airway: If the patient cannot speak or is unconscious, further evaluation of the airway should follow. Look, listen, and feel for movement of air. The team leader or Rescuer 2 should position the airway as needed. Because of the ever-present danger of spinal injury, never extend the neck to open the airway of a trauma patient. If the airway is obstructed (apnea, snoring, gurgling, stridor), use an appropriate method (reposition, sweep, suction) to open it immediately (see Figure 2-2). Failure to provide an open airway is one of two reasons to interrupt the Primary Survey. If simple positioning and suctioning fail to provide an adequate airway, or if the patient has stridor, transport the patient *immediately.*

TABLE 2-1	Levels of Mental Status (AVPU)

A—**A**lert (Awake *and* oriented)

V—Responds to **V**erbal stimuli (awake but confused or unconscious but responds in some way to verbal stimuli)

P—Responds to **P**ain (unconscious but responds in some way to painful stimuli)

U—**U**nresponsive (no gag or cough reflex)

Assess Breathing: Look, listen, and feel for movement of air. If the patient is unconscious, place your ear over the patient's mouth so you can judge both the rate and depth (tidal volume—see Chapter 4) of ventilations. Look at the movement of the chest (or abdomen), listen to the sound of the air movement, and feel both the movement of air on your cheek and the movement of the chest wall with your hand. Notice if the patient uses accessory muscles in order to breathe. If ventilation is inadequate (less than 10 per minute or too shallow), Rescuer 2 should begin to assist ventilation immediately, using his knees to restrict movement of the patient's neck, freeing his hands to apply oxygen or use a bag-valve mask to assist ventilation (see Figure 2-3). When assisting with or providing ventilation, be sure that the patient not only gets an adequate ventilatory rate (see Table 2-2), but also an adequate volume. All patients that are breathing too fast should receive supplemental high-flow oxygen. As a general rule, all patients with multisystem trauma should also receive supplemental high-flow oxygen.

Assess Circulation: As soon as you have ensured a patent airway and adequate ventilation, note the rate and quality of the pulses at the wrist (brachial in the infant). Checking the pulse in the neck is not necessary if the patient is awake and alert or if there is a palpable peripheral pulse. Quickly note whether the rate is too slow (<60 in an adult) or too fast (>120), and note also its quality (thready, bounding, weak, irregular). If pulses are absent at the neck, immediately start CPR (unless there is massive blunt trauma) and prepare for immediate transport. This is the other reason to interrupt the Primary Survey. While at the wrist, also note skin color, temperature, and condition (and capillary refill in an infant or small child). Pale, cool, clammy skin, thready radial pulse, and decreased LOC are the best early assessment of decreased perfusion (shock). Be sure the bleeding has

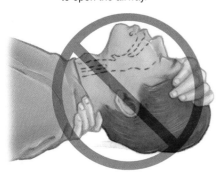
Since neck may be injured, do not extend the neck to open the airway.

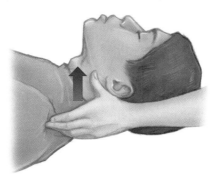
Use modified jaw thrust

Figure 2-2 Opening the airway using the modified jaw thrust. Maintain in-line stabilization while pushing up on the angles of the jaw with your thumbs.

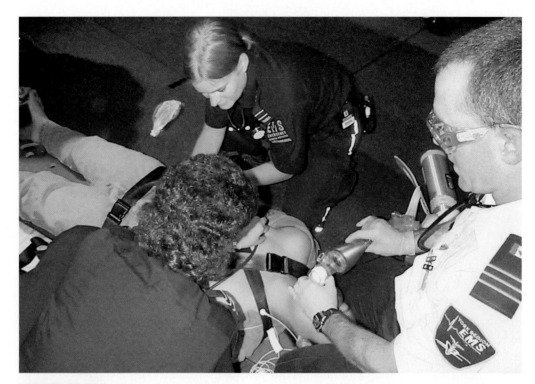

Figure 2-3 Using your knees to maintain immobilization of the neck will free your hands to assist ventilation. *(Photo courtesy of BTLS Ontario, Steve McNenly, Jennifer Lundgren, and Sheryl Jackson)*

been controlled (direct Rescuer 3 to do this). Most bleeding can be stopped by direct pressure or pressure dressings. Air splints or the pneumatic antishock garment (PASG) may be used to tamponade bleeding. Tourniquets are rarely needed. In the past it has been taught that blood-soaked dressings should only have more dressings placed on top of them, but in some cases this only allows more bleeding. If a dressing becomes blood soaked, remove the dressing and redress **once** to be sure direct pressure is being placed on the bleeding area. It is important to report such excessive bleeding to the receiving physician. Do not use clamps to stop bleeders; this may cause injuries to other structures (nerves are present alongside arteries).

Rapid Trauma Survey or Focused Exam

The choice between the Rapid Trauma Survey and the Focused Exam depends on the mechanism of injury and/or the results of the Initial Assessment. If there is a dangerous generalized mechanism of injury (auto crash, fall from a height, etc.) or if the patient is unconscious, you should perform the BTLS Rapid Trauma Survey. If there is a dangerous focused mechanism of injury suggesting an isolated injury (bullet wound of thigh, stab

TABLE 2-2	Normal and Abnormal Respiratory Rates	
	Normal	**Abnormal**
Adult	10–20	<10 and >24
Small child	15–30	<15 and >35
Infant	25–50	<25 and >60

wound to the chest, etc.), you may perform the Focused Exam limited to the area of injury. If there is no significant mechanism of injury (dropped rock on toe) and the Initial Assessment was normal (alert with no history of loss of consciousness, breathing normally, radial pulse less than 120, not complaining of dyspnea, chest, abdominal, or pelvic pain), you may move directly to the Focused Exam based on the patient's chief complaint.

If you identify a priority patient, you need to find the cause of the abnormal findings and to identify if this is a load-and-go patient.

You have identified a priority patient if there is:

1. A dangerous mechanism of injury
2. A history that reveals:
   a. Loss of consciousness
   b. Difficulty breathing
   c. Severe pain of head, neck, or torso
3. An abnormal Initial Assessment:
   a. Altered mental status
   b. Difficulty breathing
   c. Abnormal perfusion
   d. High-risk group (very young, very old, chronically ill, etc.)

RAPID TRAUMA SURVEY

Assessment of the Head, Neck, Chest, Abdomen, Pelvis, and Extremities: This is a *brief* exam done to find all life-threats. (A more thorough, detailed exam will follow later if time permits.) You should obtain a SAMPLE history (see Table 2-3) as you are doing your assessment. You are the only one who gets to see the scene and you may be the only one who gets to take a history. Many patients who are initially alert lose consciousness before arriving at the hospital. You are not only making interventions to deliver a living patient to the hospital; you must be the detective that figures out what happened and why. Pay special attention to the chief complaint and the events prior to the incident (the "S" and "E" of the SAMPLE history). The patient's symptoms may suggest other injuries, and this will affect further examination. It is important to know as much about the mechanism as possible (Was she restrained? How far did she fall? What caused her to fall?). Look for clues to serious injury such as history of loss of consciousness (LOC), shortness of breath, or pain in the neck, back, chest, abdomen, or pelvis.

Briefly assess (look and feel) the head and neck for injuries and to see if the neck veins are flat or distended and the trachea is in the midline. You may apply a rigid cervical

TABLE 2-3	SAMPLE History
S—symptoms **A**—allergies **M**—medications **P**—past medical history (Other illnesses?) **L**—last oral intake (When was the last time there was any solid or liquid intake?) **E**—events preceding the incident (Why did it happen?)	

extrication collar at this time. *Note:* If the team leader elected to stabilize the neck, this duty should be transferred to another rescuer at this time.

Now look, feel, and listen to the chest. Look for both asymmetrical and paradoxical movement. Note if the ribs rise with respiration or if there is only diaphragmatic breathing. Look for signs of blunt trauma or open wounds. Feel for tenderness, instability, and crepitation (TIC). Now listen to see if breath sounds are present and equal bilaterally. Listen with the stethoscope over the lateral chest about the fourth interspace in the midaxillary line on both sides. If breath sounds are not equal (decreased or absent on one side), you should percuss the chest to determine whether the patient is just splinting from pain or if a pneumothorax or a hemothorax is present. If abnormalities are found during the chest exam (open chest wound, flail chest, tension pneumothorax, hemothorax), delegate the appropriate intervention (seal open wound, stabilize flail). Very briefly notice the heart sounds so you will have a baseline for changes such as development of muffled heart sounds.

Rapidly expose and look at the abdomen (distension, contusions, penetrating wounds), and gently palpate the abdomen for tenderness, guarding, and rigidity.

Check the pelvis. Look for deformity or penetrating wounds. Feel for tenderness, instability, and crepitation by *gently* pressing down on the symphysis and *gently* squeezing in on the iliac crests. If the pelvis is unstable, do not check again!

Check the extremities. Assess both upper legs, looking for deformity and feeling for TIC. Remember that bilateral femur fractures can produce enough blood loss to be life threatening. Scan for obvious wounds or deformities of the arms and lower legs. Note whether the patient can move her fingers and toes before transferring to the backboard.

At this point, transfer the patient to a long backboard, *checking the back* as you do this. If the patient has an unstable pelvis or bilateral femur fractures, to prevent further injuries, use a scoop stretcher (see Figure 2-4) to transfer the patient to a long backboard. You have now obtained enough information to determine critical trauma situations that should be treated by immediate transport to the hospital (load-and-go). If a critical situation is present, transport now and obtain baseline vital signs and the rest of the SAMPLE history during transport.

If there is altered mental status, do a brief neurological exam to identify possible increased intracranial pressure (ICP). This exam should include the pupils, Glasgow Coma Score (GCS), and signs of cerebral herniation (see Chapter 10). Also look for medical identification devices. Head injury, shock, and hypoxia are not the only things that cause altered mental status; think about nontraumatic causes such as hypoglycemia and drug or alcohol overdose. Obtain finger-stick glucose at this time.

CRITICAL INTERVENTIONS AND TRANSPORT DECISION

Upon completion of the Initial Assessment and Rapid Trauma Survey, enough information is available to decide if a critical situation is present. *Patients with critical trauma situations are transported immediately.* Most treatment will be done during transport.

To decide whether the patient falls into the load-and-go category, you need to determine whether the patient has any of the following critical injuries or conditions:

1. Initial Assessment reveals:

   a. Altered mental status

   b. Abnormal respiration

   c. Abnormal circulation (shock or uncontrolled bleeding)

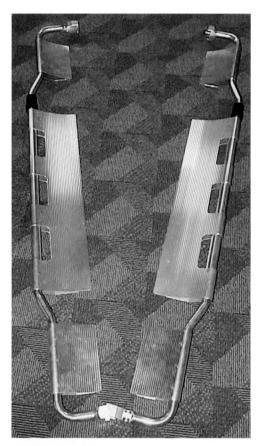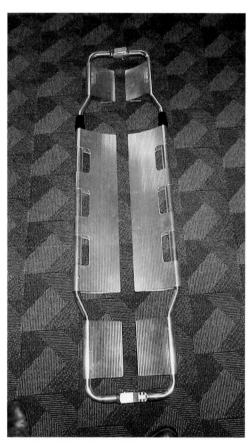

Figure 2-4 Scoop stretcher is useful for transferring to the backboard patients who should not be log-rolled.

2. Signs discovered during the Rapid Trauma Survey of conditions that rapidly lead to shock:

   a. Abnormal chest exam (flail chest, open wound, tension pneumothorax, hemothorax)

   b. Tender, distended abdomen

   c. Pelvic instability

   d. Bilateral femur fractures

3. Significant mechanism of injury and/or poor general health of patient. As you consider mechanisms, age, general appearance, chronic illnesses, etc., you may decide that the patient is at higher risk than the primary survey would suggest. This may have more to do with deciding on where to transport the patient (trauma center versus closest hospital) than necessarily whether to load and go, but is just to remind you that there are more considerations than just the physical exam.

   If the patient has one of the critical conditions listed above, after the Rapid Trauma Survey or Focused Exam, immediately load her into an ambulance, and transport rapidly to the nearest *appropriate* emergency facility. When in doubt, transport early. There are only a few procedures that are done at the scene and *these can be delegated to team members during the BTLS Primary Survey:*

1. Initial airway management

2. Assist ventilation

3. Administer oxygen

4. Begin CPR

5. Control of major external bleeding

6. Seal sucking chest wounds

7. Stabilize flail chest

8. Stabilize impaled objects

9. Complete packaging of the patient

Procedures that are not lifesaving, such as splinting or bandaging must not hold up transport of the critical patient. Be sure to call Medical Direction early so that the hospital is prepared for the patient's arrival.

FOCUSED EXAM

If the mechanism is limited to a certain area of the body (stab wound of the chest), then you may only need to focus your exam on the affected area (chest and possibly the abdomen), obtain a SAMPLE history (may suggest further exam), and check baseline vital signs (defer until after transport if radial pulse is not present). You would then have enough information to make a decision about urgency of transport and what interventions need to be done immediately.

ONGOING ASSESSMENT AND MANAGEMENT

This includes the critical procedures performed on scene and during transport, the Ongoing Exam, and also communication with Medical Direction. The Ongoing Exam is an abbreviated exam to assess for changes in the patient's condition. In some critical cases with short transport times, this exam may take the place of the Detailed Exam.

The Ongoing Exam should be recorded every five minutes in critical patients and every 15 minutes in stable patients. The Ongoing Exam also should be performed each time the patient is moved, an intervention is performed, or her condition changes. This exam is to find any changes in the patient's condition, so concentrate on reassessing only those things that may change.

🖐 PROCEDURE

❋ The Ongoing Exam should be performed in the following order:

1. Ask the patient about any changes in how she feels.

2. Reassess mental status (LOC and pupils, recheck GCS if altered mental status).

3. Reassess the ABCs.

    a. Reassess the airway.

        (1) Recheck patency.

        (2) If burn patient, assess for signs of inhalation injury.

    b. Reassess breathing and circulation.

        (1) Recheck vital signs.

        (2) Note skin color, condition, temperature.

        (3) Check the neck for jugular venous distention (JVD) and tracheal deviation. (If collar has been applied, remove the front.)

(4) Recheck the chest. Notice the quality of breath sounds. If breath sounds are unequal, evaluate for splinting, pneumothorax, or hemothorax. Listen to the heart to see if the sounds have become muffled.

4. Reassess the abdomen (if mechanism suggests possible injury). Note the development of tenderness, distention, or rigidity.

5. Check each of the identified injuries (lacerations for bleeding, PMS distal to all injured extremities, flails, pneumothorax, open chest wounds, etc.).

6. Check interventions.

   a. Check oxygen for flow rate.

   b. Check seals on sucking chest wounds.

   c. Check splints and dressings.

   d. Check impaled objects to be sure they are well stabilized.

   e. Check position of pregnant patients.

   f. Check cardiac monitor and pulse oximeter (if available).

Accurately record what you see and what you do. Record changes in the patient's condition during transport. Record the times that interventions are performed. Extenuating circumstances or significant details should be recorded in the comments or remarks section of the written report (review documentation in Appendix C).

CONTACTING MEDICAL DIRECTION

When you have a critical patient, it is extremely important to contact Medical Direction as early as possible. It takes time to get the appropriate surgeon and the operating room team in place, and the critical patient has no time to wait. Always notify the receiving facility of your estimated time of arrival (ETA), the condition of the patient, and any special needs on arrival (see Appendix B).

DETAILED EXAM

This is a more comprehensive exam to pick up additional injuries that might have been missed in the brief BTLS Primary Survey. This assessment also establishes the baseline from which treatment decisions will eventually be made. It is important to record the information discovered in this assessment. *Critical patients should always have this assessment done during transport.* If there is a short transport and you must perform interventions, you may not have time to do the Detailed Exam. If the Primary Survey does not reveal a critical condition, the Detailed Exam may be performed on the scene. Even though the patient appears to be stable, if there is a dangerous mechanism or other dangers (age, poor general health, death of another passenger, etc.), reconsider early transport. "Stable" patients may become unstable quite rapidly. Stable patients with no dangerous mechanism of injury (dropped rock on toe) do not require a Detailed Exam.

You should have obtained most of the pertinent history during the BTLS Primary Survey, but now you can obtain further information if needed. You should perform your detailed physical exam while you are obtaining the rest of the SAMPLE history (if the patient is conscious).

✋ PROCEDURE

✴ The exam should contain the following elements:

1. *Record vital signs again:* Record pulse, respiration, and blood pressure. Remember, the pulse pressure is as important as the systolic pressure. Many people now consider the pulse oximetry reading one of the vital signs.

2. *Do a neurological exam:* It gives important baseline information that is used in later treatment decisions. This exam should include the following:

   a. Level of consciousness: If the patient is conscious, describe her orientation and emotional status. If she has an altered mental status, record her level of coma (Glasgow Coma Score—see Table 2-4). *If there is altered mental status, you should check the blood glucose and check the oxygen saturation by pulse oximetry.*

   b. Pupils: Are they equal or unequal? Do they respond to light?

   c. Motor: Can the patient move fingers and toes?

   d. Sensation: Can she feel you when you touch her fingers and toes? Does the unconscious patient respond when you pinch her fingers and toes?

3. *Think about monitors (cardiac, pulse oximeter):* These are usually applied during transport.

4. *Perform a head-to-toes exam in more detail:* Pay particular attention to the patient's complaints and also recheck the injuries that you found previously. The exam should consist of inspection, auscultation, palpation, and sometimes percussion.

   a. Begin at the head examining for deformities, contusions, abrasions, penetrations, burns, tenderness, lacerations, or swelling (DCAP-BTLS), raccoon eyes, Battle's sign, and drainage of blood or fluid from the ears or nose. Assess the mouth. Assess the airway again.

   b. Check the neck for DCAP-BTLS, distended neck veins, or deviated trachea.

   c. Check the chest for DCAP-BTLS. Also check for paradoxical movement of the chest wall and for instability and crepitation of the ribs. Be sure that breath sounds are present and equal on each side (checking four [4] fields).

TABLE 2-4		Glasgow Coma Score			
Eye Opening		**Verbal Response**		**Motor Response**	
	Points		Points		Points
Spontaneous	4	Oriented	5	Obeys commands	6
To voice	3	Confused	4	Localizes pain	5
To pain	2	Inappropriate words	3	Withdraws	4
None	1	Incomprehensible sounds	2	Abnormal flexion	3[*]
		Silent	1	Abnormal extension	2[**]
				No movement	1

[*]Decorticate posturing to pain
[**]Decerebrate posturing to pain

Note rales, wheezing, or "noisy" breath sounds. Notice if heart sounds are as loud as before. (A noticeable decrease in heart sounds may be an early sign of cardiac tamponade.) Recheck seals over open wounds. Be sure flails are well stabilized. If you detect decreased breath sounds, percuss to determine whether the patient has a pneumothorax or hemothorax.

d. Perform an abdominal exam. Look for signs of blunt or penetrating trauma. Feel all four quadrants for tenderness or rigidity. Do not waste time listening for bowel sounds. If the abdomen is painful to gentle pressure during examination, you can expect the patient to be bleeding internally. If the abdomen is both distended and painful, you can expect hemorrhagic shock to occur very quickly.

e. Assess pelvis and extremities (unstable pelvis noted in Rapid Trauma Survey is <u>not rechecked</u>). Check for DCAP-BTLS. Be sure to check and record pulse, motor function, and sensation (PMS) on all fractures. Do this before and after straightening any fracture. Angulated fractures of the upper extremities are usually best splinted as found. Most fractures of the lower extremities are gently straightened and then stabilized using traction splints or air splints. Critical patients have all splints applied during transport.

Transport immediately if the Detailed Exam reveals the development of any of the critical trauma situations.

When you finish the Detailed Exam, you should finish bandaging and splinting.

PEARLS

1. *Do not approach the patient before doing a Scene Size-up:* Foolish haste may subtract a rescuer and add a patient.

2. The team leader should delegate any intervention required during the BTLS Primary Survey and should not interrupt the completion of the survey except for airway obstruction or cardiac arrest.

3. Critical trauma patients need definitive care in the operating room. Limit on-scene time. Survival of the critical trauma patient is time dependent. Most interventions should be performed in the ambulance during transport to an appropriate facility.

4. Use the same systematic BTLS approach for each trauma patient.

CASE STUDY

Dan, Joyce, and Buddy of the Emergency Transport System have been called to the scene of a construction accident where a man fell from a scaffold onto a pile of lumber. Their Scene Size-up reveals that the scene is safe and that there is only one male victim who is awake and appears to be about fifty years old (high-risk group). The initial impression is poor because the patient is pale and diaphoretic and appears to be having some trouble breathing. He is clutching a two-foot

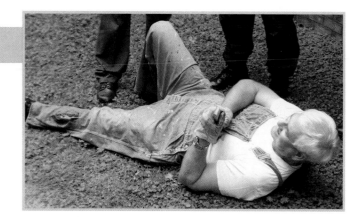

piece of wood that is protruding from his left chest. The bone can be seen in an open wound of his left lower leg. Buddy is acting as team leader. The team dons personal protective equipment, gathers the essential equipment and approaches the patient.

Buddy begins his Initial Assessment by introducing the team as Joyce stabilizes the patient's neck with her knees and prepares to apply a non-rebreather oxygen mask. Dan places the long backboard beside the patient and checks the pulse in his left foot before splinting the lower leg. When questioned about what happened, Mr. Cuthbert Mulford states he was building a concrete wall and was on a scaffold about 10 feet high. He was lifting a concrete block when he felt a "fluttering" in his chest and the next thing he knew his friends were bending over him asking him what happened. They state he was unconscious for about two to three minutes. Buddy notes that Mr. Mulford has a good airway but his breathing is rapid and shallow. He has a rapid, thready pulse at the wrist. Dan has applied a compression dressing to the open wound on the left lower leg and is applying a splint at this time. There is no bleeding now. Because of the mechanism of injury, Buddy chooses to perform a Rapid Trauma Survey. He has already determined that this is a priority patient because of the abnormal Initial Assessment and this is also a load-and-go situation because of the loss of consciousness and the respiratory difficulty.

Brief exam of the head and face reveals no evidence of head trauma and Joyce notes that the pupils are 4 mm and react equally. The neck veins are flat and the trachea is midline. There is no tenderness or deformity of the neck. At this time Buddy and Joyce choose the correct-size rigid cervical collar and apply it while maintaining motion-restriction of the cervical spine in a neutral position. Buddy notes the two-inch-wide piece of wood that enters from the front of the left chest but does not protrude from the back. There is no paradoxical movement of the chest. The breath sounds are markedly decreased on the left and the left chest is dull to percussion. The heart sounds are good but slightly irregular. The abdomen is negative for DCAP-BTLS and is soft and nontender. The pelvis is stable and nontender. Exam of the extremities is normal except for the left lower leg, which has an open fracture that has been splinted and dressed. The patient is able to move his fingers and toes and has sensation in all extremities. Because of the history of loss of consciousness, a brief neurological exam is done. It reveals normal level of consciousness with good PMS in all extremities. The Glasgow coma score is 15.

After stabilizing the impaled piece of wood, the patient is carefully log-rolled onto the long backboard and strapped securely in place to provide spinal motion restriction (SMR). He is then immediately moved to the ambulance and transported. Dan drives while Buddy and Joyce provide patient care. While Buddy obtains the rest of the SAMPLE history and obtains vital signs, Joyce attaches a cardiac monitor and performs a rapid blood-glucose check. Mr. Mulford states that he hurts in his chest and left lower leg and feels short of breath. He has no allergies. His past medical history is positive for hypertension but he has never had any heart disease or palpitations in the past. He takes one aspirin tablet each day (has taken his dose today) and medication for hypertension but is not sure of the name. His last oral intake was breakfast (it is now 11:00 AM).

The vital signs are: blood pressure 70/40, pulse 130 and irregular, respiratory rate 30 and shallow. The pulse oximeter reading is 92% on 100% oxygen, the blood glucose is normal, and the monitor shows an irregular heart rhythm.

Buddy notifies Medical Direction that he is transporting a patient who had syncope after cardiac palpitations and fell about 10 feet, sustaining a penetrating wound of his left chest and an open fracture of his left lower leg.

The trauma team is waiting upon their arrival and the patient is taken to surgery where the impaled wood is removed (no cardiac damage from the wood) and the open fracture is irrigated and repaired. An EKG done in the emergency department showed an acute myocardial infarction. A balloon angioplasty and stent insertion is performed and the patient receives three units of blood. After a stormy course he eventually recovers.

CASE STUDY WRAP-UP

This is a complex case in which a medical event (acute myocardial infarction with arrhythmia) causes syncope that in turn causes serious traumatic injury. By following the BTLS assessment and management protocol they obtained the best possible outcome in this case.

SUMMARY

Patient assessment is the key to trauma care. The interventions required are not difficult; their timing often is critical. If you know what questions to ask and how to perform the exam, you will know when to perform the lifesaving interventions. This chapter has described a rapid, orderly, and thorough examination of the trauma patient with examination and treatment priorities always in mind. The continuous practice of approaching the patient in the way described here will allow you to concentrate on the patient, rather than on what to do next. Optimum speed is achieved by teamwork. Teamwork is achieved by practice. You should plan regular exercises in patient evaluation to perfect each team member's role in the priority plan.

TABLE 2-5	Acronyms

ATV—all terrain vehicle

AVPU—**A**lert, responds to **V**erbal stimuli, responds to **P**ainful stimuli, **U**nresponsive

BSI—body substance isolation

BVM—bag-valve mask

DCAP-BTLS—deformities, contusions, abrasions, penetrations, burns, tenderness, lacerations, swelling

EMS—emergency medical services

ETA—estimated time of arrival

GCS—Glasgow Coma Score

IPPV—intermittent positive pressure ventilation

LOC—level of consciousness

MCI—multiple casualty incident

MVC—motor vehicle collision

PMS—pulse, motor, sensory

PWC—personal watercraft

SAMPLE—**S**ymptoms, **A**llergies, **M**edicines, **P**ast medical history, **L**ast meal, **E**vents preceding the injury

SMR—spinal motion restriction

TIC—tenderness, instability, crepitation

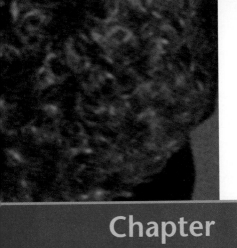

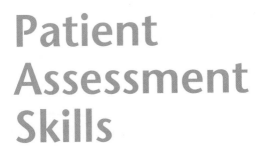

Chapter 3

Patient Assessment Skills

Donna Hastings, EMT-P

Objectives

Upon completion of these Skill Stations, you should be able to:

BTLS Primary Survey

1. Correctly perform the BTLS Primary Survey.
2. Identify within two minutes which patients require load-and-go.
3. Describe when to perform critical interventions.

Ongoing Exam and Detailed Exam

1. Correctly perform the Ongoing (reassessment) Exam.
2. Describe when to perform critical interventions.
3. Demonstrate proper communications with Medical Direction.
4. Correctly perform the Detailed Exam.

Assessment and Management of the Trauma Patient

1. Demonstrate the proper sequence of rapid assessment and the management of the multiple-trauma patient.

(Photo courtesy of BTLS Ontario).

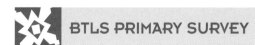

BTLS PRIMARY SURVEY

Objectives

Upon completion of this skill station, you should be able to:

1. Correctly perform the BTLS Primary Survey (see Figure 3-1).
2. Identify within two minutes which patients require load-and-go.
3. Describe when to perform critical interventions.

PROCEDURE

Short written scenarios will be used along with a model (to act as the patient). You will divide into teams to practice performing the Initial Assessment, critical interventions, and transfer decisions. Each member of the team must practice being team leader at least once. The Critical Information represents the answers you should be seeking at each step of the survey. The Treatment Decision Tree at the end of the chapter represents the actions that should be taken (personally or delegated) in response to your assessment.

CRITICAL INFORMATION—BTLS PRIMARY SURVEY

If you ask the right questions, you will get the information you need to make the critical decisions necessary in the management of your patient. The following questions are presented in the order in which you should ask them to yourself as you perform patient assessment. This is the minimum information that you will need as you perform each step of the Initial Assessment.

Scene Size-up

Which BSI precautions do I need to take?

Do I see, hear, smell, or sense anything dangerous?

Are there any other patients?

Are additional personnel or resources needed?

Do we need special equipment?

What is the mechanism of injury here?

Is it generalized or focused?

Is it potentially life-threatening?

Initial Assessment

What is my general impression of the patient as I approach?

Level of Consciousness (AVPU)
Introduce yourself and say: "We are here to help you. Can you tell us what happened?"

Airway
Is the airway open and clear?

Breathing
Is the patient breathing?

What is the rate and quality of respiration?

Patient Assessment Using Priority Plan

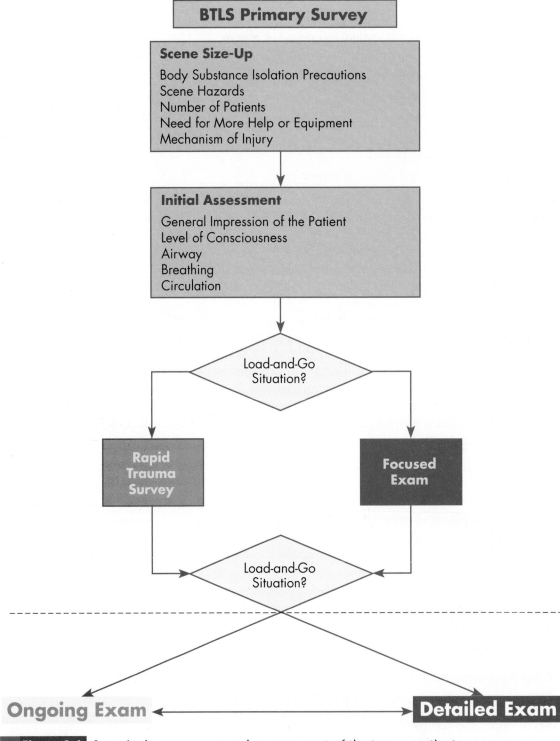

Figure 3-1 Steps in the assessment and management of the trauma patient.

Ventilation Instructions

Order oxygen for any patient with abnormal respiration, altered mental status, shock, or major injuries.

Delegate assisted ventilation if the patient is hypoventilating (<10 per minute) or if there is inadequate movement of air.

Hyperventilate only those head injury patients who are unresponsive and show signs of cerebral herniation.

Circulation

What is the rate and quality of the pulse at the wrist (and at the neck, if not palpable at the wrist)?

Is major external bleeding present?

What are the skin color, condition, and temperature?

Decision

Is this a critical situation?

Are there interventions that I must make now?

Rapid Trauma Survey

Head and Neck

Are there obvious wounds of the head or neck?

Are the neck veins distended?

Does the trachea look and feel midline or deviated?

Is there deformity or tenderness of the neck?

Chest

Is the chest symmetrical? Is there paradoxical movement? Is there any obvious blunt or penetrating trauma?

Are there any open wounds or paradoxical movement?

Is there TIC of the ribs?

Are the breath sounds present and equal?

If breath sounds are not equal, is the chest hyperresonant or dull?

Are heart sounds normal or decreased?

Abdomen

Are there obvious wounds?

Is the abdomen soft, rigid, or distended?

Is there tenderness?

Pelvis

Are there obvious wounds or deformity?

Is there TIC?

Upper Legs

Are there obvious wounds, swelling, or deformity?

Is there TIC?

Scan of Lower Legs and Arms

Are there obvious wounds, swelling, or deformity?

Is there TIC?

Can the patient feel/move fingers and toes?

Exam of the Posterior (done during transfer to the backboard)
Is there any deformity, contusions, abrasions, penetrations, burns, tenderness, lacerations, or swelling (DCAP-BTLS) of the patient's posterior side?

Decision
Is there a critical situation?

Are there interventions that I must make now?

History
What is the SAMPLE history? (may have been obtained during the exam)

Vital Signs
Are the vital signs abnormal?

Disability
(Perform this exam now if there is altered mental status. Otherwise, postpone this exam until you perform the Detailed Exam.)

Are the pupils equal and reactive?

What is the Glasgow Coma Score?

Are there signs of cerebral herniation (unconscious, dilated pupil(s), hypertension, bradycardia, posturing)?

Does the patient have a medical identification device?

ONGOING EXAM AND DETAILED EXAM

Objectives
Upon completion of this skill station, you should be able to:
1. Correctly perform the Ongoing (reassessment) Exam.
2. Describe when to perform critical interventions.
3. Demonstrate proper communications with Medical Direction.
4. Correctly perform the Detailed Exam.

PROCEDURE

Short written scenarios will be used along with a model (to act as the patient). You will divide into teams to practice performing the Ongoing Exam, making critical decisions and interventions, and performing the Detailed Exam. Each member of the team must practice being team leader at least once. The Critical Information represents the answers you should be seeking at each step of the exam.

CRITICAL INFORMATION—ONGOING EXAM

The following questions are presented in the order in which you should ask them to yourself as you perform the Ongoing (reassessment) Exam. This is the minimum information that you will need as you perform each step of the exam.

Subjective Changes
Are you feeling better or worse now?

Mental Status

What is the LOC?

What is pupillary size? Are they equal? Do they react to light?

If altered mental status, what is the Glasgow Coma Score now?

Reassess ABCs

Airway

Is the airway open and clear?

If there are burns of the face, are there signs of inhalation injury?

Breathing and **C**irculation

What is the rate and quality of respiration?

What is the rate and quality of the pulse?

What is the blood pressure?

What are the skin color, condition, and temperature (capillary refill in children)?

Neck

Is the trachea midline or deviated?

Are the neck veins normal, flat, or distended?

Is there increased swelling of the neck?

Chest

Are the breath sounds present and equal?

If breath sounds are unequal, is the chest hyperresonant or dull?

Are heart sounds still normal or have they become muffled?

Abdomen (if mechanism suggests possible injury)

Is there any tenderness?

Is the abdomen soft, rigid, or distended?

Assessment of Identified Injuries

Have there been any changes in the condition of any of the injuries that I have found?

Check Interventions

Ask the appropriate question for your patient.

    Is the oxygen rate correct?

    Is the oxygen tubing connected?

    Is the open chest wound still sealed?

    Are any of the dressings blood soaked?

    Are the splints in good position?

    Is the impaled object still well stabilized?

    Is the pregnant patient tilted to the left?

    Is the cardiac monitor attached and working?

    Is the pulse oximeter attached and working?

CRITICAL INFORMATION—DETAILED EXAM

If you ask the right questions, you will get the information you need to make the critical decisions necessary in the management of your patient. The following questions are presented in the order in which you should ask them to yourself as you perform the Detailed Exam. This is the minimum information that you will need as you perform each step of the exam.

SAMPLE History (complete if not already done)
What is the patient's history?

Vital Signs
What are the vital signs?

Neurological Exam
What is the LOC?

What is the blood glucose (if altered mental status)?

Are the pupils equal? Do they respond to light?

Can the patient move his fingers and toes?

Can the patient feel me touch his fingers and toes?

What is the Glasgow Coma Score (if altered mental status)?

Head
Is there DCAP-BTLS of the face or head?

Are Battle's sign or raccoon eyes present?

Is there blood or fluid draining from the ears or nose?

Is there pallor, cyanosis, or diaphoresis?

Airway
Is the airway open and clear?

If there are burns of the face, are there signs of burns in the mouth or nose?

Breathing
What is the rate and quality of respiration?

Neck
Is there DCAP-BTLS of the neck?

Are the neck veins normal, flat, or distended?

Is the trachea midline or deviated?

Circulation
What is the rate and quality of the pulse?

What is the skin color, condition, and temperature (capillary refill in children)?

Is all external bleeding still controlled?

Chest
Is there DCAP-BTLS of the chest?

Are there any open wounds or paradoxical movement?

Are the breath sounds present and equal?

    If breath sounds are not equal, is the chest hyperresonant or dull?

Are heart sounds normal or decreased?

Abdomen
Is there DCAP-BTLS of the abdomen?

Is the abdomen soft, rigid, or distended?

Pelvis
(already examined in the initial assessment—no further exam should be done)

Lower Extremities
Is there DCAP-BTLS of the legs?

Is there normal PMS?

Is range of motion normal? (optional)

Upper Extremities
Is there DCAP-BTLS of the arms?

Is there normal PMS?

Is range of motion normal? (optional)

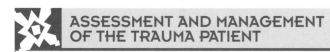

ASSESSMENT AND MANAGEMENT OF THE TRAUMA PATIENT

Objective

Upon completion of this skill station, you should be able to:

1. Demonstrate the proper sequence of rapid assessment and the management of the multiple-trauma patient.

PROCEDURE

Short written trauma scenarios will be used along with a model (to act as the patient). You will be divided into teams to practice the management of simulated trauma situations using the principles and techniques taught in the course. You will be evaluated in the same manner on the second day of the course. You will be expected to use all the principles and techniques taught in this course while managing these simulated patients. To familiarize yourself with the evaluation procedure, you will be given a copy of a scenario and a grade sheet. Review Chapter 2 and the previous surveys in this chapter.

Ground Rules for Teaching and Evaluation

1. You will be allowed to stay together in three-member groups (different-sized groups are optional) throughout the practice and evaluation stations.

2. You will have three practice scenarios. This allows each member of the team to be team leader once.

3. You will be evaluated as team leader once.

4. You will assist as a member of the rescue team during two scenarios in which another member of your team is being evaluated as team leader. You may assist, but the team leader must do all assessments. This gives you a total of six scenarios from which to learn: three practices, one evaluation, and two assists while others are evaluated.

5. Wait outside the door until the instructor comes out and gives you your scenario.

6. You will be allowed to look over your equipment before you start your exam.

7. Be sure to ask about scene safety if not provided in the scenario.

8. Be sure to apply your personal protective gear.

9. If you have a live model for a patient, you must talk to that person just as you would a real patient. It is best to explain what you are doing as you examine the patient. Be confident and reassuring.

10. You must ask your instructor for things you cannot find out from your patient. Examples: blood pressure, pulse, breath sounds.

11. Wounds and fractures must be dressed or splinted just as if they were real. Procedures must be done correctly (blood pressure, log-rolling, strapping, splinting, etc.).

12. If you need a piece of equipment that is not available, ask your instructors. They may allow you to simulate the equipment.

13. During practice and evaluation, you may be allowed to go (or may be directed) to any station, but you cannot go to the same station twice.

14. You will be graded on the following:

    a. Assessment of the scene

    b. Assessment of the patient

    c. Management of the patient

    d. Efficient use of time

    e. Leadership

    f. Judgment

    g. Problem-solving ability

    h. Patient interaction

15. When you finish your testing scenario, there is to be no discussion of the case. If you have any questions, they will be answered after the faculty meeting at the end of the course.

Patient Assessment Pearls

1. Do not approach the patient until you have done a Scene Size-up.

2. Do not interrupt the BTLS Primary Survey except for:

    a. Airway obstruction

    b. Cardiac arrest

    Your team members may perform other critical interventions while you complete the Primary Survey.

3. Give ventilation instructions as soon as you assess the airway and breathing.

4. Prophylactic hyperventilation is no longer recommended for patients with decreased LOC. It is only used for the head injury patient who shows signs of the cerebral herniation syndrome.

5. Assist ventilations for anyone who is hypoventilating (<10 per minute).

6. Give oxygen to all multiple-trauma patients. If in doubt, give oxygen.

7. Transfer the patient to the backboard as soon as the BTLS Primary Survey is completed.

8. When the BTLS Primary Survey is completed, decide if the patient is critical or stable. Critical trauma situations are characterized by any of the following:

    a. Decreased level of consciousness

    b. Difficulty with airway or breathing

    c. Shock

    d. Tender abdomen

    e. Unstable pelvis

    f. Bilateral femur fractures

    g. High risk group

9. If the BTLS Primary Survey reveals that the patient has a critical trauma situation, load the patient in the ambulance and transport.

10. If absolutely necessary, certain interventions may have to be done before transport. Remember that you are trading minutes of the patient's golden hour for those procedures. Use good judgment.

11. Critical patients get a Detailed Exam en route to the hospital if time permits.

12. Stable patients may get a Detailed Exam at the scene (on the backboard).

13. Transport immediately if your Detailed Exam reveals any of the critical trauma situations.

14. Critical patients should not have traction splints applied at the scene (it takes too long).

15. Call Medical Direction early if you have a critical patient (other physicians may have to be called from home to treat the patient).

16. Repeat the Ongoing Exam:

    a. If the patient's condition changes

    b. If you make an intervention

    c. If you move the patient (scene to ambulance, ambulance to emergency room)

17. Unconscious patients with no gag reflex cannot protect their airways. Have suction ready

18. Transport pregnant patients with the backboard tilted slightly to the left. Do not let them roll over onto the floor.

19. Remain calm and think. Your knowledge, training, and concern are the most important tools you carry.

Trauma Assessment—Treatment Decision Tree

Initial Assessment	Action
SCENE SIZE-UP	
Safety	Put on gloves, protective clothing. Remove hazards or patient from hazards.
Number of patients	Call for help if needed.
Extrication needed	Call for special equipment if needed.
Mechanisms of injury	Suspect appropriate injuries (e.g., cervical spine).
GENERAL IMPRESSION	Begin to establish priorities.
Age, sex, weight	
Position (in surroundings, body position/posture)	
Activity	
Obvious major injuries; major bleeding	
LEVEL OF CONSCIOUSNESS	
Alert/responsive to voice	Maintain cervical-spine motion restriction.

Unresponsive to voice ....Modified jaw thrust prn.

AIRWAY

Snoring...Modified jaw thrust.

Gurgling ....Suction.

Stridor ....Check for airway obstruction

Silence ....Attempt to ventilate—if unsuccessful:
                Reposition; extricate immediately.
                Visualize.
                Suction.
                Consider Heimlich maneuver.

BREATHING

Absent ....Ventilate twice (check pulse before continuing ventilation at 10–20 + oxygen).

<10...Assist ventilation at 10–20 + oxygen.

Low tidal volume ....Assist ventilation.

Labored ....Oxygen by non-rebreather at 15 L/min.

Normal or rapid..Consider oxygen.

RADIAL PULSE

Absent ....Check carotid pulse (see below).
                Note late shock.

Present ....Note rate and quality.

Bradycardia..Consider spinal shock, head injury.

Tachycardia...Attempt to calm to reduce rate; consider shock.

CAROTID PULSE (done if no radial pulse)

Absent ....CPR + BVM + oxygen, load-and-go.

Present ....Note rate and quality.
  Bradycardia   Consider spinal shock, head injury.
  Tachycardia   Consider shock.

SKIN

Color and condition

Pale, cool, clammy...Consider shock.

Cyanosis ....Give 100% oxygen; consider assisted ventilation.

MAJOR BLEEDING..Direct pressure, pressure dressing.

Rapid Trauma Survey	Action

HEAD

Major facial injuries..Consider airway obstruction.

NECK

Swelling, bruising, retracting ....Consider airway obstruction.

Neck vein distention ....Consider tamponade, tension pneumothorax.

Tracheal deviation...Consider tension pneumothorax.

Deformity, tenderness.......................................**APPLY CERVICAL COLLAR NOW.**

INSPECT/PALPATE CHEST

Symmetrical, stable...Continue exam.

Bruises, crepitus..Consider early cardiac monitoring.

Penetrating wounds..Occlusive dressing.

Paradoxical motion..Stabilize flail.

BREATH SOUNDS

Present and equal ....Continue exam.

Unequal..Percuss chest to determine pneumothorax versus hemothorax.

HEART TONES ....Note for comparison later.

Muffled with JVD and bilateral ....Consider pericardial tamponade.
breath sounds

ABDOMEN, PELVIS, UPPER LEGS

If tender abdomen, unstable pelvis, or ....Expect development of shock.
bilateral femur fractures

MOVEMENT/SENSATION IN EXTREMITIES

Present ....Record.

Decreased or absent ....Suspect spinal injury.

BACK ....Appropriate management of identified injuries.

Transfer to backboard.

TRANSPORT IMMEDIATELY IF CRITICAL TRAUMA SITUATION IS PRESENT.

SAMPLE HISTORY ....RECORD.

VITAL SIGNS

Measure pulse, respirations...............................Record.

Auscultate blood pressure

Systolic < 80 ....Consider PASG per local protocol.

Systolic < 60 ....Consider PASG inflation per local protocol

Neurological Exam to Be Done If Patient Has Altered Mental Status

PUPILS

Unequal..Suspect head injury unless patient is alert, then suspect eye injury. Give 100% oxygen.

GLASGOW COMA SCORE (for decreased LOC)

≤8...Give 100% oxygen.

Consider hyperventilation only if patient shows signs of cerebral herniation:

a. GCS ≤8 with extensor posturing,

b. GCS ≤8 with pupillary asymmetry or nonreactivity

c. GCS ≤8 with a subsequent drop of more than 2 points

ALL PATIENTS WITH DECREASED LOC..............Check for medical identification devices. Do blood glucose check.

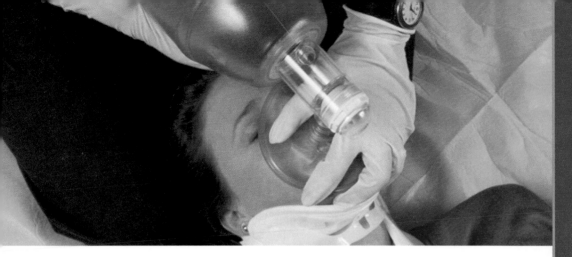

Initial Airway Management

Ronald D. Stewart, M.D., F.A.C.E.P.
John E. Campbell, M.D., F.A.C.E.P.

Objectives

Upon completion of this chapter, you should be able to:

1. Describe the anatomy and physiology of the respiratory system.
2. Define the following terms:
   a. Hyperventilation
   b. Hypoventilation
   c. Tidal volume
   d. Minute volume
   e. Delivered volume
   f. Compliance
3. Explain the importance of observation as it relates to airway control.
4. Describe methods to deliver supplemental oxygen to the trauma patient.
5. Briefly describe the indications and contraindications and the advantages and disadvantages of the following airway adjuncts:
   a. Nasopharyngeal airways
   b. Oropharyngeal airways
   c. Bag-valve masks
   d. Flow-restricted oxygen-powered ventilation devices
6. Describe the Sellick maneuver.
7. Describe the essential contents of an airway kit.

(Photo courtesy of Bonnie Meneely, EMT-P)

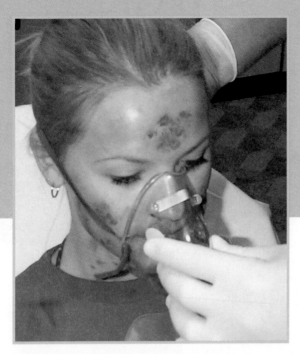

(Photo courtesy of Buddy Denson, EMT-P)

CASE STUDY

Dan, Joyce, and Buddy of the Emergency Transport System have been called to the scene of a house fire. Their Scene Size-up reveals that the fire department is present, the scene is safe and there is only one victim. She had been asleep in a back bedroom and the firemen pulled her out of the window. She is covered in soot and is coughing. How would you approach this patient? What is the mechanism of injury? What type of assessment would you perform? What would you do first? Is this a load-and-go situation? Keep these questions in mind as you read the chapter. The case study will continue at the end of the chapter.

Of all the tasks expected of field teams caring for the trauma patient, none is more important than that of airway control. Maintaining an open airway and adequate ventilation in the trauma patient can be a challenge in any setting, but it can be almost impossible in the adverse environment of the field, with its poor lighting, the chaos that often surrounds an accident, the position of the patient, and perhaps hostile onlookers.

Airway control is a task that you must master, since it frequently cannot wait until you get to the hospital. Patients who are cyanotic, or underventilated, or both, are in need of immediate help—help that only you can give them in the initial stages of their care. It falls to you, then, to be fully versed in the basic structure and function of the airway, in how to achieve and maintain an open airway, and in how to oxygenate and ventilate a patient.

Because of the unpredictable nature of the field environment, you will be called on to manage patients' airways in almost every conceivable situation: in wrecked cars, dangling above rivers, in the middle of a shopping center, at the side of a busy highway. You therefore need *options* and alternatives from which to choose. What will help one patient may not work for another. One patient may require a simple jaw thrust to open an airway, while another may require a surgical procedure to prevent impending death.

Whatever the methods required, you must always start with the basics. It is of little value—and in some cases downright dangerous—to apply "advanced" techniques of airway control before beginning basic maneuvers. The discussion of airway control in the trauma patient will be rooted in several fundamental truths: Air should go in and out, oxygen is good, and blue is bad. Everything else follows from this.

ANATOMY

The airway begins at the tip of the nose and the lips and ends at the *alveolocapillary membrane,* through which gas exchange takes place between the air sacs of the lung (the *alveoli*) and the lung's capillary network. The airway consists of chambers and pipes that conduct air and its 21% oxygen content to the alveoli during inspiration and carry away the waste *carbon dioxide* that diffuses from the blood into the alveoli.

The beginning of the respiratory tract, the *nasal cavity* and *oropharynx,* perform important functions (see Figure 4-1). Lined with moist *mucous membranes,* these areas serve to warm and filter inhaled gases. They are highly vascular and contain protective lymphoid tissue. Bypassing this portion of the respiratory tract through the use of an endotracheal tube will reduce the natural protection of the vulnerable lung, and you will have to provide some of these protective tasks. That is why suctioning of the airway, as well as the warming and humidification of gases, becomes of such importance in intubated patients.

The lining of the respiratory tract is delicate and highly vascular. It deserves all the respect that you can give it, and that means preventing undue trauma, using liberally lubricated tubes, and avoiding unnecessary poking about. The *nasal cavity* is divided by a very vascular midline *septum,* and on the lateral walls of the nose are "shelves" called the *turbinates.* These projections, which increase the surface area of the mucosa, can get in the way of tubes or other devices that it may be necessary to insert into the nostrils. Carefully sliding a well-lubricated tube's bevel along the floor or the septum of the nasal cavity will usually prevent traumatizing the turbinates.

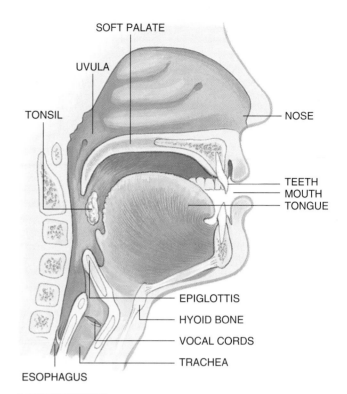

Figure 4-1 Anatomy of the upper airway. Note that the tongue, hyoid bone, and epiglottis are attached to the mandible by a series of ligaments. Lifting forward on the jaw will therefore displace all these structures anteriorly.

The teeth are the first obstruction we meet in the oral part of the airway. They may be more obstructive in some patients than in others. In any case, the same general principle always applies: **Patients should have the same number and condition of teeth at the end of an airway procedure as they had at the beginning.**

The tongue is a large chunk of muscle and represents the next potential obstruction. These muscles are attached to the jaw anteriorly and through a series of muscles and ligaments to the *hyoid bone,* a wishbone-like structure just under the chin from which the cartilage skeleton (the larynx) of the upper airway is suspended. The *epiglottis* is also connected to the hyoid, and elevating the hyoid will lift the epiglottis upward and open the airway further.

The epiglottis is one of the main anatomic landmarks in the airway. You must be familiar with it and be able to identify it by sight and by touch. It looks like a floppy piece of cartilage covered by mucosa—which is exactly what it is—and it feels like the tragus, the cartilage at the opening of the ear canal. Its function is unclear; it may be a "leftover" (i.e., vestigial) piece of anatomy, but it is nonetheless important to you when you must assume control of the airway. The epiglottis is attached to the hyoid and thence to the mandible by a series of ligaments and muscles. In the unconscious patient, the tongue can produce some airway obstruction by falling back against the soft palate and even the posterior pharyngeal wall. However, it is the epiglottis that will produce complete airway obstruction in the supine unconscious patient whose jaw is relaxed and whose head and neck are in the neutral position. In such patients the epiglottis will fall down against the glottic opening and prevent ventilation.

It is essential to understand this crucial fact in the management of the airway. To ensure an open (patent) airway in an unconscious supine patient, you can displace

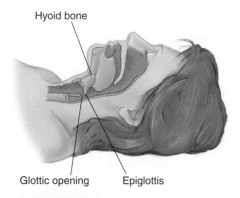

Figure 4-2a

The epiglottis is attached to the hyoid and then to the mandible. When the mandible is relaxed and falls back, the tongue falls upward and against the soft palate and the posterior pharyngeal wall, while the epiglottis falls over the glottic opening.

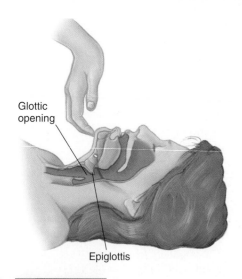

Figure 4-2b

Extension of the head and lifting the chin will pull the tongue and the epiglottis upward and forward, exposing the glottic opening and ensuring the patent airway. In the trauma patient, only the jaw, or chin and jaw, should be displaced forward, while the head and neck should be kept in alignment.

the hyoid anteriorly by lifting forward on the jaw (chin lift, jaw thrust) or by pulling on the tongue. This will lift the tongue out of the way and keep the epiglottis elevated and away from the posterior pharyngeal wall and glottic opening (see Figure 4-2a and b).

The vocal cords are protected by the *thyroid cartilage,* a boxlike structure shaped like a "C," with the open part of the "C" representing its posterior wall, which is covered with muscle. When the cords vibrate, sound is produced. In some patients, the cords can close entirely in *laryngospasm,* producing complete airway obstruction. The thyroid cartilage can easily be seen in most people on the anterior surface of the neck as the laryngeal prominence.

Inferior to the thyroid cartilage is another part of the larynx, the *cricoid,* a cartilage shaped like a signet ring with the ring in front and the signet behind. It can be palpated as a small bump on the anterior surface of the neck inferior to the laryngeal prominence. The esophagus is just behind the posterior wall of the cricoid cartilage. Pressure on the cricoid at the front of the neck will close off the esophagus to pressures as high as 100 cm H_2O. This maneuver (the *Sellick maneuver*) can be used to reduce the risk of gastric regurgitation during the process of intubation and to prevent insufflation of air into the stomach during positive pressure ventilation by mouth-to-mouth, bag-valve mask, or flow-restricted oxygen-powered ventilator (see Figure 4-3 and 4-4). If there is any danger of cervical spine injury, you must carefully support and stabilize the neck while performing the Sellick maneuver.

The *tracheal rings,* C-shaped cartilaginous supports for the trachea, continue beyond the cricoid cartilage, and the trachea soon divides into the *left* and *right mainstem bronchi* (see Figure 4-5). The open part of the C-shaped rings lies posterior against the esophagus. An impacted swallowed foreign body that remains in the esophagus, or a misplaced esophageal airway or endotracheal tube cuff, can create tracheal obstruction by pressing against the soft posterior tracheal wall and narrowing the lumen. The point at which the trachea divides is called the *carina.* It is important to note that the right mainstem bronchus takes off at an angle that is slightly more in line with the trachea. As a result, tubes or other foreign bodies that are poked or that trickle down the airway usually end up in the right mainstem bronchus.

To help protect the airway from becoming blocked and to reduce the risk of aspiration, the body has developed brisk reflexes that will attempt to expel any offending foreign material from the oropharynx, the glottic opening, or the trachea. These areas are well supplied by sensitive nerves that can activate the swallowing, gag, and cough reflex. Activation of swallowing, gagging, or coughing by stimulation of the upper airway can cause significant cardiovascular stimulation as well as elevation in intracranial pressure.

The *lungs* are the organs through which this gas exchange takes place. They are contained within a "cage" formed by the ribs, and usually fill up the *pleural space*—the *potential space* between the internal chest wall and the lung surface. The lungs have only one opening to the outside, the *glottic opening,* the space between the vocal cords. Expansion of the chest wall (the cage) and movement of the diaphragm downward cause the lungs to expand (since the pleural space is airtight), and air rushes in through the *glottis.* The air travels down the smaller and smaller tubes to the *alveoli,* where gas exchange (respiration) takes place.

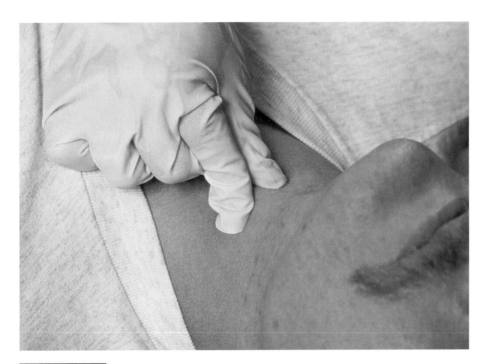

Figure 4-3 The Sellick maneuver.

THE PATENT AIRWAY

One of the first maneuvers essential to caring for a patient is ensuring a *patent* or *open airway*. Without this, all other care is of little use. This must be done quickly, for patients cannot tolerate hypoxia for more than a few minutes. The effect of hypoxia on an unconscious injured patient can be devastating, and if hypoxia is compounded by the absence of adequate perfusion, the patient is in even more difficult straits. Patients suffering from head trauma not only may have hypoxic brain damage from airway compromise but may also build up high levels of carbon dioxide that can increase blood flow to the injured brain, causing swelling and increased intracranial pressure.

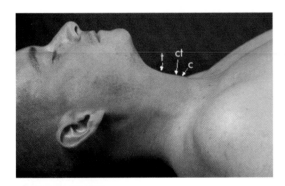

Figure 4-4a External view of the anterior neck, showing the surface landmarks for the thyroid cartilage (laryngeal) prominence, the cricothyroid membrane, and the cricoid cartilage.

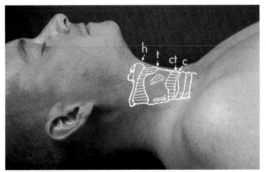

Figure 4-4b Cut-away view showing the important landmarks of the larynx and upper airway: hyoid, thyroid cartilage, cricothyroid membrane, and cricoid cartilage.

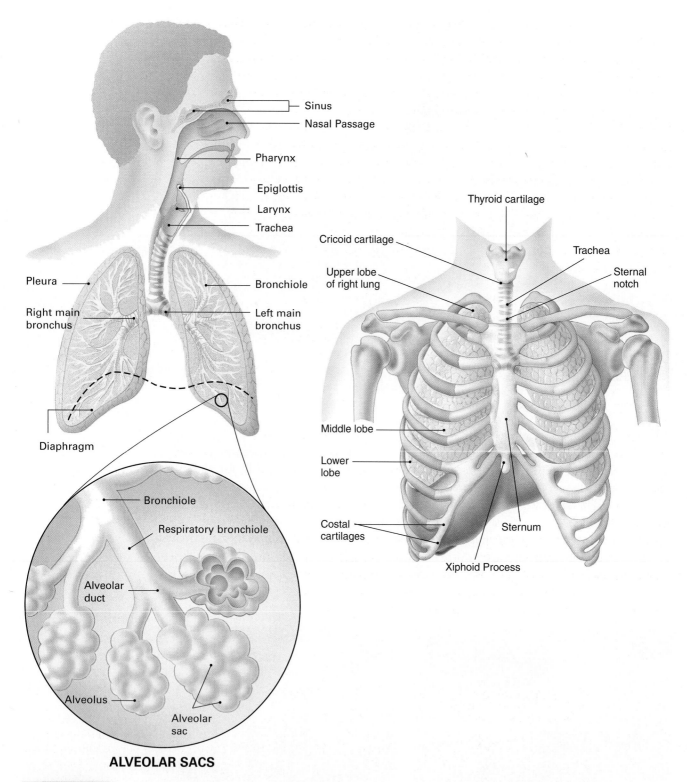

Figure 4-5 Anatomy of the respiratory tract.

Ensuring an open airway in a patient can be a major challenge in the prehospital setting. Not only can trauma disrupt the anatomy of the face and airway, but also resultant bleeding can lead to airflow obstruction and can obscure airway landmarks. Add to this the risk of cervical spine injury, and the challenge is readily apparent. You must also remember that some airway maneuvers, including suction and insertion of nasopharyngeal and oropharyngeal airways, may stimulate a patient's protective reflexes and increase the likelihood of vomiting and aspiration, cardiovascular stimulation, and increased intracranial pressure. The first step in providing a patent airway in the unconscious patient is to ensure that the tongue and epiglottis are lifted forward and maintained in that position. This is done by either the modified jaw thrust (see Figure 4-6a) or the jaw lift (see Figure 4-6b). Either of these maneuvers will prevent the tongue from falling backward against the soft palate or posterior pharyngeal wall. Either will pull forward on the hyoid, lifting the epiglottis up out of the way. These are essential maneuvers for both basic and advanced airway procedures. Done properly, they will open the airway without tilting the head backward or moving the neck.

Constant vigilance and care are required to maintain a patent airway in your patient. There are several essentials for this task:

1. Continual observation of the patient in order to anticipate problems
2. An adequate suction device with large-bore tubing and attachment
3. Airway adjuncts

Observation

The patient who is injured is at risk of airway compromise even if completely conscious and awake. This is partially due to the fact that many patients have full stomachs, are anxious, and are prone to vomiting. Some patients will also be bleeding into their oropharynx and thus swallowing blood.

In view of these facts, you should constantly observe your patient for airway problems following injury. One team member must be responsible for both airway control and adequate ventilation for any patient who might be at risk of airway compromise.

The general appearance of the patient, the respiratory rate, and any complaints must be noted and addressed. In a patient who is breathing spontaneously, you must check frequently for adequate tidal volume by feeling over the mouth and nose and by observing chest wall movements. Check the supplemental oxygen line periodically to ensure that oxygen is being

Since neck may be injured, do not extend the neck to open the airway.

Use modified jaw thrust

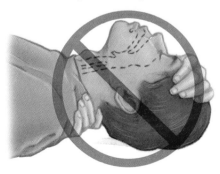 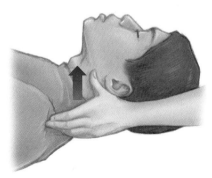

Figure 4-6a

Opening the airway using modified jaw thrust. Maintain in-line stabilization while pushing up on the angle of the jaw with your thumbs.

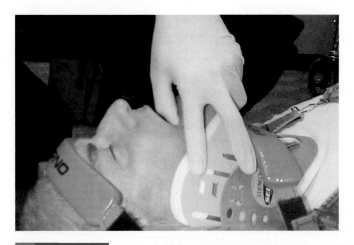

Figure 4-6b Jaw lift. *(Photo courtesy of Buddy Denson, EMT-P)*

delivered to the patient at a given flow rate or percentage. You should always immediately clear blood and secretions. You must be alert for sounds that indicate trouble. Be alert for this danger sign: *noisy breathing is obstructed breathing.* Consider combative patients to be hypoxic until a systematic and rapid evaluation rules this out. Use of pulse oximetry is strongly recommended in all trauma patients (see Chapter 5).

Suction

All patients who are injured and who have cervical motion-restriction devices in place should be considered at high risk for airway compromise. One of the greatest threats to the patent airway is that of vomiting and aspiration, particularly in patients who have recently eaten a large meal washed down with large quantities of alcohol. As a result, portable suction devices should be considered basic equipment for field trauma care and should have the following characteristics (see Figure 4-7):

1. They should be carried in a kit with an oxygen cylinder and other airway equipment; they should not be separated or stored remote from oxygen; otherwise, they represent an "extra" piece of equipment requiring extra hands.

2. They should be hand-powered or battery-powered rather than oxygen-driven. Hand-powered is preferred. You should always have a hand-powered suction as a backup if you use a battery-powered suction.

3. They should generate sufficient pressure and volume displacement to suction pieces of food, blood clots, and thick secretions from the oropharynx.

4. They should have tubing of sufficient diameter (0.8–1 cm) to handle whatever is suctioned from the patient.

Suction tips of more recent design are of large bore, particularly the new rigid "tonsil-tip" suckers that can handle most clots and bleeding. In some cases the suction tubing

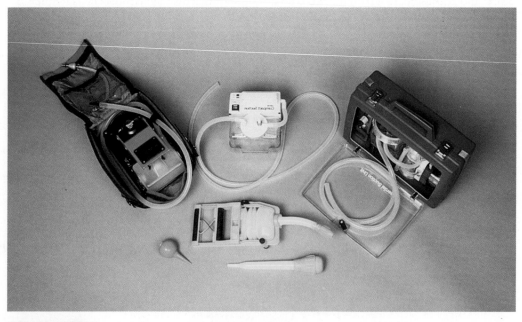

Figure 4-7 Examples of suction apparatus.

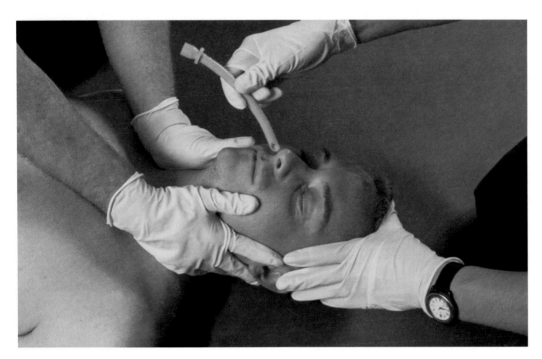

Figure 4-8a The nasopharyngeal airway is inserted with the bevel slid along the septum or floor of the nasal cavity.

itself can be used to withdraw large amounts of blood or gastric contents. A 6-mm endo-tracheal tube can be used with a connector as a suction tip. The tube's side hole removes the necessity for a proximal control valve to interrupt suction. Usually Rescuer 2 (see Chapter 2) assumes responsibility for the airway. As the "V.O." (vomit officer), he must be constantly alert to prevent the patient from aspirating.

Airway Adjuncts

Equipment to help ensure a patent airway will include various nasopharyngeal, oropharyngeal, and blind insertion airway devices (BIAD). Insertion of these devices must be reserved for patients whose protective reflexes are sufficiently depressed to tolerate them. Care must be taken not to provoke vomiting or gagging, since both occurrences are bad for these patients.

Nasopharyngeal airways should be soft and of appropriate length. They are designed to prevent the tongue and epiglottis from falling against the posterior pharyngeal wall (see Chapter 5 for insertion technique). In a pinch, a 6-mm or 6.6-mm endotracheal tube can be cut and serve as a nasopharyngeal airway. With gentle insertion there should be few problems with this airway (see Figures 4-8a and b). However, bleeding and trauma to the nasal mucosa are not infrequent. Mild hemorrhage from the nose after insertion of the airway is not an indication to remove it. In fact, it is probably better to keep the nasopharyngeal airway in place so as not to disturb the clot or reactivate the bleeding. The nasopharyngeal airway will be better tolerated than the oropharyngeal one and thus can usually be used in patients who still have a gag reflex.

Oropharyngeal airways are designed to keep the tongue off the posterior pharyngeal wall and thereby help maintain a patent airway (see Figure 4-9; see Chapter 5 for insertion techniques). Special oropharyngeal airways are available. Some are designed as intuba-

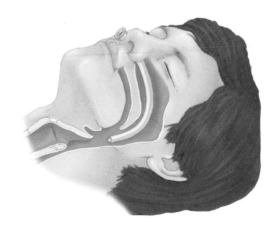

Figure 4-8b The nasopharyngeal airway rests between the tongue and the posterior pharyngeal wall.

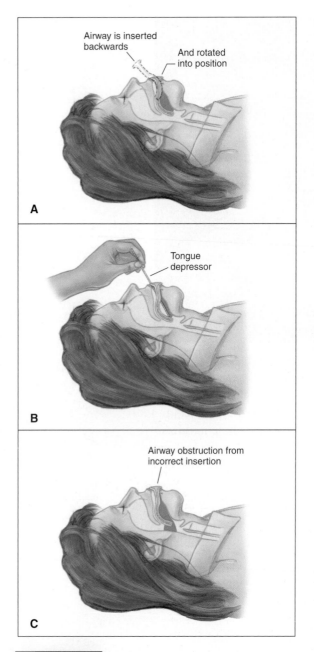

Figure 4-9 Insertion of oropharyngeal airway.

tion guides, while others have proximal ends that protrude from the lips and are designed to be used with balloon masks that seal the mouth and nose.

Esophageal obturator airways, pharyngotracheal airways, esophageal tracheal combitube (Combitube®), and the *laryngeal mask airway* are all blind insertion airway devices.

The esophageal qastric tube airway (EGTA) is designed to be inserted into the esophagus at a level beyond the carina. A cuff is then inflated to reduce the likelihood of gastric distension or regurgitation during bag-valve mask or demand-valve mask ventilation. The tube has an opening that allows for the placement of a nasogastric tube for decompression of the stomach (See Appendix A, Optional Skills).

The pharyngotracheal airway is a combination of the EGTA and an endotracheal tube and represents an attempt to solve the problem of possible intratracheal placement of the EGTA. It also seeks to provide for tracheal ventilation should blind insertion result in intratracheal positioning. This is an airway device that incorporates two tubes and a balloon that can be inflated to fill the oropharynx (see Appendix A. Optional Skills).

The esophageal tracheal combitube (Combitube®) is a double-lumen tube like the pharyngotracheal airway. It has both a distal balloon to seal the esophagus to help prevent regurgitation and a proximal balloon to seal the pharynx to help prevent air from escaping from the mouth and nose. The pharyngeal balloon can also help prevent food and other foreign material from being aspirated (see Appendix A, Optional Skills).

SUPPLEMENTAL OXYGEN

Patients who are injured need supplemental oxygen, especially if they are unconscious. It is well recognized that patients suffering from head injury are frequently hypoxic. Supplemental oxygen can be supplied by a simple face-mask run at 10 to 12 L/min. This will provide the patient with about 40 to 50% oxygen. Non-rebreathing masks with a reservoir bag with oxygen flow rates into the bag of 12 to 15 L/min can provide 60 to 90% oxygen to the patient. These are recommended for all trauma patients requiring supplemental oxygen. Nasal oxygen cannulae are well tolerated by most patients, but provide only about 25 to 30% oxygen to the patient. They are recommended for only those patients who refuse to accept an oxygen mask.

Supplemental oxygen must be used to ensure adequate oxygenation when you perform positive pressure ventilation. Oxygenation must be supplemented during mouth-to-mask ventilation by running oxygen at 10 to 12 L/min through the oxygen nipple attached to most masks or by placing the oxygen tubing under the mask and running it at the same rate. Alternatively, you can increase the oxygen percentage delivered during mouth-to-mask breathing by placing a nasal cannula on yourself. This increases the delivered oxygen percentage from 17% to about 30%.

Bag-valve mask (BVM) devices or resuscitator bags with a large (2.5 L) reservoir bag and an oxygen flow rate of 12 to 15 L/min will increase the delivered oxygen from

21% (air) to 90 or 100%. Adding a reservoir bag to a BVM will increase the delivered oxygen from 40–50% to 90–100% and thus should always be used.

Flow-restricted oxygen-powered ventilation devices (FROPVD) will provide 100% oxygen at a flow rate of 40 L/min at a maximum pressure of 50 ± 5 cm water.

NORMAL VENTILATION

The movement of air or gases in and out of the lungs is called *ventilation.* At rest, adults normally take in about 400 to 600 cc with each breath. This is called the *tidal volume.* Multiplying that value by the number of breaths per minute (the respiratory rate) gives the *minute volume,* the amount of air breathed in and out each minute. This is an important value and is normally 5 to 12 L/min. Normal ventilation with normal lungs will produce an oxygen level of about 100 mmHg and a carbon dioxide level of 35 to 40 mmHg. The terms *hypoventilation* and *hyperventilation* do not refer to oxygenation but rather refer to the level of carbon dioxide maintained. A carbon dioxide level below 35 mmHg is called hyperventilation, and values greater than 40 mmHg are called hypoventilation. It is easier for carbon dioxide to diffuse across the alveolocapillary membrane of the lungs than it is for oxygen to do so. This makes it easier to excrete carbon dioxide than to oxygenate the blood. Thus if the chest or lungs are injured, the body may be able to maintain normal levels of carbon dioxide and yet be hypoxic. A patient with a contused lung might have a respiratory rate of 36, a carbon dioxide level of 30 mmHg, and an oxygen level of only 80 mmHg. While this person is hyperventilating, he is still hypoxic. He does not need to breathe faster; he needs to have supplemental oxygen. When in doubt, give your patient oxygen.

Devices to measure oxygen saturation (pulse oximeters) are available for prehospital use. Pulse oximeters measure oxygen saturation and should be used on almost all trauma patients. Paulse oximeters will be discussed in Chapter 5.

POSITIVE PRESSURE (ARTIFICIAL) VENTILATION

Normal breathing takes place because the negative pressure inside the (potential) pleural space "draws" air in through the upper airway from the outside. In any patient who is unable to do this, or whose airway needs protecting, you may need to "pump" air or oxygen in through the glottic opening. This is called *intermittent positive pressure ventilation* (IPPV). IPPV in trauma patients can take various forms, from mouth-to-mouth to bag-valve-endotracheal tube. **Pumping air into the oropharynx is no guarantee that it will go through the glottic opening and into the lungs.** The oropharynx also leads to the esophagus, and pressure in the oropharynx of greater than 25 cm H_2O will open the esophagus and lead to air being pumped into the stomach (gastric insufflation). Bag-valve masks and FROPVD can produce pressures greater than this. This is why the Sellick maneuver (posterior pressure on the cricoid cartilage) is so very important as a basic airway procedure. When you need to ventilate a patient using IPPV, you should know approximately how much volume you are delivering with each breath you give (*delivered volume*). You can estimate the minute volume by multiplying this volume by the ventilatory rate. A flow-restricted oxygen-powered ventilator that delivers oxygen at the rate of 40 L/min will have a delivered volume of about 700 cc each second that the valve is activated. Unless the Sellick maneuver is used, delivering this volume at a pressure of 50 cm H_2O will almost guarantee gastric insufflation and all the complications resulting from it. BVM breathing is no better, since pressures generated by squeezing the bag may equal or exceed 60 cm H_2O.

Delivered volumes are usually less with bag resuscitators than with FROPVD. There are two reasons for this. The average resuscitator bag holds only 1,800 cc of gas, and that is the absolute limit to the volume that could be delivered if you were able to squeeze the bag completely. Using one hand, the best an average adult can squeeze is approximately

1,200 cc. Most people will squeeze only 800 to 1,000 cc with one hand. The other reason for greater delivered volumes with flow-restricted oxygen-powered ventilators is that a FROPVD has a trigger that allows the rescuer to hold a mask on the face with both hands, thus decreasing mask leak. Keep in mind that these volumes, delivered from the ventilating port of these devices, equal the volumes delivered to the patient only if an endotracheal tube is in place. In other words, they do not take into account mask leak. When performing IPPV with a mask, keep the following essentials in mind:

1. Supplemental oxygen must be provided for the patient during IPPV.
2. Suction must be **immediately** available.
3. Ventilation must be done carefully to avoid gastric distension and to reduce the risk of regurgitation and possible aspiration. You can help prevent these complications by using the Sellick maneuver.
4. Careful attention must be paid in estimating the minute volume being delivered to the trauma patient. A minute volume of at least 12 to 15 L should be provided. If an adult's hand squeezes approximately 800 cc from a bag, "bagging" the patient every 3 or 4 seconds (15 to 20 times per minute) would provide a minute volume of from 12 to 16 L. This should be enough to provide for the patient's increased ventilatory needs. However, in the case of bag-mask breathing, up to 40% mask leak can be expected. Balloon mask designs can reduce this, and a two-person technique, in which one rescuer holds the mask in place with both hands while a second squeezes the bag, may better ensure adequate delivered volumes. During the stress of an emergency situation you will tend to ventilate patients at an increased rate, but delivered volumes are often deficient. Normal rates should be 18 to 24 times per minute. Pay attention to delivered volumes as well, since rate alone cannot compensate for grossly inadequate ventilatory volumes.

COMPLIANCE

When air, or air containing oxygen, is delivered by positive pressure into the lungs of a patient, the "give" or elasticity of the lungs and chest wall will influence how easily it will be for the patient to breathe. If you are performing mask ventilation, a normal elasticity of the lungs and chest wall will allow air to enter the glottic opening and little gastric distension should result. However, if the elasticity is poor, ventilation will be harder to achieve. The ability of the lungs and chest wall to expand and therefore ventilate a patient is known as *compliance.* It is simpler to speak of "good compliance" or "bad compliance" rather than "high" or "low" compliance, since the latter terms can be somewhat confusing.

Compliance is an important concept, since it governs whether you can adequately ventilate a patient. Compliance can become bad (i.e., low) in some disease states of the lung or in patients who have an injury to the chest wall. In cardiac arrest, compliance will also become bad, due to poor circulation to the muscles. This makes ventilating the patient all the more difficult.

VENTILATION TECHNIQUES
Mouth-to-Mouth

This is a most reliable and effective method of ventilation, with the advantage of requiring no equipment and a minimum of experience and training. In addition, delivered volumes are consistently adequate since mouth seal is effectively and easily maintained. In addition, compliance can be "felt" more accurately, and high oropharyngeal pressures are therefore less likely. This method is almost never used because of the danger of disease transmission. Even though you should rarely have to use mouth-to-mouth ventilation, it is an option.

Mouth-to-Mask

Most of the disadvantages of mouth-to-mouth ventilation can be overcome by interposing a face-mask between your mouth and that of the patient. Commercially designed pocket-masks (folds into a small case that can be carried in your pocket) are particularly suited for the initial ventilation of many types of patients, and some have a side port for supplemental oxygen. Pocket-ventilating-masks have consistently been shown to deliver larger volumes than bag-mask devices and do so with a greater percentage of oxygen than mouth-to-mouth ventilation. Mouth-to-mask ventilation has significant advantages over other methods, and should be more widely used (see Chapter 5).

Flow-Restricted Oxygen-Powered Ventilating Device

In the past, the high-pressure, oxygen-powered ventilators (demand valves) were considered too dangerous to use in multiple-trauma patients. Experience with the newer flow-restricted oxygen-powered ventilators (FROPVD) that

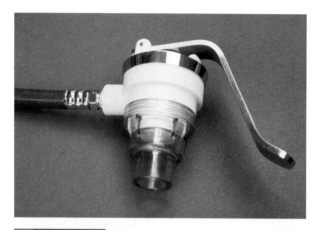

The flow-restricted oxygen-powered ventilation device. This valve delivers a set flow of 40 L/min at maximum pressure of 50 ± 5 cm H_2O. Do not use unless it meets these standards and your Medical Director approves.

meet American Heart Association guidelines (oxygen flow rate of 40 L/min at a maximum pressure of 50 ± 5 cm H_2O) suggests that these may now be the equal of bag-valve devices for ventilation (Figure 4-10). They have the advantage of delivering 100% oxygen and allowing use of two hands while using face-mask ventilation. FROPVDs are no worse than BVMs at producing gastric distention. However, because it is more difficult to feel lung compliance when ventilating with the FROPVD, there is still some controversy about its use. Follow your Medical Director's advice on the use of a FROPVD.

Bag-Valve Mask

This descendant of the anesthetic bag is a fixed-volume ventilator with an average delivered volume of about 800 cc. With a two-handed squeeze, over 1 L can be delivered to the patient. They should be used with a reservoir bag or tubing. Plain BVMs without reservoir bag or tubing can only deliver 40 to 50% oxygen and thus should be replaced with reservoir bags.

The most important problem associated with the bag-valve mask devices is the volumes delivered. Mask leak is a serious problem, decreasing the volume delivered to the oropharynx by sometimes 40% or more. In addition, old masks of conventional design have significant dead space beneath them, thus increasing the challenge to provide an adequate volume to the patient. The newer balloon mask has a design that eliminates dead space beneath the mask and provides an improved seal over the nose and mouth. It has been shown in mannequin studies to decrease mask leak and to improve ventilation. It is recommended particularly for trauma patients (see Figure 4-11).

A better seal can sometimes be obtained, and larger volumes delivered, in either the balloon or conventional mask, with the use of extension tubing

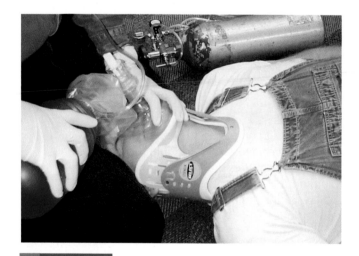

The inflated balloon mask has been shown to reduce mask leak and provide greater volumes during ventilation with bag-mask devices. *(Photo courtesy of Buddy Denson, EMT-P)*

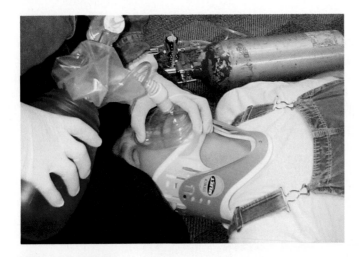

Figure 4-12

A ventilating port extension attached to a ventilating bag permits a better mask seal and therefore greater delivered volumes. When the bag is compressed against the thigh, as shown here, delivered volumes may be increased further. *(Photo courtesy of Buddy Denson, EMT-P)*

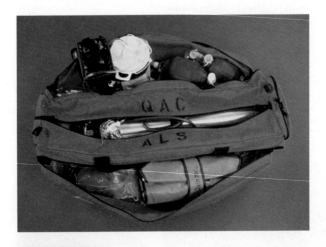

Figure 4-13

An airway kit containing the essentials for airway management. Note that portable suction is included in this design. The total weight of (with aluminum "D" oxygen cylinder) is approximately 10 kg (22 lbs), about the same as a steel "E" oxygen cylinder.

attached to the ventilating port of the bag-valve device. This permits the mask to be better seated on the face without a levering effect from the rigid ventilating port connector that tends to unseat the mask. With the extension in place, the bag can be more easily compressed, even against the knee or thigh, thus increasing the delivered volume and overcoming any mask leak (see Figure 4-12).

Airway Equipment

The most important rule to follow in regard to airway equipment is that it should be in good working order and immediately available. It will do the patient no good if you have to run to get the suction apparatus. In other words, be prepared. This is not difficult. Five basic pieces of equipment are necessary for the initial response to all prehospital trauma calls:

1. Personal protection equipment (see Chapter 1)
2. Long backboard with attached head motion-restriction device
3. Appropriately-sized rigid cervical extrication collar
4. Airway kit (see below)
5. Trauma box (see Chapter 1)

The *airway kit* should be completely self-contained and should contain everything needed to secure an airway in any patient. Equipment now available is lightweight and portable. Oxygen cylinders are aluminum, and newer suction devices are less bulky and lighter. It is no longer acceptable to have suction units that are bulky and stored separate from a source of oxygen. Suction units should be contained in a kit with oxygen and other essential airway tools. A lightweight airway kit should consist of the following (see Figure 4-13):

1. Oxygen D cylinder, preferably aluminum
2. Portable battery-powered and hand-powered suction units
3. Oxygen cannulae and masks
4. Bag-valve mask ventilating device (with reservoir bag)
5. Pocket mask with supplemental oxygen intake
6. Pulse oximeter

The contents of the airway kit are critical; you should check all equipment each shift and the kit should have a card attached to be initialed by the person checking it.

CASE STUDY

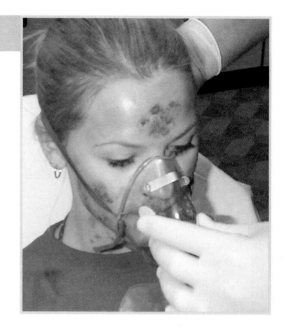

Dan, Joyce, and Buddy of the Emergency Transport System have been called to the scene of a house fire. Their Scene Size-up reveals that the fire department is present, the scene is safe and there is only one victim. She had been asleep in a back bedroom and the firemen pulled her out of the window. She is covered in soot and is coughing. The initial impression is poor because the patient is coughing and appears to be having some trouble breathing. Buddy is acting as team leader. The team dons personal protective equipment, gathers the essential equipment and approaches the patient.

Buddy begins his initial assessment by introducing the team as Joyce prepares to apply a non-rebreather oxygen-mask. When questioned about what happened, Ms. Von Huffenpuffen states she had some food simmering on the stove and had decided to take a brief nap. When she awakened the room was full of smoke and when she opened the bedroom door the hallway was engulfed in flames. She slammed the door and was trying to climb out the window when the fire department arrived. She denies any history of asthma or lung disease and does not smoke. She complains of headache, persistent cough, and some dyspnea. Buddy notes that Ms. Von Huffenpuffen has a hoarse voice and her breathing is rapid and shallow. She has a strong rapid pulse at the wrist. Dan has the stretcher ready and she climbs onto it. Because of the mechanism of injury Buddy chooses to perform a Rapid Trauma Survey. He has already determined that this is a priority patient because of the abnormal initial assessment and this is also a load-and-go situation because of the respiratory difficulty.

Brief exam of the head and face reveals erythema and blistering of the face and lips. Her hair is singed. There is also soot in the nose and mouth with singed hairs in her nose. Joyce notes that the pupils are 4 mm and react equally. The neck veins are flat and the trachea is midline. There is also erythema of the skin of the neck. There is no tenderness or deformity of the neck. There are no burns of the chest. The breath sounds are present and equal bilaterally but there is a slight expiratory wheeze. The heart sounds are good. The abdomen is negative for DCAP-BTLS and is soft and nontender. The pelvis is stable and nontender. Exam of the extremities reveals erythema (but no blistering) of the exposed surfaces of her arms, with some singeing of the hair. The patient is able to move her fingers and toes and has sensation in all extremities

She is immediately moved to the ambulance and transported. Dan drives while Buddy and Joyce provide patient care. While Buddy obtains the rest of the SAMPLE history and obtains vital signs, Joyce applies a pulse oximeter. Ms. Von Huffenpuffen states that the oxygen helps her dyspnea but Buddy notes that her voice is more hoarse. She has no allergies. Her past medical history is negative for any serious illnesses and she takes no medications. Her last oral intake was noon (it is now 6:00 PM).

The vital signs are: blood pressure 120/70, pulse 130, respiratory rate 36 with expiratory wheezing. The pulse oximeter reading is 100% on 100% oxygen, but Buddy realizes that it is not reliable in this situation. Buddy notifies Medical Direction that he has a patient who was asleep in a closed space with smoke and was briefly exposed to flames. She is now dyspneic and coughing with bilateral expiratory wheezing and a hoarse voice. She also has a headache.

After arrival at the emergency department the patient is found to have a carboxyhemoglobin level of 25% and also upper airway burns. She was immediately intubated and required several days of endotracheal intubation until her airway swelling decreased.

(Photo courtesy of Buddy Denson, EMT-P)

PEARLS

Preventing deaths from airway problems:

1. Become skilled at recognizing:

   a. When active airway management is necessary

   b. When the patient needs assistance with ventilation

   c. When an airway device is placed incorrectly

   d. When an airway device that was placed correctly has become displaced. Pulse oximeters are very useful for this.

2. Prevent aspiration of gastric contents. Suction must be immediately available. Be prepared for equipment failure by having backup equipment available.

3. Failure to manage the airway is a fatal error.

CASE STUDY WRAP-UP

This is a case of upper airway burns and smoke inhalation. The carbon monoxide poisoning can be treated with 100% oxygen; hyperbaric oxygen can be used if available. Protecting the airway and maintaining oxygenation are the keys to recovery. The pulse oximeter is worthless in this situation, as it does not recognize carboxyhemoglobin or cyanide poisoning and will give falsely high readings. Rapid transport was critical in this patient as she was in danger of losing her airway due to swelling of the larynx from airway burns.

SUMMARY

Trauma patients provide the greatest challenge in airway management. To be successful you must have a clear understanding of the anatomy of the airway and be proficient in techniques to open and maintain your patient's airway. You must have the correct equipment organized in a kit that is immediately available when you begin assessment of the trauma patient. To provide adequate ventilation for your patient, you must understand the concepts of tidal volume, minute volume, and lung compliance. Finally, you must become familiar with the various options for control of the airway and develop expertise in performing them.

BIBLIOGRAPHY

1. American Heart Association Committee on Emergency Cardiac Care. "Guidelines for Cardiopulmonary Resuscitation and Emergency Cardiac Care." *Journal of the American Medical Association,* Vol. 268 (1992), p. 2200.

2. Biebuyck, J. F. "Management of the Difficult Adult Airway." *Anesthesiology,* Vol. 75 (1991), pp. 1087–1110.

3. Boidin, M. P. "Airway Patency in the Unconscious Patient." *British Journal of Anaesthesiology,* Vol. 57 (1985), pp. 306–310.

4. Jesudian, M. C. S., R. R. Harrison, R. L. Keenan, and others. "Bag-Valve-Mask Ventilation: Two Rescuers Are Better than One: Preliminary Report." *Critical Care Medicine,* Vol. 14 (1985), pp. 403–406.

5. Martin, S. E., G. Ochsner, and others. "Laryngeal Mask Airway in Air Transport When Intubation Fails: Case Report." *The Journal of Trauma: Injury, Infection, and Critical Care,* Vol. 42, No. 2 (1997), pp. 333–336.

6. Salem, M. R., A. Y. Wong, M. Mani, and others. "Efficacy of Cricoid Pressure in Preventing Gastric Inflation During Bag-Mask Ventilation in Pediatric Patients." *Anesthesiology,* Vol. 40 (1974), pp. 96–98.

7. Stewart, R. D., R. M. Kaplan, B. Pennock, and others. "Influence of Mask Design on Bag-Mask Ventilation." *Annals of Emergency Medicine,* Vol. 14 (1985), pp. 403–406.

8. White, S. J., R. M. Kaplan, and R. D. Stewart. "Manual Detection of Decreased Lung Compliance as a Sign of Tension Pneumothorax" (abstr). *Annals of Emergency Medicine,* Vol. 16 (1987), p. 518.

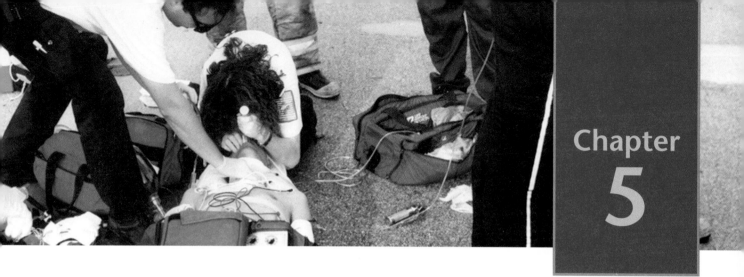

Airway Management Skills

Donna Hastings, EMT-P

Objectives

Upon completion of this chapter, you should be able to:

1. Suction the airway.
2. Insert a nasopharyngeal and oropharyngeal airway.
3. Use the pocket mask.
4. Use the bag-valve mask.
5. Use the pulse oximeter.
6. Properly prepare for endotracheal intubation.
7. Assist with laryngoscopic orotracheal intubation.
8. Assist nasotracheal intubation.
9. Confirm placement of the endotracheal tube.
10. Properly anchor the endotracheal tube.

BASIC AIRWAY MANAGEMENT
✋ PROCEDURES

❇ Suctioning the Airway

Use of the hand-powered suction device also should be taught at this time.

1. Attach the suction connecting tubing to the portable suction machine.

2. Turn the device on and test it.

3. Insert the suction tip through the nose (soft or whistle tip) or mouth (soft or rigid) without activating the suction.

4. Activate the suction and withdraw the suction tube.

5. Repeat the procedure as necessary.

Note: Although the intent is to suction foreign matter, air and oxygen are also being suctioned out of the patient. Never suction for greater than 15 seconds. After suctioning, reoxygenate the patient as soon as possible.

❇ Inserting Nasopharyngeal Airways

1. Choose the appropriate size. It should be as large as possible but still fit easily through the patient's external nares. The size of the patient's little finger can be used as a rough guide.

2. Lubricate the tube with a water-based lubricant.

3. Insert it straight back through the right nostril with the beveled edge of the airway toward the septum.

4. Gently pass into the posterior pharynx with a slight rotating motion until the flange rests against the nares.

5. To insert in the left nostril, turn the airway upside down so that the bevel is toward the septum; then insert straight back through the nostril until you reach the posterior pharynx. At this point, turn the airway over 180 degrees and insert it down the pharynx.

Note: If the tongue is occluding the airway, a jaw thrust or chin lift must be done to allow the nasopharyngeal airway to go *under* the tongue.

❇ Inserting Oropharyngeal Airways

1. Choose the appropriate size. The distance from the corner of the mouth to the lower part of the external ear is a good estimate.

2. Open the airway:

   a. Scissor maneuver

   b. Jaw lift

   c. Tongue blade

3. Insert the airway gently without pushing the tongue back into the pharynx.

   a. Insert the airway under direct vision using a tongue blade. This is the preferred method and is safe for adults or children.

   b. Insert the airway upside down or sideways and rotate into place. This method should not be used for children.

4. If the oropharyngeal airway causes gagging, remove and replace with a nasopharyngeal airway.

❄ Using a Pocket Mask with Supplemental Oxygen

1. Stabilize the patient's head in a neutral position.
2. Connect the oxygen tubing to the oxygen cylinder and the mask.
3. Open the oxygen cylinder and set the flow rate at 12 L/min.
4. Open the airway.
5. Insert the oral or nasal airway.
6. Place the mask on the face and establish a good seal.
7. Ventilate mouth-to-mask with enough volume (about 800–1,000 cc oxygen) to cause adequate chest rise. The inspiratory phase should last 1.5 to 2.0 seconds. Let the patient exhale for 1.5 to 4.0 seconds.

❄ Using the Bag-Valve Mask

1. Stabilize the patient's head in a neutral position.
2. Connect the oxygen connecting tubing to the bag-valve system and oxygen cylinder.
3. Attach the oxygen reservoir to the bag-valve mask.
4. Open the oxygen cylinder and set the flow rate at 12 L/min.
5. Select the proper size mask and attach it to the bag-valve device.
6. Open the airway.
7. Insert the oral airway (insert the nasal airway if the patient has a gag reflex).
8. Place the mask on the face and have your partner establish and maintain a good seal.
9. Using both hands, ventilate with about 800 to 1,000 cc oxygen.
10. If you are forced to ventilate without a partner, use one hand to maintain a face seal and the other hand to squeeze the bag. This decreases the volume of ventilation because less volume is produced by only one hand squeezing the bag.

Using the Pulse Oximeter: A pulse oximeter is a noninvasive photoelectric device that measures the arterial oxygen saturation and pulse rate in the peripheral circulation. It consists of a portable monitor and a sensing probe that clips onto the patient's finger, toe, or earlobe (see Figure 5-1). The device displays the pulse rate and the arterial oxygen saturation in a percentage value (% SaO_2). This is a very useful device that should be used on all patients with any type of respiratory compromise. The pulse oximeter is useful to assess the patient's respiratory status, the effectiveness of oxygen therapy, and the effectiveness of BVM or FROPVD ventilation.

Remember that the device measures % SaO_2, not the arterial partial pressure of oxygen (PaO_2). The hemoglobin molecule is so efficient at carrying oxygen that it is 90% saturated (90% SaO_2) when the partial pressure of oxygen is only 60 mmHg (100 is normal). If you are used to thinking about PaO_2 (where 90–100 mmHg is normal), then you may be fooled into thinking that a SaO_2 reading (pulse oximeter) of 90% is normal when it is actually critically low. As a general rule, any pulse oximeter reading below 92% is cause for concern and requires some sort of intervention (open airway, suction, oxygen, assisted ventilation, intubation, decompression of tension pneumothorax, etc.). A pulse oximeter reading below 90% is critical and requires *immediate* intervention to maintain adequate tissue oxygenation. Try to maintain a pulse oximeter reading of 95% or higher. However, do not withhold oxygen from a patient with a pulse oximeter reading above 95% who also shows signs and symptoms of hypoxia or difficulty breathing.

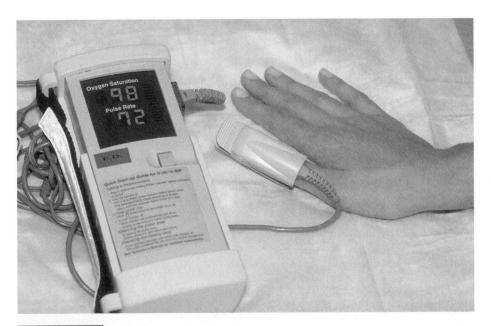

Figure 5-1 Portable pulse oximeter. *(Photo courtesy of David Effron, M.D.)*

The following are conditions that make the pulse oximeter reading unreliable:

1. Poor peripheral perfusion (shock, vasoconstriction, hypotension). Do not attach the sensing probe onto an injured extremity. Try not to use the sensing probe on the same arm that you are using to monitor the blood pressure. Be aware that the pulse oximeter reading will go down while the blood pressure cuff is inflated.

2. Severe anemia.

3. Carbon monoxide poisoning. This will give falsely high readings because the sensing probe cannot distinguish between oxyhemoglobin and carboxyhemoglobin.

4. Hypothermia.

5. Excessive patient movement.

6. High ambient light (bright sunlight, high-intensity light on area of the sensing probe).

7. Nail polish or a dirty fingernail if you are using a finger probe. Use acetone to clean the nail before attaching the probe.

To use the pulse oximeter, turn on the device, clean the area that you are to monitor (earlobe, fingernail, or toenail), and attach the sensing clip to the area.

Remember that while very useful, the pulse oximeter is just another tool to help you assess the patient. Like all tools, it has limitations and should not replace careful physical assessment.

ASSISTING WITH ADVANCED AIRWAY MANAGEMENT
Preparations

Whatever the method of intubation used, both patients and rescuers should be prepared for the procedure. The following equipment is considered basic to all intubation procedures (see Figure 5-2):

1. *Gloves:* Rubber examining (not necessarily sterile) gloves should be worn for all intubation procedures.

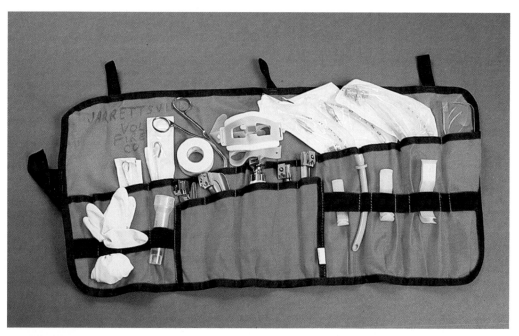

Figure 5-2 An intubation wrap contains the essentials for carrying out endotracheal intubation. The kit folds on itself and is compact and portable. When opened, it provides a clean working surface.

2. *Eye protection:* Goggles or face shield.

3. *Oxygenation:* All patients should be ventilated or should breathe high-flow oxygen (12 L/min) for several minutes prior to the attempt.

4. *Equipment:* Check all equipment, and keep at hand in an organized kit. For laryngoscopic intubation, the endotracheal tube should be held in a "field hockey stick" or open "J" shape by a malleable stylet that is first lubricated and inserted until the distal end is just *proximal* to the side hole of the endotracheal tube. Check the cuff of the endotracheal tube by inflating it with 10 cc of air. *Completely* remove the air and leave the syringe filled with air attached to the pilot tube. Lubricate the cuff and distal end of the tube.

5. *Suction:* Suction must be immediately at hand.

6. *Assistant:* You should assist with the procedure. Apply the Sellick maneuver during ventilation and the subsequent intubation attempt. You may also help hold the head and neck in a neutral position and count aloud to 30 during the intubation procedure.

Intubation Techniques

Laryngoscopic Orotracheal Intubation: In this method, the upper airway and the glottic opening are visualized, and the tube is slipped gently through the cords. The advantages of this method include the ability to see obstructions and to visualize the accurate placement of the tube. It has the disadvantage of requiring a relatively relaxed patient without anatomic distortion and with minimal bleeding or secretions.

Equipment

1. A straight (Miller) or curved (Macintosh) blade and laryngoscope handle. All in good working order (checked daily).

2. A transparent endotracheal tube, 28 to 33 cm in length and 7.0, 7.5, or 8.0 mm in internal diameter for the adult patient.

3. A stylet to help mold the tube into a field hockey stick shape.

4. A water-soluble lubricant—there is no need for it to contain a local anesthetic.

5. A 10 or 12 cc syringe.

6. Magill forceps.

7. Tape and tincture of benzoin or endotracheal tube holder.

8. Suction equipment in good working order.

9. Pulse oximeter and CO_2 detector or monitor.

10. If available, a bougie for difficult intubations.

✋ PROCEDURE

Intubation in the trauma patient differs from usual endotracheal intubation in that the patient's neck must be stabilized during the procedure. Following ventilation and initial preparations, the following steps should be carried out:

1. You should hold the head, perform the Sellick maneuver, and count slowly aloud to 30 as the ALS provider performs the intubation.

2. When the tube is inserted, inflate the cuff and check the tube for placement using the confirmation protocol below.

Nasotracheal Intubation: The nasotracheal route of endotracheal intubation in a prehospital setting may be justified when you cannot open the adult patient's mouth because of clenched jaws and when you cannot ventilate the patient by other means. The greatest disadvantage of this method is its relative difficulty, depending as it does upon the appreciation of the intensity of the breath sounds of spontaneously breathing patients. It is a blind procedure and as such requires extra skill and care to successfully perform proper intratracheal placement.

The success of this method will also depend upon an anterior curve to the tube that will prevent its passing into the esophagus. Prepare two tubes prior to carrying out the intubation attempt. Insert the distal end of the 7-mm tube into its proximal opening, thus molding it into a formed circle. Preparing two tubes permits the immediate use of the second, more rigid tube should the first plastic tube become warm with body temperature, thus losing its anterior curve. You may assist by lifting the tongue and jaw forward, since this maneuver lifts the epiglottis anteriorly out of the way of the advancing tube.

✋ PROCEDURE

1. Perform routine preparation procedures.

2. Hold the head, perform the Sellick maneuver, and count slowly aloud to 30 as the ALS provider performs the intubation.

3. Confirm tube placement using the confirmation protocol below.

Confirmation of Tube Placement: One of the greatest challenges of intubation is ensuring the correct intratracheal placement of endotracheal tubes. An unrecognized esophageal intubation is a lethal complication of this lifesaving procedure. Even in the context of prehospital care, it is inexcusable. Every effort must be made to avoid this catastrophe, and a strict protocol must be followed to reduce the risk.

A simple yet effective protocol for tube confirmation is possible and practical. Such a protocol should recognize the unreliable nature of auscultation as the sole method of confirming intratracheal placement. Correct intratracheal placement should be suspected from the following initial signs:

1. An anterior displacement of the laryngeal prominence as the tube is passed distally.

2. Coughing, bucking, or straining on the part of the patient. Note: Phonation—any noise made with the vocal cords—is absolute evidence that the tube is in the esophagus, and the tube should be removed immediately.

3. Breath condensation on the tube with each ventilation—not 100% reliable, but very suggestive of intratracheal placement.

4. Normal compliance with bag ventilation—the bag does not suddenly "collapse," but rather there is some resilience to it and resistance to lung inflation.

5. No cuff leak after inflation—persistent leak indicates esophageal intubation until proven otherwise.

6. Adequate chest rise with each ventilation.

The following procedure should then be carried out *immediately* to prove correct placement:

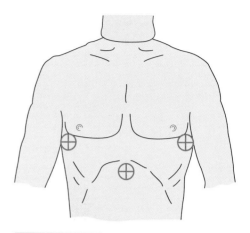

Figure 5-3

Sites to auscultate when initially checking placement of the endotracheal tube.

🖐 PROCEDURE

1. Auscultate three sites as shown in Figure 5-3:

   a. The epigastrium—the most important; it should be silent, with no sounds heard.

   b. Right and left midaxillary lines.

2. Inspect for full movement of the chest with ventilation.

Watch for any change in the patient's color or in the pulse oximeter reading. Also observe the EKG monitor for changes.

Commercial suction bulbs or syringes are available for confirming tube placement (See Figure 5-4a and b). They are at least as reliable as CO_2 detectors for confirming initial tube placement (CO_2 detectors are better for constant monitoring of tube position). To use a bulb detector, squeeze the bulb and insert the end into the 15-mm adapter on the endotracheal tube. Release the bulb. If the tube is in the trachea the bulb will expand immediately. If the tube is in the esophagus, the bulb will remain collapsed. If you are

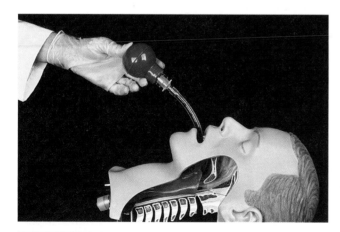

Figure 5-4a Esophageal intubation detector device, bulb style.

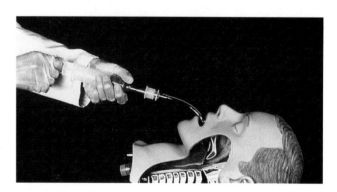

Figure 5-4b Esophageal intubation detector device, syringe style.

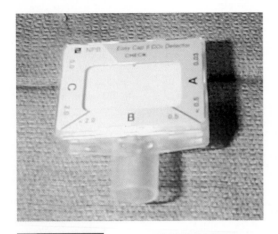

Figure 5-5

Commercial CO_2 detector.

using the detector syringe you will be able to withdraw the syringe plunger easily if the tube is in the trachea but you will not be able to withdraw the plunger if the tube is in the esophagus.

Commercial CO_2 detectors are also available to attach in-line between the ET tube and the BVM or FROPVD. There are two different kinds available. There are relatively inexpensive but also relatively insensitive devices (see Figure 5-5) that indicate by a color change that there is CO_2 in the expired air and thus indicate that the tube is in the trachea rather than the esophagus. Recently CO_2 monitors have become available (often combined with a pulse oximeter—see Figure 5-6) that directly measure expired CO_2. These are very sensitive and are the best way to continuously monitor endotracheal tube placement. If the endotracheal tube becomes dislodged and goes into the esophagus there will no longer be CO_2 in the expired air and the CO_2 monitor will detect the change immediately. As CO_2 monitors become less expensive they will become the gold standard for monitoring endotracheal intubation. They are extremely useful in the prehospital setting, where there is frequently too much noise to monitor breath sounds.

Apply the protocol for confirmation of tube placement immediately following intubation and again after several minutes of ventilation. Thereafter, repeat the protocol after movement of the patient from the floor to the stretcher, after loading onto the ambulance, each time you perform the Ongoing Exam, and immediately prior to arrival at the hospital.

When you perform the Detailed Exam, or when there is a question of correct tube placement after the above confirmation protocol, you should:

✋ PROCEDURE

1. Auscultate six sites as shown in Figure 5-7:
   a. The epigastrium; it should be silent with no sounds heard.
   b. Right and left apex.
   c. Right and left midaxillary lines.
   d. The sternal notch—"tracheal" sounds should be readily heard here.
2. Inspect the chest for full movement of the chest with ventilation.
3. Gently palpate the tube cuff in the sternal notch while compressing the pilot balloon between the index finger and thumb; a pressure wave should be felt in the sternal notch.
4. Use adjuncts such as a suction bulb or CO_2 detectors to help confirm placement.

Any time placement is still in doubt in spite of the above protocol, visualize directly or remove the tube. Never assume that the tube is in the right place—always be sure and record that the protocol has been carefully followed.

Anchoring the Tube: This can be a frustrating exercise. Not only does it require some fine movements of the hands when we appear to be all thumbs,

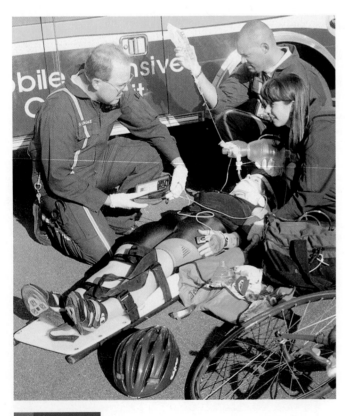

Figure 5-6

Combined CO_2 monitor and pulse oximeter. *(Photo courtesy of Nonin Medical, Inc.)*

but it is difficult to perform this task when ventilation, movement, or extrication is being carried out. There is one thing to keep in mind: **There is no substitute for the human anchor.** That is, one person should be held responsible for ensuring that the tube is held fast and that it does not migrate in or out of the airway. To lose a tube can be a catastrophe, especially if the patient is rather inaccessible or the intubation was a difficult one to begin with.

Fixing the endotracheal tube in place is important for several reasons. First, movement of the tube in the trachea will produce more mucosal damage and may increase the risk of postintubation complications. In addition, movement of the tube will stimulate the patient to cough, strain, or both, leading to cardiovascular and intracranial pressure changes that could be detrimental. Most important, there is a greater risk in the prehospital setting of dislodging a tube and losing control of the airway if it is not anchored solidly in place.

The endotracheal tube can be secured in place by either tape or a commercially available holder. While taping a tube in place is convenient and relatively easily done, it is not always effective. There is often a problem with the tape sticking to skin wet with rain, blood, airway secretions, or vomitus. If you are using tape, several principles should be followed:

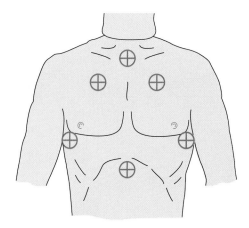

Figure 5-7

Sites to auscultate when performing the Detailed Exam, or if there is doubt about the placement of the endotracheal tube.

1. Insert an oropharyngeal airway to prevent the patient from biting down on the tube.

2. Dry the patient's face and apply tincture of benzoin to better ensure proper adhesion of the tape.

3. Carry the tape right around the patient's neck when anchoring the tube. Do not move the neck. Do not tie it so tight that it occludes the external jugular veins.

4. Anchor the tube at the corner of the mouth, not in the midline.

Because of the difficulty of fixing the tube in place with tape, it may be better to use a commercial endotracheal tube holder that uses a strap to fix the tube in a plastic holder that also acts as a bite block (see Figure 5-8). Since flexion or extension of the patient's head can move the tube in or out of the airway by 2 or 3 cm, it is good practice to restrict head and neck movement of any patient who has an endotracheal tube in place (even more important in children). If the patient is spinal motion-restricted because of the risk of cervical spine injury, flexion and extension should be less of a concern.

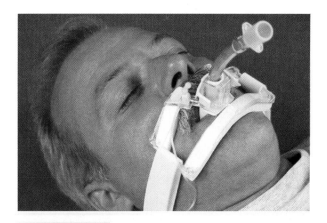

Figure 5-8

A commercial endotracheal tube holder.

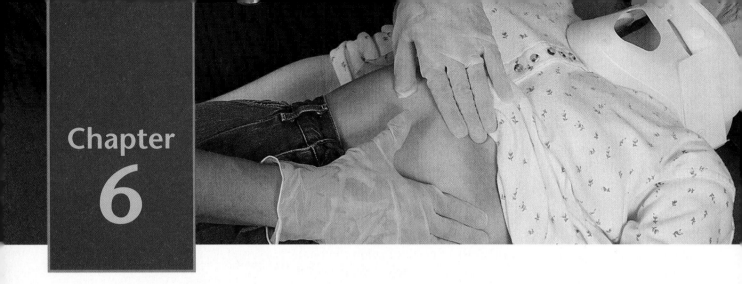

Chapter 6

Thoracic Trauma

Andrew B. Peitzman, M.D., F.A.C.S.
Paul Paris, M.D., F.A.C.E.P.

Objectives

Upon completion of this chapter, you should be able to:

1. Identify the major symptoms of thoracic trauma.
2. Describe the signs of thoracic trauma.
3. State the immediate life-threatening thoracic injuries.
4. Explain the pathophysiology and management of an open pneumothorax.
5. Describe the clinical signs of a tension pneumothorax in conjunction with appropriate management.
6. Explain the hypovolemic and respiratory compromise pathophysiology and management in massive hemothorax.
7. Define flail chest in relation to associated physical findings and management.
8. Identify the triad of physical findings in the diagnosis of cardiac tamponade.
9. Explain the cardiac involvement and management associated with blunt injury to the chest.
10. Summarize other injuries and their appropriate management.

CASE STUDY

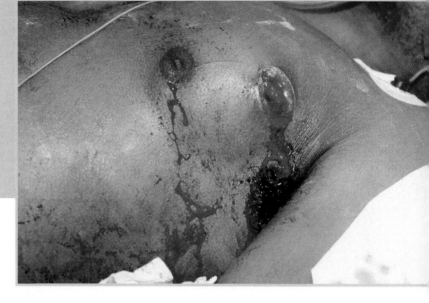

(Photo courtesy of Roy Alson, M.D.)

Dan, Joyce, and Buddy of the Emergency Transport System have been called to a local bar where a patron has been stabbed. The Scene Size-up reveals that the police are on-scene and have cleared the bar and are questioning bystanders outside. There is a single male victim who is sitting in a chair and holding his chest. Since the scene is safe and the mechanism of injury (stab wound) is readily apparent, the team dons personal protective equipment and each carries their essential trauma care equipment as they approach the patient. How would you approach this patient? What type of assessment would you perform? What would you do first? Is this a load-and-go situation? Keep these questions in mind as you read the chapters. The case study will continue at the end of the chapter.

INTRODUCTION

Twenty-five percent of trauma deaths are due entirely to thoracic injuries, and half of trauma patients with multiple injuries have an associated chest injury. Two-thirds of these patients with potentially fatal thoracic trauma are alive when they reach the emergency department and only 15% require surgery. Thus, these are salvageable trauma patients who can usually be saved by procedures done in the prehospital phase and the emergency department. The goal of this chapter is to enable you to recognize signs and symptoms of major thoracic injury and provide appropriate care. Major thoracic injury may result from MVCs, falls, gunshot wounds, crush injuries, stab wounds, or other mechanisms.

ANATOMY

The thorax is a bony cavity that is formed by 12 pairs of ribs that join posteriorly with the thoracic spine and anteriorly with the sternum. The intercostal neurovascular bundle runs along the inferior surface of each rib (see Figure 6-1).

The inner side of the thoracic cavity and the lung itself are lined with a thin layer of tissue, the pleura. The space between the two pleural layers is normally only a potential space. However, this space may be occupied by air, forming a pneumothorax, or blood, forming a hemothorax. This potential space can hold three liters of fluid on each side in an adult.

As shown in Figure 6-2, one lung occupies each thoracic cavity. Between the two chest cavities is the mediastinum, which contains the heart, aorta, superior and inferior vena cava, trachea, major bronchi, and esophagus. The spinal cord is protected by the vertebral column. The diaphragm separates the thoracic organs from the abdominal cavity. The

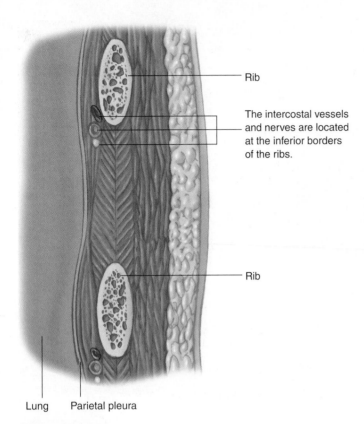

Figure 6-1

Rib with intercostal vessels and nerve.

Rib

The intercostal vessels and nerves are located at the inferior borders of the ribs.

Rib

Lung   Parietal pleura

upper abdominal organs, including the spleen, liver, kidneys, pancreas, and stomach, are protected by the lower rib cage (see Figure 6-3). Any patient with a penetrating thoracic wound at the level of the nipples (fourth intercostal space) or lower should be assumed to have an abdominal injury as well as a thoracic injury. Similarly, blunt deceleration injuries such as steering wheel injuries often injure both thoracic and abdominal structures.

Penetrating wounds that traverse the mediastinum have a particularly high potential for life-threatening injury because of the vital cardiovascular and tracheobronchial structures within this area.

PATHOPHYSIOLOGY

When evaluating a patient with probable thoracic trauma, always follow the BTLS assessment priorities (Chapter 2) to avoid missing life-threatening injuries. During the BTLS primary survey, search for the most dangerous injuries first to give your patient the best chance for survival. As with any trauma patient, the mechanism of injury is very important in caring for the thoracic trauma patient. Thoracic injuries may be the result of blunt or penetrating trauma. With blunt trauma, the force is distributed over a large area, and visceral injuries occur from deceleration, shearing forces, compression, or bursting. Penetrating injuries, usually gunshot wounds or stab wounds, distribute the forces of injury over a smaller area. However, the trajectory of a bullet is often unpredictable, and all thoracic structures are at risk.

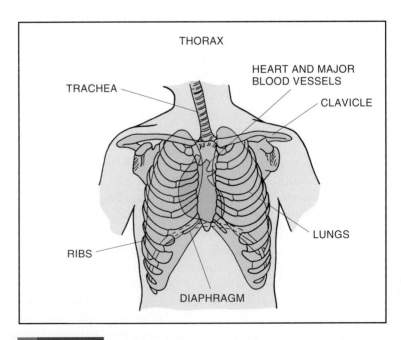

THORAX

TRACHEA

HEART AND MAJOR BLOOD VESSELS

CLAVICLE

LUNGS

RIBS

DIAPHRAGM

Figure 6-2 Thorax.

The common end point in thoracic injury is tissue hypoxia. Tissue hypoxia may result from the following:

1. Inadequate oxygen delivery to the tissues secondary to airway obstruction

2. Hypovolemia from blood loss

3. Ventilation/perfusion mismatch from lung parenchymal injury

4. Changes in pleural pressures from tension pneumothorax

5. Pump failure from severe myocardial injury

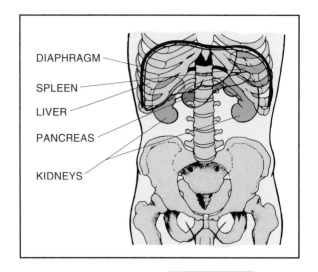

Figure 6-3

Intrathoracic abdomen.

ASSESSMENT

The major symptoms of chest injury include shortness of breath, chest pain, and respiratory distress. The signs indicative of chest injury include shock, hemoptysis, cyanosis, chest wall contusion, flail chest, open wounds, distended neck veins, tracheal deviation, or subcutaneous emphysema. Check the lung fields for the presence and equality of breath sounds. Life-threatening thoracic injuries should be identified immediately. Major thoracic injuries to identify may be remembered as the "deadly dozen."

The following injuries must be detected and treated during the BTLS Primary Survey:

1. Airway obstruction

2. Open pneumothorax

3. Tension pneumothorax

4. Massive hemothorax

5. Flail chest

6. Cardiac tamponade

Life-threatening injuries that are more likely to be detected during the Detailed Exam or during hospital evaluation are the following:

7. Traumatic aortic rupture

8. Tracheal or bronchial tree injury

9. Myocardial contusion

10. Diaphragmatic tears

11. Esophageal injury

12. Pulmonary contusion

Airway Obstruction

Airway management remains a major challenge in the care of any multiple-trauma patient. This has been discussed in Chapter 4. Always assume that there is an associated cervical-spine injury when securing the airway.

Open Pneumothorax

This is caused by a penetrating thoracic injury and may present as a sucking chest wound. The signs and symptoms are usually proportional to the size of the chest wall defect (see Figure 6-4).

Normal ventilation involves a negative pressure being generated inside the chest by diaphragmatic contraction. As air is drawn through the upper airway, the lungs expand.

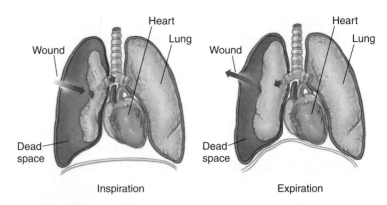

Figure 6-4 Open pneumothorax. If the wound is larger than the opening to the trachea, air will preferentially go into dead space rather than the lung.

On inspiration, dressing seals wound, preventing air entry

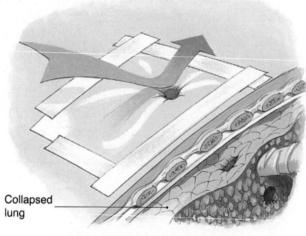

Collapsed lung

Expiration allows trapped air to escape through untaped section of dressing

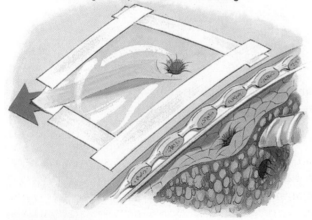

Figure 6-5 Treatment of sucking chest wound.

With a large open wound of the chest (larger than the trachea—about the size of the patient's little finger), the path of least resistance for airflow is through the chest wall defect. Air going in and out of this opening makes a sucking sound, from which the term "sucking chest wound" comes. This air will only enter the pleural dead space. It will not enter the lung and therefore will not contribute to oxygenation of the blood. Ventilation is impaired and hypoxia results.

✋ PROCEDURE

✳ Management of Open Pneumothorax

1. Ensure an airway.
2. Promptly close the chest wall defect by any available means. You may accomplish this with a defibrillation pad, Vaseline gauze, a rubber glove, or plastic dressing. Placing an occlusive dressing carries the risk of a tension pneumothorax. To circumvent this problem, tape the occlusive dressing on three sides to produce a flutter valve: Air can escape from the chest but will not enter (see Figure 6-5). A commercial chest seal (Asherman Chest Seal®) with a one-way valve is now available and is currently the best thing with which to close an open chest wound (see Figure 6-6). A chest tube will be needed ultimately, followed by operative closure of the chest wall defect.
3. Administer oxygen.
4. Monitor the heart if you have monitoring equipment.

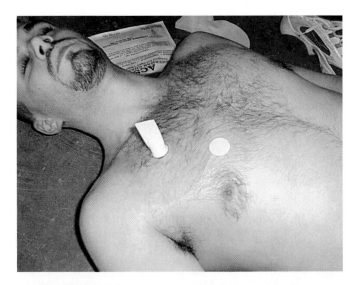

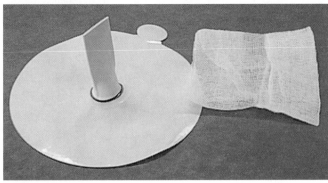

Figure 6-6

Sealing a sucking chest wound with Asherman Chest Seal®.

5. Monitor oxygen saturation with a pulse oximeter.

6. Transport rapidly to the appropriate hospital.

Tension Pneumothorax

This injury occurs when a one-way valve is created from either blunt or penetrating trauma. Air can enter but not leave the pleural space (see Figure 6-7). This causes an increase in the intrathoracic pressure which will collapse the affected lung and will then exert pressure on the mediastinum. This pressure will eventually collapse the superior and inferior vena cava, resulting in a loss of venous return to the heart. A shift of the trachea and mediastinum away from the side of the tension pneumothorax will also compromise ventilation of the other lung, although this is a late phenomenon.

Clinical signs of a tension pneumothorax include dyspnea, anxiety, tachypnea, diminished breath sounds and hyperresonance to percussion on the affected side, hypotension, and distended neck veins. Tracheal deviation is a late (and rare) finding and its absence does not rule out the presence of a tension pneumothorax. In a review of 108 field patients diagnosed with tension pneumothorax and requiring needle decompression, none were recorded as having a deviated trachea. The development of decreased lung compliance (difficulty in squeezing the bag-valve device) should always alert you to the possibility of a tension pneumothorax.

✋ PROCEDURE

⚕ Management of Tension Pneumothorax

1. Establish an open airway.
2. Administer high-concentration oxygen.
4. Monitor oxygen saturation with a pulse oximeter
5. Rapidly transport to the appropriate hospital.
6. Notify Medical Direction.

The patient must be transported rapidly to the hospital so that chest decompression can be performed. A chest tube will also be necessary upon arrival to the hospital.

Massive Hemothorax

Blood in the pleural space is a hemothorax (see Figure 6-8). A *massive hemothorax* occurs as a result of at least a 1,500-cc blood loss into the thoracic cavity. Each thoracic cavity may contain up to 3,000 cc of blood. Massive hemothorax is more often due to penetrating than blunt trauma, but either injury may disrupt a major pulmonary or systemic vessel. As blood accumulates within the pleural space, the lung on the affected side is compressed. If enough blood accumulates (rare), the mediastinum will be shifted away from

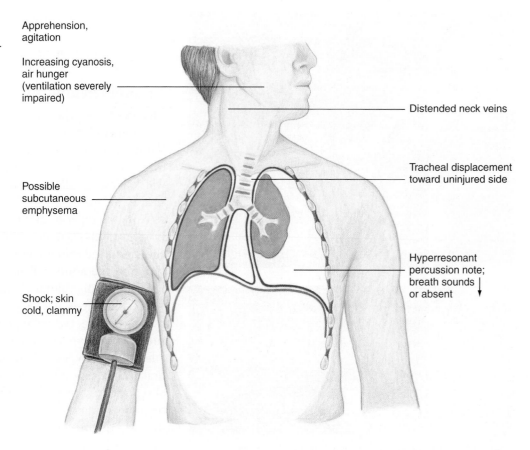

Figure 6-7

Physical findings of tension pneumothorax.

Apprehension, agitation

Increasing cyanosis, air hunger (ventilation severely impaired)

Distended neck veins

Tracheal displacement toward uninjured side

Possible subcutaneous emphysema

Hyperresonant percussion note; breath sounds ↓ or absent

Shock; skin cold, clammy

the hemothorax. The inferior and superior vena cava and the contralateral lung are compressed. Thus the ongoing blood loss is complicated by hypoxemia.

Signs and symptoms of massive hemothorax are produced by both hypovolemia and respiratory compromise. The patient may be hypotensive from blood loss and compression of the heart or great veins. Anxiety and confusion are produced by hypovolemia and hypoxemia. Clinical signs of hypovolemic shock may be apparent. The neck veins are usually flat secondary to profound hypovolemia, but may *rarely* be distended due to mediastinal compression. Other signs of hemothorax include decreased breath sounds and dullness to percussion on the affected side. See Table 6-1 for comparison of tension pneumothorax and massive hemothorax.

✋ PROCEDURE

✳ Management of Massive Hemothorax

1. Secure an airway.
2. Apply high-flow oxygen.
3. Rapidly transport to the appropriate hospital.
4. Monitor oxygen saturation with a pulse oximeter.
5. Notify Medical Direction.

Flail Chest

This occurs when three or more adjacent ribs are fractured in at least two places (see Figure 6-9). The result is a segment of the chest wall that is not in continuity with the tho-

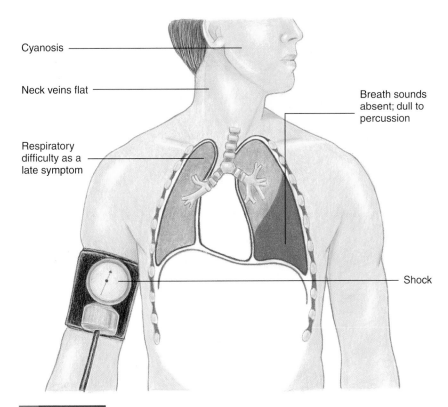

Cyanosis

Neck veins flat

Respiratory difficulty as a late symptom

Breath sounds absent; dull to percussion

Shock

Figure 6-8 Physical findings of massive hemothorax.

rax. A lateral flail chest or anterior flail chest (sternal separation) may result. With posterior rib fractures, the heavy musculature usually prevents the occurrence of a flail segment. The flail segment moves with paradoxical motion relative to the rest of the chest wall (see Figures 6-10 and 6-11). The force necessary to produce this injury also bruises the underlying lung tissue, and this pulmonary contusion also will contribute to the hypoxia. The patient is at risk for the development of a hemothorax or pneumothorax. With a large flail segment, the patient may be in marked respiratory distress. Pain from the chest wall injury exacerbates the already impaired respiration from paradoxical

TABLE 6-1	Comparison of Tension Pneumothorax and Hemothorax.	
	Tension Pneumothorax	**Hemothorax**
Primary presenting symptom	Difficulty breathing, then shock	Shock, then difficulty breathing
Neck veins	Usually distended	Usually flat
Breath sounds	Decreased or absent on side of injury	Decreased or absent on side of injury
Percussion of chest	Hyperresonant	Dull
Tracheal deviation away from the side of the injury	Rarely present as a late sign	Usually not present

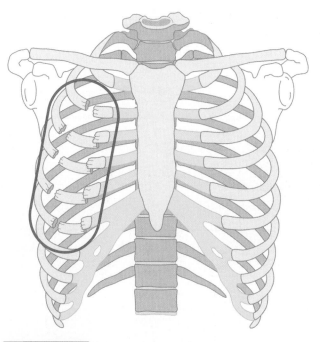

Figure 6-9 Flail chest occurs when three or more adjacent ribs fracture in two or more places.

motion and the underlying lung contusion. Palpation of the chest wall may reveal crepitus in addition to the abnormal respiratory motion (see Figure 6-12).

✋ PROCEDURE

✳ Management of Flail Chest

1. Ensure an airway.
2. Administer oxygen.

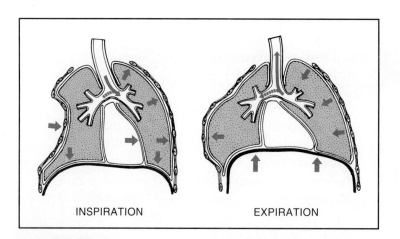

INSPIRATION   EXPIRATION

Figure 6-10

Pathophysiology of flail chest.

3. Assist ventilation if required. Remember that pneumothorax is commonly associated with a flail chest.

4. Monitor oxygen saturation with a pulse oximeter.

5. Rapidly transport to the appropriate hospital.

6. Stabilize the flail segment with manual pressure, then with bulky dressings taped to the chest wall (see Figure 6-13). This is usually not necessary until the patient is stabilized on a backboard. Trying to maintain manual pressure on a flail segment while performing log-rolling may compromise maintaining a stable spine.

8. Notify Medical Direction.

9. Monitor the heart if you have monitoring equipment. Associated myocardial trauma is frequent.

Cardiac Tamponade

This injury is usually due to penetrating injury. The pericardial sac is an inelastic membrane that surrounds the heart. If blood collects rapidly between the heart and pericardium from a cardiac injury, the ventricles of the heart will be compressed. A small amount of pericardial blood may compromise cardiac filling. As the compression of the ventricles increases, the heart is less able to refill and cardiac output falls.

Diagnosis of cardiac tamponade classically relies upon the triad of hypotension, distended neck veins, and muffled heart sounds (Beck's triad). Muffled heart sounds may be very difficult to appreciate in the prehospital setting, but if you briefly listen to the heart when you perform the primary survey you may notice a change later. The patient may have a paradoxical pulse. If the patient loses his peripheral pulse during inspiration, this is suggestive of a paradoxical pulse and the presence of cardiac tamponade. The major differential diagnosis in the field is tension pneumothorax. With cardiac tamponade, the patient will be in shock with a midline trachea and equal breath sounds (see Figure 6-14) unless there is an associated pneumothorax or hemothorax.

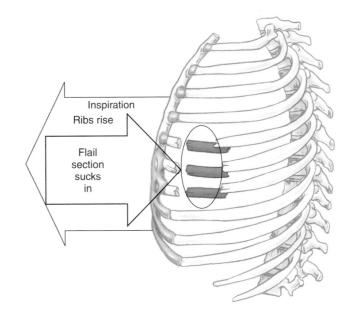

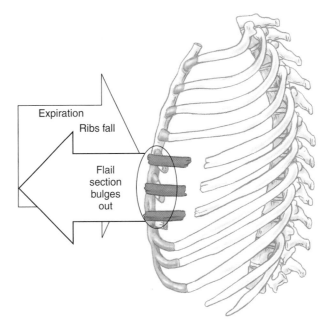

Figure 6-11

Paradoxical motion.

✋ PROCEDURE

❇ Management of Cardiac Tamponade

1. Ensure an airway and administer oxygen.

2. This lesion is rapidly fatal and cannot be readily treated in the field. Load the patient and proceed rapidly to the appropriate hospital.

3. Notify Medical Direction.

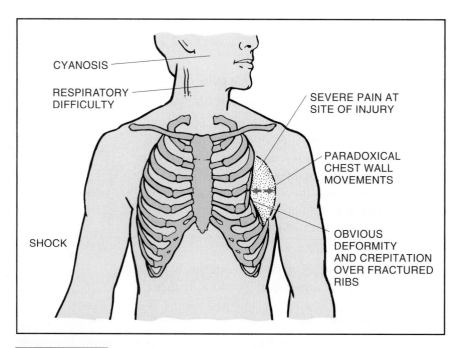

Figure 6-12 Physical findings of flail chest.

4. Monitor the oxygen saturation with a pulse oximeter.

6. Monitor the heart if you have monitoring equipment.

Traumatic Aortic Rupture

This is the most common cause of immediate death in motor vehicle accidents or falls from heights. Ninety percent of these patients die immediately. For the survivors, salvage is feasible with prompt diagnosis and surgery. Traumatic thoracic aortic tears usually are due to deceleration injury with the heart and aortic arch moving suddenly anteriorly (third collision), transecting the aorta where it is fixed at the ligamentum arteriosum. In the 10% of patients who do not exsanguinate promptly, the aortic tear will be contained temporarily by surrounding tissues and the adventitia. However, this will usually rupture within hours unless surgically repaired.

The diagnosis of a contained thoracic aortic laceration is impossible in the field and may be missed even in the hospital. The history from the scene is critically important, since many of these patients have no obvious signs of chest trauma. Information about damage to the car or steering wheel with a deceleration injury or the height from which the patient fell is vital. Infrequently, the patient may present with upper extremity hypertension and diminished lower extremity pulses.

Tape pad in place, extending tape to both sides of chest

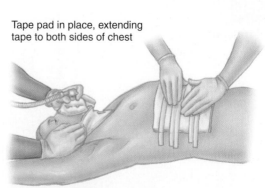

Intubation and positive pressure ventilation is the best stabilization

Figure 6-13 Stabilizing flail chest.

✋ PROCEDURE

✳ Management of Potential Aortic Tears

1. Ensure an airway.

2. Administer oxygen.

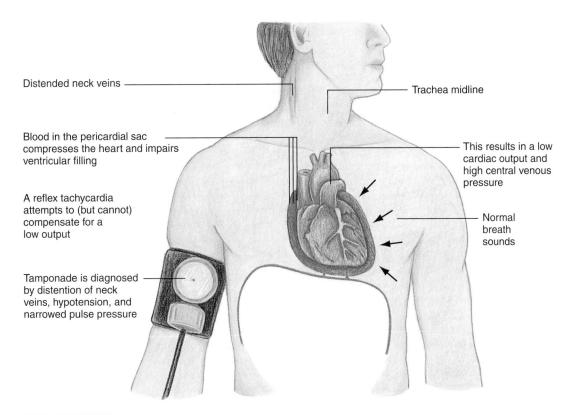

Distended neck veins

Trachea midline

Blood in the pericardial sac compresses the heart and impairs ventricular filling

This results in a low cardiac output and high central venous pressure

A reflex tachycardia attempts to (but cannot) compensate for a low output

Normal breath sounds

Tamponade is diagnosed by distention of neck veins, hypotension, and narrowed pulse pressure

Figure 6-14 Pathophysiology and physical findings of cardiac tamponade.

3. Rapidly transport to the appropriate hospital.
4. Notify Medical Direction.
5. Monitor oxygen saturation with a pulse oximeter
6. Monitor the heart if you have monitoring equipment.

Tracheal or Bronchial Tree Injury

These injuries may be the result of penetrating or blunt trauma. Penetrating upper airway injuries often have associated major vascular injuries and extensive tissue destruction. Blunt trauma may present with subtle findings. Blunt injury usually ruptures the trachea or mainstem bronchus near the carina. Presenting signs of blunt or penetrating injury include subcutaneous emphysema of the chest, face, or neck or an associated pneumothorax or hemothorax Give 100% oxygen and transport immediately.

Myocardial Contusion

This is a potentially lethal lesion resulting from blunt chest injury. Blunt injury to the anterior chest is transmitted via the sternum to the heart, which lies immediately posterior to it (see Figure 6-15). Cardiac injuries from this mechanism may include valvular rupture, pericardial tamponade, or cardiac rupture, but contusion of the right atrium and right ventricle occurs most commonly (see Figure 6-16). This bruising of the heart is basically the same injury as an acute myocardial infarction and likewise presents with chest pain, dysrhythmia, or cardiogenic shock (rare). In the field, cardiogenic shock cannot be distinguished from cardiac tamponade. The chest pain may be difficult to differentiate

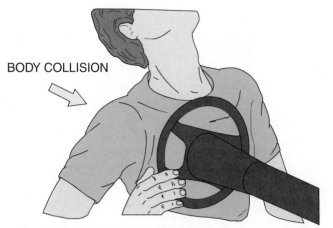

Collision 2 – Body hits steering wheel, causing broken ribs

Figure 6-15 Pathophysiology of myocardial contusion.

from the associated musculoskeletal discomfort that the patient also suffers as a result of the injury. All patients with blunt anterior chest trauma should be presumed to have a myocardial contusion.

✋ PROCEDURE

✳ Management of Myocardial Contusion

1. Administer oxygen.
2. Transport the patient to the appropriate hospital.
3. Monitor the heart if you have monitoring equipment.
4. Monitor oxygen saturation with a pulse oximeter.

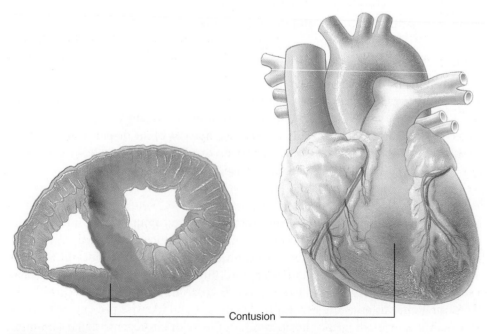

— Contusion —

Figure 6-16 Myocardial contusion most frequently affects the right atrium and ventricle as they collide with the sternum.

Diaphragmatic Tears

Tears in the diaphragm may result from a severe blow to the abdomen. A sudden increase in intra-abdominal pressure, such as a seat belt injury or kick to the abdomen, may tear the diaphragm and allow herniation of the abdominal organs into the thoracic cavity. This occurs more commonly on the left than the right, since the liver protects the right hemidiaphragm. Blunt trauma produces large radial tears in the diaphragm. Penetrating trauma may also produce holes in the diaphragm, but these tend to be small.

Traumatic diaphragmatic hernia is difficult to diagnose even in the hospital. The herniation of abdominal contents into the thoracic cavity may cause marked respiratory distress. On examination, the breath sounds may be diminished, and infrequently bowel sounds may be heard when the chest is auscultated. The abdomen may appear scaphoid if a large quantity of abdominal contents is in the chest.

✋ PROCEDURE

✳ Management of Diaphragmatic Rupture

1. Ensure an airway.
2. Administer oxygen.
3. Transport the patient to the appropriate hospital.
4. Monitor the oxygen saturation with a pulse oximeter.
5. Notify Medical Direction.

Esophageal Injury

This injury is usually produced by penetrating trauma. Management of associated trauma including airway or vascular injuries is generally more pressing than the esophageal injury. However, esophageal injury is lethal if unrecognized in the hospital. Operative repair is required.

Pulmonary Contusion

This very common chest injury results from blunt trauma. Contusion of the lung may produce marked hypoxemia. Management consists of assisted ventilation if indicated, oxygen administration, and transport.

Other Chest Injuries

Any penetrating object, usually a knife, may cause *impalement injuries* of the chest. As in other areas of the body, the object should not be removed in the field. Stabilize the object, ensure an airway, insert an IV, and transport the patient.

Traumatic asphyxia is an important set of physical findings. The term is a misnomer since the condition is not caused by asphyxia. The syndrome results from a severe compression injury to the chest, such as from a steering wheel, a conveyor belt, or a heavy object. The sudden compression of the heart and mediastinum transmits this force to the capillaries of the neck and head. The patients appear similar to those of strangulation, with cyanosis and swelling of the head and neck. The tongue and lips are swollen, and conjunctival hemorrhage is evident. The skin below the level of the crush injury to the chest will be pink unless there are other problems.

Traumatic asphyxia indicates that the patient has suffered a severe blunt thoracic injury, and major thoracic injuries are likely to be present. Management includes airway maintenance, IV treating other injuries, and rapid transport.

Similarly, *sternal fractures* indicate that the patient has suffered marked blunt trauma to the anterior chest. These patients should be presumed to have a myocardial contusion. Diagnosis can be made by palpation.

Scapular fractures and *first or second rib fractures* require a significant force. The incidence of associated major thoracic vascular injury is high, and these patients should be promptly transported.

Simple pneumothorax may result from blunt or penetrating trauma. Fractured ribs are the usual cause in blunt trauma. Pneumothorax is caused by accumulation of air within the potential space between the visceral and parietal pleura. The lung may be totally or partially collapsed as the air continues to accrue in the thoracic cavity. In a healthy patient this should not acutely compromise ventilation, if a tension pneumothorax does not evolve. Patients with less respiratory reserve may not tolerate even a simple pneumothorax.

Diagnosis of a pneumothorax is based on pleuritic chest pain, dyspnea, decreased breath sounds on the affected side, and hypertympany to percussion. Close observation is required in anticipation of the patient developing a tension pneumothorax.

Simple rib fracture is the most frequent injury to the chest. If the patient does not have an associated pneumothorax or hemothorax, the major problem is pain. This pain will prohibit the patient from breathing adequately. On palpation, the area of rib fracture will be tender and may be unstable. Give oxygen and monitor for pneumothorax or hemothorax while encouraging the patient to breathe deeply.

CASE STUDY

Dan, Joyce, and Buddy of the Emergency Transport System have been called to a local bar where a patron has been stabbed. The Scene Size-up reveals that the police are on-scene and have cleared the bar and are questioning bystanders outside. There is a single male victim who is sitting in a chair and holding his chest. Since the scene is safe and the mechanism of injury (stab wound) is readily apparent, the team dons personal protective equipment and each carries their essential trauma care equipment as they approach the patient. The patient (Doobie Mullengrabber) states that he was stabbed twice in the left chest but has no other injuries. He states that during an argument his friend JoJo stabbed him twice in the left anterior chest before bystanders could take the knife away from him. The patient denies falling or any other injuries.

Joyce is acting as team leader and as she begins the initial assessment her general impression is good. The patient is a young man who is sitting in a chair and is awake and answering appropriately. He does not appear to be in any distress. Respiration appears to be fast and shallow and when his hand is removed from his left chest there are two stab wounds. One of the wounds is small but the other is about 5 centimeters long and obviously sucks when he inhales. The radial pulse is rapid but strong. Joyce immediately asks Dan to apply a non-rebreather oxygen mask and then clean the chest and apply an Asherman Chest Seal®. Because of the nature of the injury she decides to do a focused exam. Exam of the airway is normal, with good movement of air and a normal speaking voice. The neck veins are flat and the trachea is in the midline. The breath sounds are not present on the left (except for the sucking sound) but are normal on the right. Respiration is rapid and shallow. The two wounds (no longer bleeding) are as mentioned above. Percussion of the chest reveals dullness to percussion on the left. Heart sounds are normal but rapid. The abdomen is soft and nontender. There are no other wounds. Vital signs: pulse 140, respiration 36/minute, blood pressure 90/60. As soon as Dan seals the sucking chest wound the patient is placed on a stretcher (no backboard or packaging) and moved to the ambulance.

He is treated with 100% oxygen by non-rebreather mask.

The History reveals:

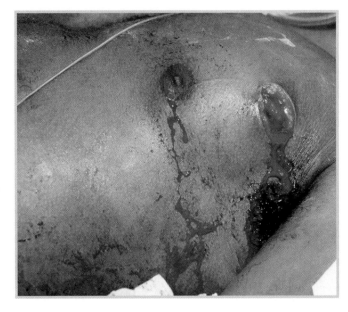

(Photo courtesy of Roy Alson, M.D.)

S—Pain in left chest, shortness of breath, and weakness

A—None

M—None

P—No history of serious illness

L—Just ate some Slim Jims and pickled eggs. Admits to drinking "three beers."

E—States he was drinking with his friend JoJo, who became upset when he said that Alabama football players are the best that money can buy. In a snit, JoJo stabbed him with a large pocketknife. JoJo is now outside talking to the police and is crying and protesting that he never meant to hurt Doobie.

Buddy applies a cardiac monitor and a pulse oximeter (98% on 100% oxygen). Joyce notifies Medical Direction that they will be arriving in five minutes with a young male with a sucking chest wound, a hemothorax, and early shock. Joyce performs the Detailed Exam and finds everything normal except what was noted on the Focused Exam. The Ongoing Exam was not performed, since they arrived at the emergency department before she had time to do one. While in the emergency department the patient had a chest tube inserted and 1,000 cc of blood evacuated. There was no further bleeding, so the patient did not have to go to surgery. He was in the hospital for five days and had an uneventful recovery. JoJo picked him up and gave him a ride home when he was discharged.

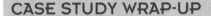

CASE STUDY WRAP-UP

This is one of the few examples of a Focused Exam being adequate for a trauma patient. Note that even a Focused Exam requires that both the chest and the abdomen be examined because the diaphragm rises so high in the chest that a mid-chest stab wound may go through the diaphragm and cause abdominal injuries. A sucking chest wound can be closed using an occlusive dressing taped on only three sides so that air can escape (preventing development of a tension pneumothorax) but air cannot enter the chest. The commercially available Asherman Chest Seal® has a built-in flutter valve and is currently the best way to seal a sucking chest wound.

Studies have found that for penetrating wounds of the chest, the pneumatic anti-shock garment or IV fluids may significantly worsen survival (See Chapter 8). Thus the PASG is contraindicated.

SUMMARY

Chest injuries are common and often life-threatening in the multiple-trauma patient. If you follow the BTLS assessment priorities, you will identify the injuries while performing the BTLS Primary Survey. These are often load-and-go patients. The primary goals in treating the patient with chest trauma are the following:

1. Ensuring an airway while protecting the cervical spine
2. Administering high-flow oxygen
3. Early transport to the appropriate hospital
4. Monitoring the oxygen saturation and the heart rhythm if equipment is available)

The thoracic injuries discussed are life threatening, but treatable by prompt intervention and transport to the appropriate hospital. It is mandatory that the injuries presented are recognized in the field and treated appropriately to salvage these patients.

BIBLIOGRAPHY

1. Blair, E., C. Topuzulu, and R. S. Deane. "Major Chest Trauma." *Current Problems in Surgery* (May 1969), pp. 2–69.

2. Jones, K. W. "Thoracic Trauma." *Surgical Clinics of North America* (1980), pp. 60–95.

3. Richardson, J.D., L. Adams, and L. M. Flint. "Selective Management of Flail Chest and Pulmonary Contusion." *Annals of Surgery,* Vol. 196, No. 4 (1982), pp. 481–487.

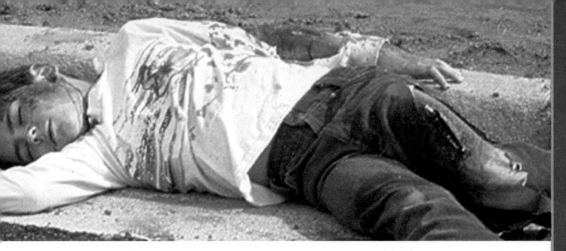

Chapter 7

Shock Evaluation and Management

Raymond L. Fowler, M.D., F.A.C.E.P.

Paul E. Pepe, M.D., M.P.H., F.A.C.E.P., F.C.C.M.

Roger J. Lewis, M.D., Ph.D., F.A.C.E.P.

Objectives

Upon completion of this chapter, you should be able to:

1. List the four components necessary for normal tissue perfusion.

2. Describe symptoms and signs of hemorrhagic shock.

3. Explain the pathophysiology of hemorrhagic shock and compare to the pathophysiology of high-space shock.

4. Describe the three common clinical shock syndromes.

5. Describe the management of the following:

   a. Hemorrhage that can be controlled

   b. Hemorrhage that cannot be controlled

   c. Nonhemorrhagic shock syndromes

6. Discuss the routine priorities in the prehospital management of shock.

7. Discuss the current indications and contraindications for the use of the antishock garment in the treatment of traumatic shock.

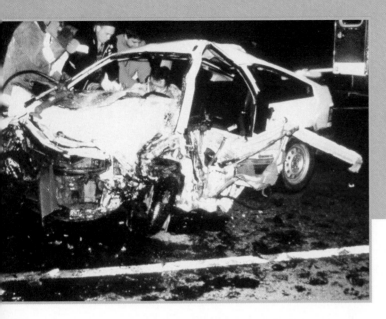

(Photo courtesy of David Effron, M.D.)

CASE STUDY

Dan, Joyce, and Buddy of the Emergency Transport System have been called to the scene of a high-speed side-impact auto collision. What injuries should they expect in a collision of this type? Would the victim likely develop shock? What type of interventions might they likely have to make? Keep these questions in mind as you read the chapter. The case study will continue at the end of the chapter.

The management of shock has been the subject of intensive research during the past few years, and changes have been made in the recommendations for prehospital treatment of the patient with hemorrhagic shock. Some excellent studies on the treatment of hemorrhagic shock secondary to penetrating trauma have suggested new thinking in this area, while research in the treatment of the patient with blunt trauma has been less revealing. This chapter will review the present knowledge about the pathophysiology and treatment of shock in the traumatized patient.

BASIC PATHOPHYSIOLOGY

The normal perfusion of body tissues requires four intact components:

1. An intact vascular system to deliver oxygenated blood throughout the body
2. Adequate air exchange in the lungs to allow oxygen to enter the blood
3. An adequate volume of fluid in the vascular system, including blood cells and plasma
4. A functioning pump: the heart

The preservation of these components can be related to the basic rules of emergency care, which are:

1. Maintain the airway.
2. Control oxygenation and ventilation.
3. Control bleeding.
4. Maintain circulation.

The term *shock* describes a condition that occurs when the perfusion of the body's tissues with oxygen, electrolytes, glucose, and fluid becomes inadequate. Several processes cause this drop in perfusion. The loss of red blood cells in hemorrhaging patients results in less oxygen transport to the body tissues. Decreased circulating blood volume leads to lowered glucose, fluid volume, and electrolytes to the cells. The above circulatory disturbances result in the cells of the body becoming "shocked," and grave changes in body tissue begin to occur. Eventually, cell death follows.

Deprived of oxygen, cells begin to use "backup" processes that utilize energy sources less efficiently, producing toxic by-products such as lactic acid. Although these backup (anaerobic) processes may postpone cellular death for a time, the lack of oxygen is compounded by these toxic by-products because they can poison certain cellular functions such as the production of energy by mitochondria. Eventually, accumulating lactic acid in the blood and organs creates a systemic acidosis that further disrupts cellular activity. Respiratory muscle function also weakens, and respiratory failure develops, which worsens hypoxia.

In response to inadequate oxygen delivery, the body responds with increased sympathetic tone and release of circulating catecholamines (epinephrine and norepinephrine). These increase the heart rate and constrict peripheral blood vessels. The midbrain responds to the progressive hypoxia with an increase in the respiratory rate.

As you can see, shock is a condition that begins with an injury, spreads throughout the body as a multisystem insult to major organs, and results in specific symptoms at the bedside as the patient becomes progressively sicker.

Shock is a cellular process with clinical manifestations. The patient with shock may be pale, diaphoretic, and tachycardic. At the cellular level, the patient's cells are starving for oxygen and nutrients. Shock, therefore, is a condition in which poor tissue perfusion can severely and possibly permanently damage the organs of the body, causing disability or death. The clinical signs and symptoms of the patient in shock imply that critical processes are threatening every vulnerable cell in the patient's body, particularly those in vital organs.

ASSESSMENT: SIGNS AND SYMPTOMS OF SHOCK

When first considering the concept of shock, you must understand that shock produces signs and symptoms that you can observe during patient assessment. The initial diagnosis of the shock state can be made from the physical assessment findings. Although blood pressure should be monitored frequently to help determine whether organ perfusion is adequate, *remember that assessment tools other than measuring the blood pressure must also be used to recognize shock in the trauma patient.*

Humans vary as to the blood pressure required to maintain adequate perfusion. The question "How low can you go?" while maintaining adequate perfusion has not yet been answered. We know that the healthy young patient can often maintain adequate perfusion in the face of hypotension whereas older patients, hypertensive patients, and those with head injury often cannot tolerate hypotension for even short periods. You must rely on physician Medical Direction and your own study of current research on shock.

While this text is about trauma, shock is a clinical condition associated with more medical problems than just trauma. Following is a discussion of shock syndromes, many of which are caused by traumatic conditions. The take-home point, though, is that the shock state is one of low tissue perfusion (from many causes) in which the body *usually* demonstrates similar signs of its response to this perfusion-deprived condition. The body may not always demonstrate similar signs; see the discussion of high-space shock that follows. Therefore, the stabbed and bleeding patient often shows many of the same signs as the burned or dehydrated patient. The classic symptoms and signs associated with hemorrhagic shock include the following:

1. *Weakness:* caused by tissue hypoxia and acidosis
2. *Thirst:* caused by hypovolemia (especially with relatively low fluid amounts in the blood vessels)

3. *Pallor* (pale, white color of the skin): caused by catecholamine-induced vasoconstriction and/or loss of circulating red blood cells

4. *Tachycardia:* caused by catecholamines' effect on the heart

5. *Diaphoresis* (sweating): caused by catecholamines' effect on sweat glands

6. *Tachypnea* (elevated respiratory rate): caused by stress, catecholamines, acidosis, and hypoxia

7. *Decreased urinary output:* caused by hypovolemia, hypoxia, and circulating catecholamines (important to remember in interhospital transfers)

8. *Weakened strength of peripheral pulses:* the thready pulse; caused by vasoconstriction, tachycardia, and loss of blood volume

9. *Hypotension:* caused by hypovolemia, either absolute or relative (see later paragraphs for a discussion of relative hypovolemia)

10. *Altered mental status* (confusion, restlessness, combativeness, unconsciousness): caused by decreased cerebral perfusion, acidosis, and catecholamine stimulation

11. *Cardiac arrest:* caused by critical organ failure secondary to blood or fluid loss, hypoxia, and occasionally arrhythmia caused by catecholamine stimulation

To summarize, many of the symptoms of shock of any etiology, including the classic hemorrhagic shock picture, are caused by the release of catecholamines. When the brain senses that perfusion to the tissues is insufficient, it sends messages down the spinal cord to the sympathetic nervous system and the adrenal glands, causing a release of catecholamines (epinephrine and norepinephrine) into the circulation. The circulating catecholamines cause the tachycardia, anxiousness, diaphoresis, and vasoconstriction. The vasoconstriction in the arterioles shunts blood away from the skin and intestines to the heart, lungs, and brain. Close monitoring early in the shock syndrome may detect an initial rise in the blood pressure due to this shunting. There will almost always be an initial narrowing of the pulse pressure because vasoconstriction raises the diastolic pressure more than the systolic. The shunting of blood from the skin causes the pallor of shock.

Decreased perfusion causes weakness and thirst initially, and then later, a decreased level of consciousness (confusion, restlessness, or combativeness) and worsening pallor. As shock continues, the prolonged tissue hypoxia leads to worsening acidosis. This acidosis can cause a loss of response to catecholamines, worsening the drop in blood pressure. This is often the point at which the patient in "compensated" shock suddenly "crashes." Eventually, the hypoxia and acidosis cause cardiac dysfunction, including cardiac arrest, and ultimately death.

Although the individual response to post-traumatic hemorrhage may vary, many patients will have the following classic patterns of "early" and "late" shock:

Early shock (loss of approximately 15 to 25% of the blood volume): enough to stimulate slight to moderate tachycardia, pallor, narrowed pulse pressure, thirst, weakness, and possibly delayed capillary refill

Late shock (loss of approximately 30 to 45% of the blood volume): enough to cause hypotension as well as the other symptoms of hypovolemic shock listed earlier

Note that during the Initial Assessment, early shock presents as a fast pulse with pallor and diaphoresis, while late shock may present as weak pulse or loss of the peripheral pulse.

Prolonged capillary refill was previously thought to be useful for detecting early shock. Low blood volume and catecholamine-induced vasoconstriction cause decreased perfusion of the capillary bed in the skin. Capillary refill is tested by pressing on the palm of the hand or, in a child, squeezing the whole foot. The test is suspicious for shock if the blanched area remains pale for longer than 2 seconds. Scientific evaluation of this test has shown it to have a high correlation with late shock but of little value for detecting early shock. The test was associated with both frequent false positive as well as false negative results. Measurement of capillary refill is useful for small children in whom it is difficult to get an accurate blood pressure, but it is of little use for detecting early shock in adults.

EVALUATION OF TACHYCARDIA

One of the first signs of illness, and arguably one of the most common, is that of tachycardia. You will frequently be confronted with the patient with an elevated pulse rate and must make some sort of distinction as to the cause. First, remember that you must always attempt to explain why a patient has tachycardia. An elevated pulse rate is never normal. Humans can transiently raise their pulses in the setting of anxiety, but such elevation quickly returns to normal or fluctuates in rate depending on the waxing and waning of the anxiety state. *A persistently elevated pulse rate while at rest is always an indication of something medically wrong with the patient, including the possibility of occult hemorrhage.*

Second, remember that an elevated pulse rate is one of the first signs of shock. Any adult trauma patient with a sustained pulse rate above 100 must be suspected as having occult hemorrhage until proven otherwise. However, during the brief Initial Assessment, a pulse rate greater than 120 should be a red flag for possible shock.

THE SHOCK SYNDROMES

While the most common shock states seen in trauma patients are associated with hemorrhage and the accompanying hypovolemia, there are actually three major classifications of shock. These three shock states can be categorized according to their causes as follows:

1. *Low-volume shock* (absolute hypovolemia): caused by hemorrhage or other major body fluid loss
2. *High-space shock* (relative hypovolemia): caused by spinal injury, vasovagal syncope, sepsis, and certain drug overdoses
3. *Mechanical (obstructive) shock:* caused by pericardial tamponade, tension pneumothorax, or myocardial contusion

There are notable differences in the appearance of patients with these conditions, and it is critical that you be aware of the signs and symptoms that accompany each one.

Low-Volume Shock (Absolute Hypovolemia)

Loss of blood from injury is called *post-traumatic hemorrhage* and, in addition to head injury, hemorrhagic shock is the number one cause of *preventable* death from injury. The amount of volume that the blood vessels *can* hold is many liters more than that which actually flows through the vasculature. The sympathetic nervous system keeps the vessels constricted, reducing their volume and maintaining blood pressure high enough to perfuse vital organs. If blood volume is lost, "sensors" in the major vessels signal the adrenal gland and the nerves of the sympathetic nervous system to secrete catecholamines, which cause vasoconstriction and thus further shrink the vascular space and maintain perfusion pressure to the brain and heart. If the blood loss is minor, the sympathetic system can shrink the space enough to maintain blood pressure. If the loss is severe, the vascular space cannot be shrunk down enough to maintain blood pressure, and hypotension occurs.

Normally, the blood vessels are elastic and are distended by the volume that is in them. This produces a radial artery pulse that is full and wide. Blood loss allows the artery to shrink in width, becoming more threadlike in size; hence the term "thready" pulse in shock.

High-Space Shock (Relative Hypovolemia)

As mentioned earlier, the volume that the blood vessels can hold is many liters more than the normal blood volume. Again, it is the steady-state action of the sympathetic nervous system that keeps the vascular bed mildly constricted in order to maintain perfusion to the heart and brain. Anything that disturbs the sympathetic nervous system and causes the loss of this normal vasoconstriction allows the vascular space to become much "too large" for the usual amount of blood. If the blood vessels dilate, the 5 liters or so of blood flowing through the normal adult's vascular space may not be sufficient to maintain blood pressure and vital tissue perfusion. The condition causing the vascular space to be too large for a normal amount of blood has been called *high-space shock* or *relative hypovolemia.* Although several types of high-space shock exist (e.g., sepsis syndrome and drug overdoses), neurogenic shock, commonly called *spinal shock,* will be addressed here.

Neurogenic shock occurs most typically after an injury to the spinal cord. Although circulating catecholamines (already present) may preserve the blood pressure for a short time, the disruption of the sympathetic nervous system outflow from the spinal cord results in loss of the normal vascular tone and in the inability of the body to compensate for any accompanying hemorrhage. The clinical presentation of neurogenic shock differs from hemorrhagic shock in that there is no catecholamine release, thus no pallor, tachycardia, or sweating. The patient will have a decreased blood pressure but the heart rate will be normal or slow, the skin warm, dry, and pink. The patient may also have accompanying paralysis and/or sensory deficit corresponding to the spinal cord injury. You may also see a lack of chest wall movement and only simple diaphragmatic movement when the patient is asked to take a deep breath. The important point is that this form of shock does not have the typical picture of hemorrhagic shock, *even when associated with severe bleeding.* The neurologic assessment is therefore very important, and you should not rely on typical shock symptoms and signs to suspect internal bleeding or accompanying hemorrhage-associated shock. A neurogenic shock patient may "look better" than his or her actual condition.

Certain overdoses (including drinking alcohol) can also result in vasodilatation and relative hypovolemia. Very often injuries result after such intoxication, and their effect on typical clinical signs and symptoms (like neurogenic shock) should be considered. You may find that intoxication is an accompanying problem in many injury victims. Other examples of overdoses that produce relative hypovolemia include nitroglycerin and calcium channel blockers.

Mechanical (Obstructive) Shock

In the normal adult's resting state, the heart pumps *out* about 5 liters of blood per minute. This means, of course, that the heart also must take *in* about 5 liters of blood per minute. Therefore, any traumatic condition that slows or prevents the venous return of blood can cause shock by lowering cardiac output and thus oxygen delivery to the tissues. Likewise, anything that obstructs the flow of blood to or through the heart can cause shock. The following are traumatic conditions that can cause mechanical shock:

Tension pneumothorax is so named because of the high air tension (pressure) that develops in the pleural space (between the lung and chest wall). This very high positive pressure is transmitted back to the right heart and prevents the venous return of blood. Shifting of mediastinal structures may also lower venous return. See Figure 7-1 and turn to chapter 6 for a complete description of the signs, symptoms, and treatment of tension pneumothorax.

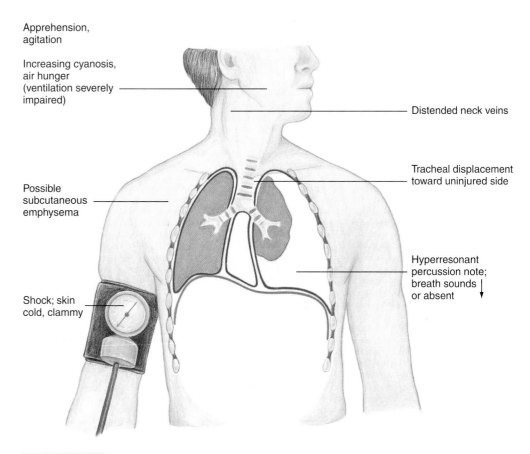

Apprehension,
agitation

Increasing cyanosis,
air hunger
(ventilation severely
impaired)

Distended neck veins

Possible
subcutaneous
emphysema

Tracheal displacement
toward uninjured side

Shock; skin
cold, clammy

Hyperresonant
percussion note;
breath sounds
or absent

Figure 7-1 Physical findings of tension pneumothorax.

Cardiac or *pericardial tamponade* occurs when blood fills the space around the heart, squeezing the heart and preventing the heart from filling or pumping well (see Figure 7-2). The net result is that the heart cannot fill properly and cardiac output falls. Pericardial tamponade may occur in more than 75% of cases of penetrating cardiac injury. *On-scene interventions should be avoided if the diagnosis is suspected because any time wasted on the scene could result in death of the patient.* Definitive surgical care in the nearest *appropriate* facility for pericardial decompression may be the only lifesaving measure available. Using intravenous fluids to increase filling pressure of the heart may possibly be of some value, but could also worsen the condition if there is thoracic vascular injury. Use of IV fluids in this situation should be during transport and only on the order of Medical Direction. See Chapter 6 for a more complete discussion.

Myocardial contusion can result in diminished cardiac output because the heart loses pumping ability due to direct injury (see Figure 7-3) or cardiac dysrhythmias (see Figure 7-4). Myocardial contusion often cannot be differentiated from cardiac tamponade in the field. Therefore, rapid transport, supportive care, and cardiac monitoring are the mainstays of therapy.

A word of caution is important here. Patients with shock from mechanical causes can be very near death. *Delay on the scene may prevent salvage of the patient.* Urban studies suggest that, in applicable cases, the time from development of a tamponade to circulatory arrest may be as little as 5 to 10 minutes. Survival following traumatic circulatory arrest, even in the best of trauma systems, is rarely achieved if surgery is not performed within 5 to 10 minutes.

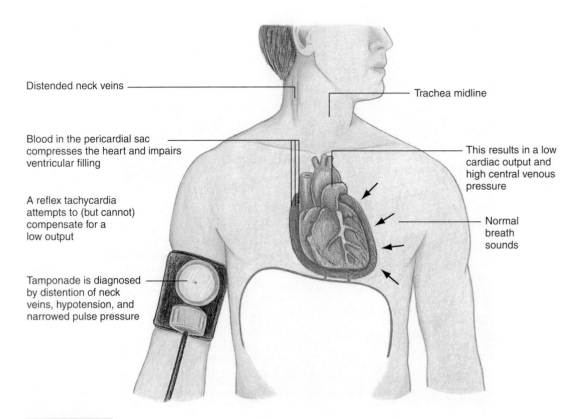

Distended neck veins

Blood in the pericardial sac compresses the heart and impairs ventricular filling

A reflex tachycardia attempts to (but cannot) compensate for a low output

Tamponade is diagnosed by distention of neck veins, hypotension, and narrowed pulse pressure

Trachea midline

This results in a low cardiac output and high central venous pressure

Normal breath sounds

Figure 7-2 Pathophysiology and physical findings of cardiac tamponade.

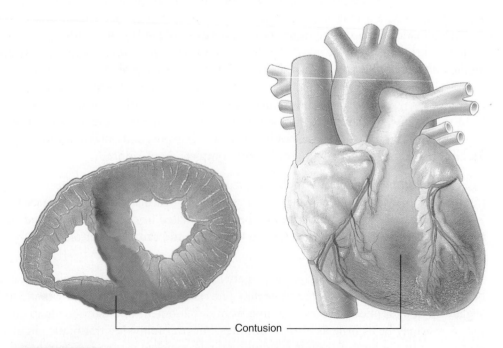

Contusion

Figure 7-3 Myocardial contusion most frequently affects the right atrium and ventricle as they collide with the sternum.

MANAGEMENT OF POST-TRAUMATIC SHOCK STATES

Control Bleeding: Red blood cells are necessary to carry oxygen. Control of bleeding must be obtained either by direct pressure or rapid transport to surgery.

Give Oxygen: Cyanosis is an extremely late sign of hypoxemia and may not occur at all if there has been extensive blood loss. Give high-flow oxygen to all patients at risk for shock. Try to maintain a pulse oximeter reading greater than 95%.

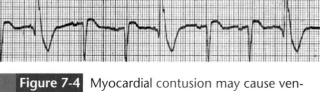

Figure 7-4 Myocardial contusion may cause ventricular ectopy.

Transport: Patients in shock are in the load-and-go category. Transport as soon as you finish the Primary Survey (Initial Survey and Rapid Trauma Survey). Almost all critical interventions should be done in the ambulance (see Chapter 2).

TREATMENT OF POST-TRAUMATIC HEMORRHAGE

Prehospital management of the patient in shock is controversial at this time. There is no question of the need for control of hemorrhage, supplemental oxygen, and early transport, but the indications for most other therapies are still being debated. Since the early days of modern shock treatment (about the middle of the 20th century), intravenous crystalloid solutions (and sometimes colloid) have been tested and/or utilized to reverse the effects of hypovolemia. In addition, it has been previously proposed that intra-abdominal and pelvic bleeding may possibly be diminished by use of the pneumatic anti-shock garment (military antishock trousers, PASG, MAST). Now, recent research suggests a modified approach. Patients in hypovolemic shock due to hemorrhage may be generally thought of as falling into one of the following two categories: those with bleeding that you can control (e.g., extremity injury) and those with bleeding that you cannot control (e.g., internal injury). We will consider each type of bleeding and discuss current concepts of therapy for each type.

Hemorrhage That Can Be Controlled

A patient with this type of injury is fairly easy to manage. Stop the bleeding by direct pressure. Only in the most extreme circumstances should a tourniquet be applied. A reasonable guide is that you should apply a tourniquet only to the extremity that you are prepared to sacrifice to save a life.

If the patient has clinical evidence of shock that persists after direct control of the bleeding, you should take the following steps:

🖐 PROCEDURE

1. Put the patient's body in a horizontal or slightly head-down position.
2. Administer high-flow oxygen.
3. Transport immediately and rapidly.
4. Apply the PASG, if local protocols recommend, until IV fluid therapy is available.
5. Monitor the heart (if equipment is available), and apply pulse oximetry.
6. Perform Ongoing Exam and observe closely.

Hemorrhage That Cannot Be Controlled

External Hemorrhage: A patient with this type of injury must be rapidly transported to an appropriate facility where necessary procedures to gain surgical hemostasis can be performed. To manage this patient, you should:

✋ PROCEDURE

1. Apply as much direct pressure as possible on the bleeding site (e.g., femoral artery, facial hemorrhage).

2. Put the patient's body in a horizontal or slightly head-down position.

3. Apply tourniquets to a bleeding extremity only as a desperate attempt to stop severe bleeding that cannot be otherwise controlled (discussed earlier).

4. Administer high-flow oxygen.

5. Transport immediately and rapidly.

6. Do not utilize the PASG in this setting unless it can be used to tamponade otherwise uncontrollable lower extremity hemorrhage.

7. Monitor the heart (if equipment is available), and apply pulse oximetry.

8. Perform Ongoing Exam and observe closely.

Note: If assistance is not available, control of hemorrhage, even if minimal, should remain the priority. Other procedures become secondary if they interrupt attempts to maintain hemorrhage control.

Internal Hemorrhage: The patient with uncontrolled internal hemorrhage is the classic critical trauma victim who will almost certainly die unless you rapidly transport to an appropriate facility where rapid operative hemostasis can be obtained. The results of the most current medical research on the management of patients with exsanguinating internal hemorrhage is that there exists no substitute for gaining surgical control of bleeding. Recent work on the use of the PASG and IV fluids in shock patients with presumed internal hemorrhage suggests the following:

1. Use of the PASG in the setting of uncontrolled internal exsanguination due to penetrating injury may increase mortality, especially in the setting of intrathoracic hemorrhage. The PASG raises blood pressure, and raising blood pressure in the setting of bleeding vessels within the thorax, abdomen, and pelvis probably increases internal bleeding, raising the chance of death due to exsanguination.

2. Any delay in providing rapid transport of such patients should not occur unless *absolutely* unavoidable, as in the case of a patient requiring prolonged extrication.

3. Moribund trauma patients (ones in very deep shock with blood pressures under 50 mmHg systolic) usually die, but the PASG may be indicated to maintain some degree of circulation. Treatment of this extreme amount of hemorrhage may override the concerns for increased hemorrhage secondary to the use of this intervention. However, this approach is still controversial. Local Medical Direction should guide such therapy.

The recommendations, therefore, for a patient with probable exsanguinating internal hemorrhage *secondary to penetrating injuries* are the following:

✋ PROCEDURE

1. Transport immediately and rapidly.

2. Put the patient's body in a horizontal or slightly head-down position.

3. Administer high-flow oxygen.

4. Do not utilize the PASG in this setting except as indicated by local Medical Direction.

5. Monitor the heart (if equipment is available), and apply pulse oximetry.

6. Perform Ongoing Exam and observe closely.

Current published research has not yet adequately addressed the treatment of the patient with presumed internal hemorrhage in the setting of blunt injuries (MVCs, falls, etc.). This creates a dilemma because many patients with blunt injuries can lose a significant amount of blood and fluid from the intravascular space into the sites of large-bone fractures (hematoma and edema). This loss can be enough to cause shock, and yet the blood loss is usually self-limited. This situation should be treated with oxygen and rapid transport.

TREATMENT OF NONHEMORRHAGIC SHOCK SYNDROMES—(MECHANICAL AND HIGH-SPACE)

Treatments for the other shock syndromes, namely, mechanical and high-space (relative hypovolemia) are somewhat different. All patients require high-flow oxygen, rapid transport, and shock positioning.

Mechanical Shock

The patient with mechanical shock must first be accurately assessed to determine the cause of the problem. The patient with tension pneumothorax needs prompt transport to the nearest appropriate hospital for emergency chest decompression.

The patient with suspected pericardial tamponade must be rapidly transported to an appropriate facility, because the time of onset of tamponade to the time of cardiac arrest can be a matter of minutes.

In two separate studies, one prospective and one retrospective, there was an increase in mortality of patients with tamponade when the PASG was applied in the prehospital setting. This may be due to the increase in field time taken to apply the PASG. By increasing peripheral resistance, the PASG also may decrease cardiac output, which may be another cause of increased mortality in such patients with an already low cardiac output. Therefore, the PASG is contraindicated in this setting.

Myocardial contusion rarely causes shock. Recent reports indicate that most contusions cause no clinical findings. However, severe contusion may cause acute heart failure, manifested by distended neck veins, tachycardia, or arrhythmias. These are the same signs seen with pericardial tamponade. These patients require rapid transport for proper care. Give high-flow oxygen and perform cardiac monitoring (if equipment is available) on the patient with suspected myocardial contusion.

High-Space Shock

High-space shock, in theory, resembles controlled hemorrhage, in that there is relative hypovolemia with an "intact" vasculature (no leak). Therefore, initial management includes possible short-term use of the PASG. In the absence of a head injury, the patient's level of consciousness is a useful monitor of the success or failure of resuscitation. Be aware of possible internal injuries, and keep in mind that raising the blood pressure may increase internal bleeding in that situation.

CURRENT USES FOR THE PNEUMATIC ANTISHOCK GARMENT (PASG OR MAST)

The PASG is an inflatable compressive device that encircles the abdomen and legs. The PASG exerts its effect by compression of the arteries of the abdomen and legs, and this increases the peripheral vascular resistance (PVR). As the PVR is a component of blood pressure, it (blood pressure) typically rises with the application and inflation of the PASG. However, as the PVR rises, cardiac output (CO) may fall. Therefore, you must be cautious about elevating the PVR in settings of low blood pressure because of the possibility of lowering the cardiac output. Furthermore, if uncontrolled bleeding is occurring within the patient, raising the blood pressure may increase bleeding.

In the past, it was commonplace to utilize the PASG for any patient with post-traumatic hypotension. Unfortunately, these well-intentioned recommendations came in the absence of real clinical proof of the effectiveness of the PASG.

Controlled clinical trials were conducted to determine if using the PASG would actually improve survival. From these studies have come the following indications and contraindications for the use of the PASG in trauma patients.

Indications for Use of the Antishock Trousers in Trauma Patients

1. Shock secondary to hemorrhage that can be controlled
2. Neurogenic shock without evidence of other internal injuries
3. Isolated fractures of legs without evidence of other internal injuries (blow up to only air-splint pressures)
4. Systolic blood pressure less than 50 mmHg (controversial)

Contraindications for Use of Antishock Trousers

1. *Absolute:*
   a. Pulmonary edema
   b. Bleeding that cannot be controlled, such as penetrating chest or abdominal trauma
2. *Conditional:* Pregnancy—may use leg compartments

(Photo courtesy of David Effron, M.D.)

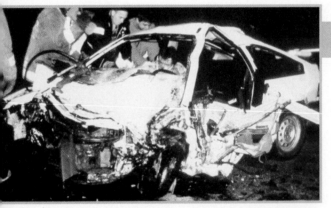

CASE STUDY

Dan, Joyce, and Buddy of the Emergency Transport System have been called to the scene of a single vehicle, high-speed, side-impact auto collision. They are informed that a rescue truck is on-scene and attempting to extricate the driver. While driving to the scene they decide that Buddy will act as team leader on this case.

On arrival Buddy gets the trauma box and cervical collars and begins the Scene Size-up. Dan gets the oxygen and airway equipment and Joyce gets the backboard. Buddy notes that the police are on-scene and the scene is safe. The team dons personal protective equipment and each carries his part of the essential equipment to the scene as they approach. The driver of the car had lost control on a wet road and hydroplaned. The car rolled over several times and then side-impacted a tree and finally came to rest upright. The driver has been extricated but is dead on-scene. The restrained front seat passenger is alert and oriented but complains of chest and abdominal pain. After extrication, Buddy's Rapid Trauma Assessment reveals facial lacerations but an open airway, tender lower ribs (no crepitation) on the right with a tender abdomen. He has deformity and instability of the right thigh. Breath sounds are present and equal and the pelvis is stable and nontender. The patient has a strong regular pulse and a normal respiratory rate with good air movement. Because of the tender abdomen they quickly package the patient and immediately load-and-go. In the ambulance the vital signs are: BP 120/90, pulse 110, respiration 22. The patient states he has no allergies, takes no medications, has always been healthy. Last food was about four hours ago. Dan applies a traction splint to the right leg. Buddy calls his on-line medical direction (OLMD) and reports that he is transporting a patient who has been in a high-speed MVC in which the driver was killed. He suspects that the patient has rib fractures, intra-abdominal injuries, and a fractured femur. They are told to transport the patient to the local level-one trauma center. The Ongoing Exam reveals that the pulse has increased to 140 and the blood pressure has dropped to 70/40. The abdomen has become distended and rigid. The lungs are still clear. The trauma team is mobilized and waiting when they arrive. The patient is found to have a fractured right femur and a ruptured spleen, but no other major injuries. He requires a splenectomy and four units of blood, but recovers uneventfully.

> **PEARLS**
>
> 1. Shock kills. Look for early signs of shock and manage appropriately.
> 2. Shock is poor perfusion, not hypotension.
> 3. Control hemorrhage. If it can't be done in the field, the patient needs to be in the operating room now!
> 4. Look for signs of mechanical or high space shock, especially if there is no bleeding.

CASE STUDY WRAP-UP

The mechanism of injury here is both rollover and lateral-impact, with the driver receiving the brunt of the forces from the lateral-impact. The driver died from major chest injuries. The passenger received serious injuries but was saved by being restrained. Though his vital signs were good when EMS arrived, they recognized the tender abdomen was suggestive of internal injuries and were prepared for the development of hemorrhagic shock. The fractured femur was also a factor here, as there is usually a loss of one or two units of blood into the soft tissue of the thigh after a femur fracture.

SUMMARY

The patient with shock is often not diagnosed early enough. Shock may not be obvious until the patient is near death. The importance of careful assessment and reassessment cannot be overemphasized. You must understand the risk of any shock state to the patient. Further, you need to study and memorize the shock syndromes, especially in regard to the rapid provision of the proper treatment for such conditions as internal hemorrhage, pericardial tamponade, and tension pneumothorax. Finally, you should be aware of the controversy on the use of IV fluid resuscitation and the PASG for cases of *uncontrolled* hemorrhage. Rely on your local Medical Direction to keep you current on the standard of care in these areas.

BIBLIOGRAPHY

1. Bickell, W. H., P. E. Pepe, M. L. Bailey, and others. "Randomized Trial of Pneumatic Antishock Garments in the Prehospital Management of Penetrating Abdominal Injury." *Annals of Emergency Medicine*, Vol. 16 (June 1987), pp. 653–658.

2. Bickell, W. H., M. J. Wall, P. E. Pepe, and others. "Immediate Versus Delayed Fluid Resuscitation for Hypotensive Patients with Penetrating Torso Injury." *New England Journal of Medicine*, Vol. 331 (October 1994), pp. 1105–1109.

3. Chestnut, R. M., L. F. Marshall, M. R. Klauber, and others. "The Role of Secondary Brain Injury in Determining Outcome from Severe Head Injury." *Journal of Trauma*, Vol. 34 (1993), pp. 216–222.

4. Domeier, R. M., R. E. O'Conner, and others. "Use of the Pneumatic Anti-Shock Garment (PASG)." *Prehospital Emergency Care*, Vol. 1, No. 1 (1997), pp. 32–44.

5. Kowalenko, T., S. Stern, S. Dronen, and X. Wang. "Improved Outcome with Hypotensive Resuscitation of Uncontrolled Hemorrhagic Shock in a Swine Mode." *Journal of Trauma*, Vol. 33 (1992), pp. 349–353.

6. Mattox, K. L., W. H. Bickell, P. E. Pepe, and others. "Prospective MAST Study in 911 patients." *Journal of Trauma,* Vol. 29 (1989), pp. 1104–1112.

7. Pigula, F. A., S. L. Wald, S. R. Shackford, and others. "The Effect of Hypotension and Hypoxia on Children with Severe Head Injuries." *Journal of Pediatric Surgery,* Vol. 28 (1993), pp. 310–316.

8. Schriger, D. L., and L. J. Baraff. "Capillary Refill—Is It a Useful Predictor of Hypovolemic States?" *Annals of Emergency Medicine,* Vol. 20 (June 1991), pp. 601–605.

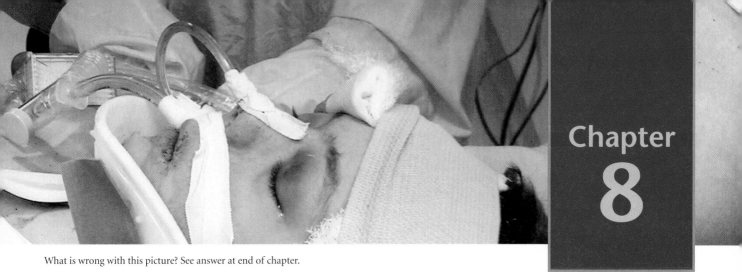

What is wrong with this picture? See answer at end of chapter.

Head Trauma

John E. Campbell, M.D., F.A.C.E.P.

Roy L. Alson, Ph.D., M.D., F.A.C.E.P.

Objectives

Upon completion of this chapter, you should be able to:

1. Describe the anatomy of the head and brain.
2. Describe the pathophysiology of traumatic brain injury.
3. Explain the difference between primary and secondary brain injury.
4. Describe the mechanisms for the development of secondary brain injury.
5. Describe the assessment of the patient with a head injury.
6. Describe the prehospital management of the patient with a head injury.
7. Recognize and describe the management of the cerebral herniation syndrome.
8. Identify potential problems in the management of the patient with a head injury.

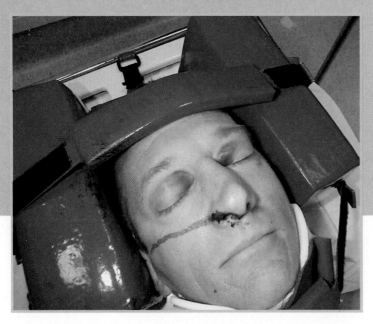

Joyce, Dan, and Buddy have been dispatched to a private home where a man has fallen off of a ladder. As they respond, they decide that Joyce will be team leader. When they arrive they find a small group of people huddled around a 40-year-old man who was taking down Christmas decorations and slipped off the ladder, landing on his head. The scene is safe and he is the only patient. His fall was witnessed by his wife who, with tears in her eyes (she nagged him into removing the decorations that day), says that when his foot slipped it caught in the rung of the ladder and he swung like a pendulum, striking his head. He was unconscious for a few minutes and she was sure that he was dead but he began to awaken and is now awake but can't remember going up the ladder at all. She says he is in good health, takes no medications and has no allergies. She prepared him lunch (hamburgers) about two hours ago. He complains of a headache and nausea and says his neck hurts. What injuries would you suspect from a mechanism such as this? Keep this in mind as you read the chapter. The case study will continue at the end of the chapter.

Head injuries or, more specifically, traumatic brain injury (TBI) is a major cause of death and disability in the multiple trauma patient. Forty percent (40%) of multisystem trauma patients have a central nervous system (CNS) injury. These patients have a death rate twice as high (35% versus 17%) as that of patients without CNS injuries. Head injuries account for an estimated 25% of all trauma deaths and up to one-half of all motor vehicle fatalities. Worldwide, the cost of TBI, in terms of lives lost, families destroyed and money spent for care, is staggering. Sadly, many head injuries are easily prevented. You can help reduce this major epidemic by encouraging the use of helmets and restraint devices in vehicles.

You may be called upon to manage head injuries that can range from the trivial to the immediately life threatening. By recognizing those injuries that need immediate intervention and providing transport to the appropriate facility, you can significantly improve the chances for a patient having a good outcome from his/her injury. Beginning with the second edition of this text, material included in this chapter has been based upon the recommendations of the Brain Trauma Foundation (a multidisciplinary organization dedicated to improving care of TBI victims by use of evidence-based treatment).

To most effectively manage the head-injured patient, you should have a working knowledge of the basic anatomy and physiology of the head and brain. Because it is not possible to perform a field clearance of the cervical spine in a patient with altered mental status and because head injury often results in the alteration of consciousness, *you must always assume that a serious head injury is accompanied by an injury to the cervical spine and spinal cord.*

ANATOMY OF THE HEAD

The head (excluding the face and facial structures) includes the following (see Figure 8-1):

1. Scalp
2. Skull
3. Fibrous coverings of the brain (meninges: dura mater, arachnoid mater, pia mater)
4. Brain tissue
5. Cerebrospinal fluid
6. Vascular compartments

The scalp is a protective covering for the skull, but it is very vascular and bleeds freely when lacerated. The skull is a closed box; the rigid and unyielding bony skull protects the brain from injury. It also contributes to several injury mechanisms in head trauma. Just like the ankle, that swells when twisted, the brain, when injured, swells. The only significant opening through which the pressure can be released is the foramen magnum at the base, where the brain stem becomes the spinal cord. Because the brain "floats" inside the cerebrospinal fluid and is anchored at its base, there is greater movement at the top of the brain than at the base. On impact, the brain is able to move within the skull and can strike bony prominences within the cranial cavity. This is the "third collision" described in mechanisms of injury in Chapter 1. The temporal bone (temple) is quite thin and easily fractured as are portions of the base of the skull. The fibrous coverings of the brain include the dura mater ("tough mother"), which covers the entire brain; the thinner pia arachnoid (called simply the arachnoid), which lies underneath the dura and in which are suspended both arteries and veins; and the very thin pia mater ("soft mother"), which lies underneath the arachnoid and is adherent to the surface of the brain. The cerebrospinal fluid (CSF) is found beneath the arachnoid and pia mater.

The intracranial volume is composed of the brain, the CSF, and the blood in the blood vessels. These three completely fill the cranial cavity. Thus the increase of any one of

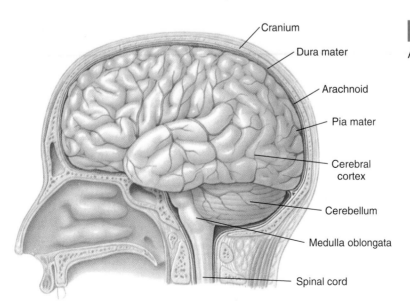

Figure 8-1

Anatomy of the head.

these is at the expense of the other two. This is of great importance in the pathophysiology of head trauma. Following injury, the brain, like all injured tissue, will swell. Because of the fixed space, as the tissue swells and the volume of fluid inside the skull increases, so does the pressure.

Cerebrospinal fluid (e.g., spinal fluid) is a nutrient fluid that bathes the brain and spinal cord. Spinal fluid is continually created within the ventricles of the brain at a rate of 0.33 mL/min. It is reabsorbed by the arachnoid membrane that covers the brain and spinal cord. Anything obstructing the flow of spinal fluid will cause an accumulation of spinal fluid within the brain (hydrocephalus) and an increase in intracerebral pressure (ICP).

PATHOPHYSIOLOGY OF HEAD TRAUMA

Head injuries are either open or closed, depending on whether the object responsible for the injury compromised the skull and exposed the brain. Brain injury can also be divided into two components, primary and secondary. Primary brain injury is the immediate damage to the brain tissue that is the direct result of the injury force and is essentially fixed at the time of injury. Management of primary brain injury is best directed at prevention with such measures as better occupant restraint systems in autos, the use of helmets in sports and cycling, firearms education, and so forth.

While penetrating wounds to the brain always cause primary injury, most primary injuries occur either as a result of external forces applied against the exterior of the skull or from movement of the brain inside the skull. In deceleration injuries the head usually strikes an object such as the windshield of an automobile, which causes a sudden deceleration of the skull. The brain continues to move forward, impacting first against the skull in the original direction of motion and then rebounding to hit the opposite side of the inner surface of the skull (a "fourth" collision). Thus, injuries may occur to the brain in the area of original impact ("coup") or on the opposite side ("contracoup"). The interior base of the skull is rough (see Figure 8-2), and movement of the brain over this area may cause various degrees of injury to the brain tissue or to blood vessels supporting the brain.

Good prehospital care can help prevent the development of secondary brain injury. Secondary brain injury is the result of hypoxia or decreased perfusion of brain tissue. Secondary injury is the result of the brain's response to the primary injury, with swelling causing a decrease in perfusion, or from complications of other injuries (hypoxia or hypotension). The initial response of the injured brain is to swell. Bruising or injury causes vasodilatation with increased blood flow to the injured area, and thus an accumulation of blood that takes up space and exerts pressure on surrounding brain tissue. There is no extra space inside the skull. Swelling of the injured area increases intracerebral pressure and eventually decreases blood flow to the brain that causes further brain injury. The increase in cerebral water (edema) does not occur immediately, but develops over hours. Early efforts to maintain perfusion of the brain can be lifesaving.

The brain normally adjusts its own blood flow in response to metabolic needs. The *autoregulation* of blood flow is adjusted based on the level of carbon dioxide (CO_2) in the blood. The normal level of CO_2 is 35 to 40 mmHg. An increase in the level of CO_2 (hypoventilation) promotes cerebral vasodilatation and increased ICP, while lowering the level of CO_2 (hyperventilation) causes vasoconstriction and decreases blood flow. In the past, it was thought that hyper-

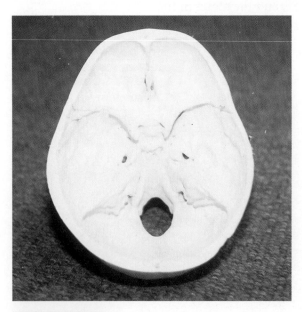

Figure 8-2 The rough inner base of the skull.

ventilation (lowering of CO_2) in the head-injured patient would decrease brain swelling and thus improve cerebral blood flow. Research has shown that hyperventilation actually has only a slight effect on brain swelling, but causes a significant decrease in cerebral perfusion from vasoconstriction, which results in cerebral hypoxia. The injured brain does not tolerate hypoxia. Thus, *both hyperventilation and hypoventilation can cause cerebral ischemia and increased mortality in the TBI patient.* Maintaining good ventilation (not hyperventilation) at a rate of about one breath every 5 to 6 seconds (10–12 per minute) with high-flow oxygen is very important. *The previously taught prophylactic hyperventilation for head injury is no longer recommended.*

Intracranial Pressure

Within the skull and fibrous coverings of the brain are the brain tissue, cerebrospinal fluid, and blood. An increase in the volume of any one of these components must be at the expense of the other two because the adult skull (a rigid box) cannot expand. Although there is some give to the volume of cerebrospinal fluid, it accounts for little space and cannot offset rapid brain swelling. Blood supply cannot be compromised, for the brain requires a constant supply of blood (oxygen and glucose) to survive. Thus, since none of the supporting components of the brain can be compromised, brain swelling can be rapidly catastrophic.

The pressure of the brain and contents within the skull is termed *intracranial pressure* (ICP). This pressure is usually very low. Intracranial pressure is considered dangerous when it rises above 15 mmHg; cerebral herniation may occur at pressures above 25 mmHg. The pressure of the blood flowing through the brain is termed the *cerebral perfusion pressure* (CPP). Its value is obtained by subtracting the intracranial (intracerebral) pressure from the mean arterial blood pressure (MAP):

$$CPP = MAP - ICP$$

If the brain swells or if bleeding occurs inside the skull, ICP increases and the perfusion pressure decreases, resulting in cerebral ischemia (hypoxia). If the swelling of the brain is severe enough, the ICP equals the MAP and blood flow to the brain ceases. The body has a protective reflex (Cushing's response or reflex) that attempts to maintain a constant perfusion pressure. When the ICP increases, the systemic blood pressure increases to try to preserve blood flow to the brain. The body senses the rise in systemic blood pressure and this triggers a drop in the pulse rate as the body tries to lower the blood pressure. With severe injury and/or ischemia, the pressure within the skull continues in an upward spiral until a critical point at which the ICP approaches the MAP and there is no cerebral perfusion. All vital signs deteriorate, and the patient dies. Because CPP depends on both the arterial pressure and the ICP, hypotension will also have a devastating effect if the ICP is high. As stated above, the injured brain loses the ability to autoregulate blood flow. In this situation perfusion of the brain is directly dependent on the CPP. You would like to maintain a cerebral perfusion pressure of at least 60 mmHg (see earlier formula), which requires maintaining a systolic blood pressure of at least 110 to 120 mmHg in the patient with a severe head injury. *This will rarely be a problem, as hypotension only occurs in about 5% of patients with severe TBI (GCS of <9).*

Cerebral Herniation Syndrome

When the brain swells, particularly after a blow to the head, a sudden rise in ICP may occur. This may force portions of the brain downward, obstructing the flow of cerebrospinal fluid and applying great pressure to the brain stem. The classic findings on exam, in this life-threatening situation, are a decreasing level of consciousness (LOC) that rapidly progresses to coma, dilation of the pupil and an outward-downward deviation of the eye on the side of the injury, paralysis of the arm and leg on the side opposite the injury, or decerebrate posturing (arms and legs extended). As the herniation is occurring the vital signs frequently reveal increased blood pressure and bradycardia (Cushing's response). The patient may soon cease all movement, stop breathing, and die. This syndrome often follows an acute epidural or subdural hemorrhage. If these signs are developing in a head injury patient, cerebral herniation is imminent and aggressive therapy is needed. As noted earlier, hyperventilation will decrease the size of the blood vessels in the brain and briefly decrease ICP. In this situation the danger of immediate herniation outweighs the risk of ischemia. The cerebral herniation syndrome is the *only* situation in which hyperventilation is still indicated. (You must ventilate every 3 seconds [20/min] for adults, every 2 seconds [30/min] for children and a little faster for infants—1.7 seconds [35/min].) To simplify knowing when to hyperventilate in the field, *the clinical signs of cerebral herniation in the patient **who has had hypoxemia and hypotension corrected** are any one (or more) of the following:*

1. **A TBI patient with a GCS <9** with extensor posturing (decerebrate posturing)
2. **A TBI patient with a GCS <9** with asymmetric (or bilateral), dilated or nonreactive pupils
3. **A TBI patient with an initial GCS <9** who then drops his GCS by more than 2 points

For the above, "asymmetric pupils" means 1 mm (or more) difference in the size of one pupil, "fixed" means no response (< 1 mm) to *bright* light. Bilateral dilated and fixed pupils usually are a sign of brainstem injury and are associated with 91% mortality. A unilateral dilated and fixed pupil has been associated with good recovery in up to 54% of patients. Remember that hypoxemia, orbital trauma, drugs, lightning strike, and hypothermia also affect pupillary reaction, so take this into account before beginning hyperventilation. Flaccid paralysis usually means spinal injury. *If the patient has signs of herniation as listed above and the signs resolve with hyperventilation, you should discontinue the hyperventilation.*

HEAD INJURIES
Scalp Wounds

The scalp is very vascular and often bleeds briskly when lacerated. Because many of the small blood vessels are suspended in an inelastic matrix of supporting tissue, the normal protective vasospasm that would limit bleeding is inhibited, which may lead to prolonged bleeding and significant blood loss. This can be very important in children who bleed as freely as adults but do not have the same blood volume. Though an uncommon cause of shock in an adult, a child may develop shock from a briskly bleeding scalp wound. As a general rule, *if you have an adult patient with a scalp injury who is in shock, look for another cause for the shock* (such as internal bleeding). However, do not underestimate the blood loss from a scalp wound. Most bleeding from the scalp can be easily controlled in the field with direct pressure if your exam reveals no unstable fractures under the wound.

Skull Injuries

Skull injuries can be linear nondisplaced fractures, depressed fractures, or compound fractures (see Figure 8-3). Suspect an underlying skull fracture in adults with a large contusion or darkened swelling of the scalp. There is very little that can be done for skull fractures in the field except to avoid placing direct pressure upon an obvious depressed or compound skull fracture. The real concern is that forces that can cause a skull fracture can also cause a brain injury. Treat the brain injury with adequate oxygenation and maintain perfusion. Open skull fractures should have the wound dressed, but avoid excess pressure when controlling bleeding. Penetrating objects in the skull should be secured in place (*not*

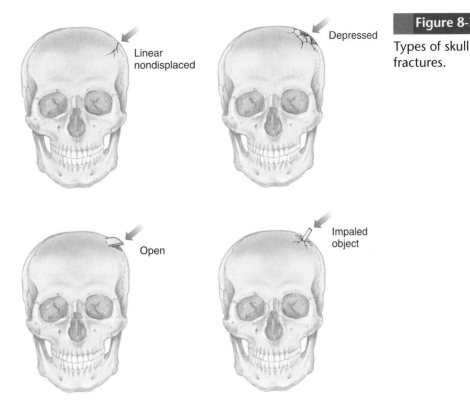

Figure 8-3

Types of skull fractures.

removed) and the patient transported immediately. If your patient has a gunshot wound to the head, unless there is a clear entrance and exit wound in a perfectly linear path, assume that the bullet may have ricocheted and is lodged in the neck near the spinal cord.

You should consider child abuse when you find a child with a head injury and no clear explanation of the cause. Suspect possible abuse if the story about the injury is inconsistent with the injury or the responsible adult suggests the child performed an activity that a child of this age is not physically capable of performing. Pay particular attention to the setting from which you rescued the child. Request police or social service assistance if the circumstances are suspicious for child abuse.

Brain Injuries

Concussion: A concussion implies no structural injury to the brain that can be demonstrated by current imaging techniques. There is a brief disruption of neural function that often results in loss of consciousness. Classically there is a history of trauma to the head with a variable period of unconsciousness or confusion and then a return to normal consciousness. There may be amnesia following the injury. This amnesia usually extends to some point before the injury (retrograde short-term amnesia), so often the patient will not remember the events leading to the injury. Short-term memory is often affected, and the patient may repeat questions over and over as if she hasn't been paying attention to your answers. Patients may also report dizziness, headache, ringing in the ears, and/or nausea.

Cerebral Contusion: A patient with cerebral contusion (bruised brain tissue) will have a history of prolonged unconsciousness or serious alteration in level of consciousness (e.g., profound confusion, persistent amnesia, abnormal behavior). Brain swelling may be rapid and severe. The patient may have focal neurological signs (weakness, speech problems) and appear to have suffered a cerebrovascular accident (stroke). Depending upon the location of the cerebral contusion, the patient may have personality changes such as inappropriately rude behavior or agitation.

Subarachnoid Hemorrhage: Blood can enter the subarachnoid space as a result either of trauma or a spontaneous hemorrhage. The subarachnoid blood causes irritation that results in intravascular fluid "leaking" into the brain and causing more edema. Severe headache, coma, and vomiting from the irritation is common. These patients may have so much brain swelling that they develop the cerebral herniation syndrome.

Diffuse Axonal Injury: This is the most common type of injury with severe blunt head trauma. The brain is injured so diffusely that there is generalized edema. Usually there is no evidence of a structural lesion. In most cases the patient presents unconscious, without focal deficits.

Anoxic Brain Injury: Injuries to the brain from lack of oxygen (e.g., cardiac arrest, airway obstruction, near-drowning) affect the brain in a serious fashion. Following an anoxic episode, perfusion of the cortex is interrupted because of spasm that develops in the small cerebral arteries. After four to six minutes of anoxia, restoring oxygenation and blood pressure will not restore perfusion of the cortex (no-reflow phenomenon), and there will be continuing anoxic injury to the brain cells. If the brain is without oxygen for a period greater than four to six minutes, irreversible damage almost always occurs.

Hypothermia seems to protect against this phenomenon, and there have been reported cases of hypothermic patients being resuscitated after almost an hour of anoxia. Current research is directed toward finding medications that either reverse the persistent postanoxic arterial spasm or protect against the anoxic injury to the cells.

Intracranial Hemorrhage: Hemorrhage can occur between the skull and dura (the fibrous covering of the brain), between the dura and the arachnoid, or directly into the brain tissue.

1. *Acute epidural hematoma.* This injury is most often caused by a tear in the middle meningeal artery that runs along the inside of the skull in the temporal region. The arterial injury is often caused by a linear skull fracture in the temporal or parietal region (see Figure 8-4). Because the bleeding is arterial (although it may be venous from one of the dural sinuses), the bleeding and rise in ICP can occur rapidly, and death may occur quickly. Symptoms of an acute epidural hematoma include a history of head trauma with initial loss of consciousness often followed by a period during which the patient is conscious and coherent (the "lucid interval"). After a period of a few minutes to several hours, the patient will develop signs of increasing ICP (vomiting, headache, altered mental status), lapse into unconsciousness, and develop body paralysis on the side opposite of the head injury (see earlier section on cerebral herniation syndrome). There is often a dilated and fixed (no response to bright light) pupil on the side of the head injury. These signs are usually followed rapidly by death. The classic example is the boxer who is knocked unconscious, wakes up, and is allowed to go home, only to be found dead in bed the next morning. If the underlying brain tissue is not injured, surgical removal of the blood and ligation of

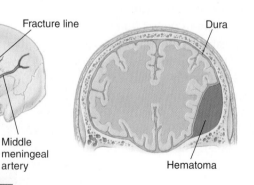

Figure 8-4

Acute epidural hematoma. This hemorrhage may follow injury to the extradural arteries. The blood collects between the fibrous dura and the periosteum.

the ruptured blood vessel often allows full recovery.

2. *Acute subdural hematoma*. This is the result of bleeding between the dura and the arachnoid and is associated with injury to the underlying brain tissue (see Figure 8-5). Because the bleeding is venous, intracranial pressure increases more slowly, and the diagnosis often is not apparent until hours or days after the injury. The signs and symptoms include headache, fluctuations in the level of consciousness, and focal neurologic signs (e.g., weakness of one extremity or one side of the body, altered deep tendon reflexes, and slurred speech). Because of underlying brain tissue injury, prognosis is often poor. Mortality is very high (60–90%) in patients who are comatose when found. Always suspect a subdural hematoma in an alcoholic with any degree of altered mental status following a fall. Elderly patients and those taking anticoagulants are also at high risk for this injury.

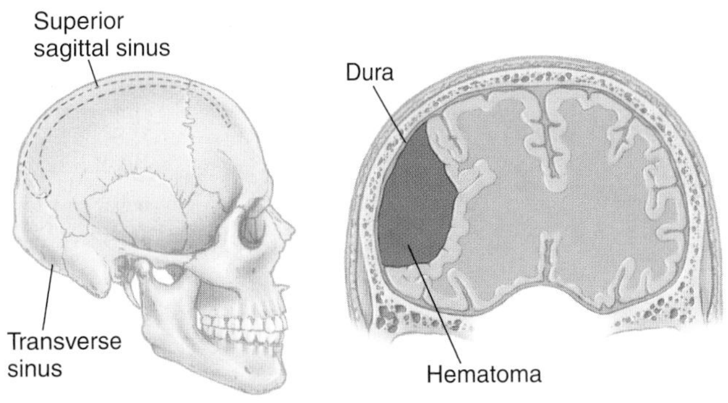

Figure 8-5 Acute subdural hematoma. This usually occurs following the rupture of dural veins. Blood collects and often severely compresses the brain.

3. *Intracerebral hemorrhage*. This is bleeding within the brain tissue (see Figure 8-6). Traumatic intracerebral hemorrhage may result from blunt or penetrating injuries of the head. Unfortunately, surgery is often not helpful. The signs and symptoms depend upon the regions involved and the degree of injury. They occur in patterns similar to those that accompany a stroke; spontaneous hemorrhages of this type may be seen in patients with severe hypertension. Alteration in the level of consciousness is commonly seen, though awake patients may complain of headache and vomiting.

EVALUATION OF THE HEAD TRAUMA PATIENT

Determining the exact type of TBI or hemorrhage cannot be done it the field, as it requires imaging techniques, such as a CAT scan. It is more important that you recognize the presence of a brain injury and be ready to provide supportive measures while transporting the patient. TBI patients may be difficult to manage because they are often uncooperative and may be under the influence of alcohol or drugs. As a rescuer, you must pay extraordinary attention to detail and never lose your patience with an uncooperative patient. Remember that every trauma patient is initially evaluated in the same sequence (see Figure 8-7).

Scene Size-Up

The results of the Scene Size-up will begin to determine if you have a priority patient. Dangerous generalized mechanisms (MVC, fall from a height) will require a complete examination (Rapid Trauma Survey) during the BTLS Primary Survey. Dangerous focused mechanisms (hit in head with baseball bat) will allow you to "focus" your exam (ABCs, with head and neurologic exams) rather than having to perform a complete exam.

Initial Assessment

The goals of the Initial Assessment are the following:

1. To determine if this is a priority patient
2. To find immediate life-threats

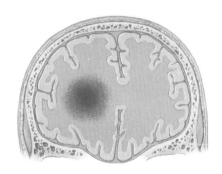

Figure 8-6

Intracerebral hemorrhage.

Patient Assessment Using Priority Plan

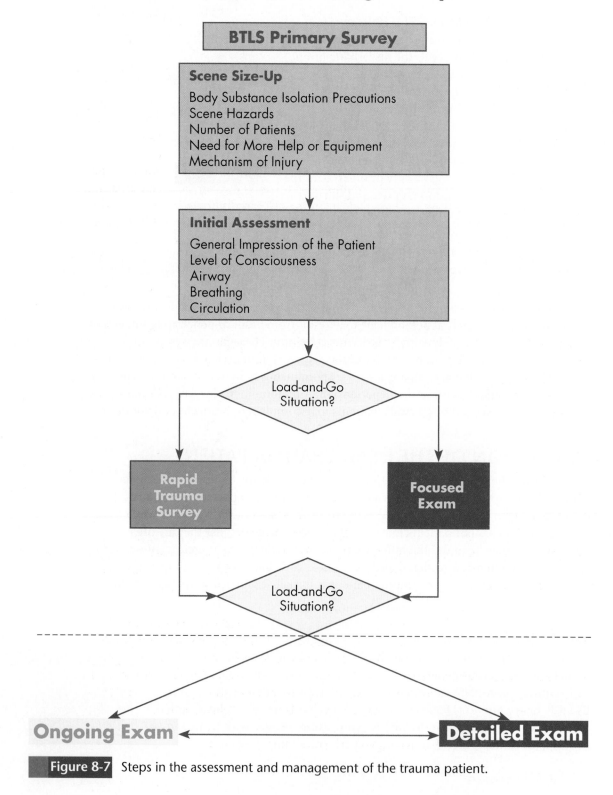

Figure 8-7 Steps in the assessment and management of the trauma patient.

The Initial Assessment in the head trauma patient is to determine quickly if the patient is brain injured and, if so, if the patient's condition is deteriorating. Obviously, a patient with a history and physical examination that indicates a loss of consciousness following a lucid period post-injury (possible epidural hematoma) should be transported with more urgency than one who is alert and oriented after being knocked out (possible concussion). It is very important that all observations be recorded (but don't interrupt patient care to do this) because later treatment is often dictated by detection of the deterioration of clinical stability.

All patients with head or facial trauma should be assumed to have a cervical spine injury until proven otherwise. Because of the alteration of LOC, it is often not possible, in this situation, to clear the cervical spine until after arrival at the hospital. Restriction of cervical spine movement should accompany airway and breathing management. Evaluation for head injury is begun as you obtain your initial level of consciousness by speaking to the patient. During the Initial Assessment your neurological exam is limited to level of consciousness and any obvious paralysis. Level of consciousness is the most sensitive indicator of brain function. Initially, the AVPU method is quite adequate (see Chapter 2). If there is a history of head trauma, or if the initial exam reveals an altered mental status, the Rapid Trauma Survey will include a more complete neurological exam. A decrease in the level of consciousness is the first indicator of a brain injury or rising ICP.

Control of the airway cannot be overemphasized. The supine, restrained, and unconscious patient is prone to airway obstruction from the tongue, blood, vomit, or other secretions. Vomiting is very common within the first hour following a head injury. *Protect the airway of the unconscious patient with no gag reflex by placement of an oral or nasal airway and constant suctioning.* Be prepared to turn the patient on his side (maintain motion-restriction of the spline) in the case of vomiting. Do not allow the head-injured patient to become hypoxic. Even one brief episode of hypoxia can increase mortality.

Rapid Trauma Survey

All patients with an abnormal level of consciousness get a Rapid Trauma Survey (see Chapter 2).

Head: Once the initial exam is completed, continue with the exam guided by the mechanism of injury. Begin with the scalp and quickly, but carefully, examine for obvious injuries such as lacerations or depressed or open skull fractures. The size of a laceration is often misjudged because of the difficulty in assessment through hair matted with blood. Feel the scalp gently for obvious unstable areas of the skull. If none are present, you may safely apply a pressure dressing or hold direct pressure upon a bandage to stop scalp bleeding.

A basilar skull fracture may be indicated by any of the following: bleeding from the ear or from the nose, clear or serosanguineous fluid running from the nose or ear, swelling and/or discoloration behind the ear (Battle's sign), and/or swelling and discoloration around both eyes (raccoon eyes) (see Figure 8-8a and b). Raccoon eyes are a sign of anterior basilar skull fracture that may go through the thin cribriform plate in the upper nasal cavity and allow spinal fluid and/or blood to leak out. *Raccoon eyes with or without drainage from the nose are an absolute contraindication to inserting a nasogastric tube or nasotracheal intubation.* The tube can go through the fractured cribriform plate and into the brain.

Pupils: The pupils (see Figure 8-9) are controlled in part by the third cranial nerve. This nerve takes a long course through the skull and is easily compressed by brain swelling, and thus may be affected by increasing ICP. Following a head injury, if both pupils are dilated and do not react to light, the patient probably has a brain-stem injury and the prognosis is grim. If the pupils are dilated but still react to light, the injury is often still reversible, so every effort should be made to transport the patient quickly to a facility capable of treating a head injury.

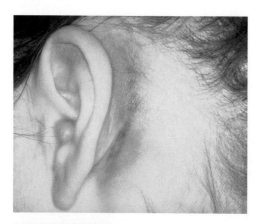

Figure 8-8a

Battle's sign—evidence of a posterior basilar skull fracture. *(Photo courtesy of David Effron, M.D., FACEP)*

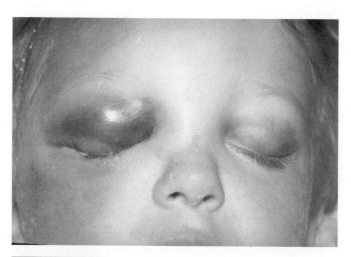

Figure 8-8b Raccoon eyes—evidence of an anterior basilar skull fracture. *(Photo courtesy of David Effron, M.D., FACEP)*

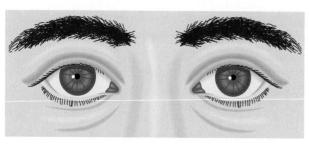

Constricted pupils

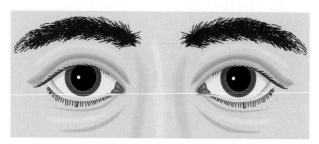

Dilated pupils

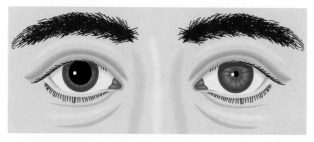

Unequal pupils

Figure 8-9

Examination of pupils.

A unilaterally dilated pupil that remains reactive to light may be the earliest sign of increasing ICP. The development of a unilaterally dilated, nonreactive pupil ("blown pupil") while you are observing the comatose patient is an extreme emergency and mandates rapid transport and hyperventilation. Other causes of dilated pupils that may or may not react to light include hypothermia, lightning strike, anoxia, optic nerve injury, drug effect (e.g., atropine), or direct trauma to the eye. *Fixed and dilated pupils signify increased intracranial pressure only in patients with a decreased level of consciousness.* If the patient has a normal level of consciousness, the dilated pupil is <u>not</u> from head injury (more likely orbital trauma or drugs such as atropine).

Fluttering eyelids are often seen with hysteria. Slow lid closure (like a curtain falling) is rarely seen with hysteria. Testing for a blink response (corneal reflex) by touching the cornea with the edge of a gauze pad or cotton swab, or by applying overly noxious stimuli to a patient to test for response to pain, are techniques that are unreliable and do not contribute to prehospital assessment.

Extremities: Note sensation and motor function in the extremities. Can the patient feel you touch her hands and feet? Can she wiggle her fingers and toes? If the patient is unconscious, note her response to pain. If she withdraws or localizes to the pinching of her fingers and toes, she has grossly intact sensation and motor function. This usually indicates that there is normal or only minimally impaired cortical function.

Both decorticate posturing or rigidity (arms flexed, legs extended) and decerebrate posturing or rigidity (arms and legs extended) are ominous signs of deep cerebral hemispheric or upper brain-stem injury (see Figure

8-10). Decerebrate posturing is worse and usually signifies cerebral herniation. It is one of the indications for hyperventilation. *Flaccid paralysis usually denotes spinal cord injury.*

Neurological Exam: To apply the Revised Trauma Score and other field triage scoring systems (see Appendix F), you should be familiar with the Glasgow Coma Score (GCS), which is simple, easy to use, and has good prognostic value for eventual outcome (see Table 8-1). **In the TBI patient, a Glasgow Coma Score of 8 or less is considered evidence of a severe brain injury.** *The GCS that is determined in the field serves as the baseline for the patient.*

Vital Signs (should be obtained by another team member while you are performing the exam): Vital signs are extremely important in following the course of a patient with head trauma. Most important, they can indicate changes in ICP (see Table 8-2). You should observe and record vital signs at the end of the BTLS Primary Survey, during the Detailed Exam, and each time you perform the Ongoing Exam.

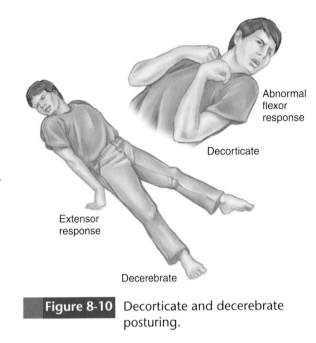

Figure 8-10   Decorticate and decerebrate posturing.

1. *Respiration*: Increasing intracranial pressure causes the respiratory rate to increase, decrease, and/or to become irregular. Unusual respiratory patterns may reflect the level of brain/brain-stem injury. Just before death the patient may develop a rapid, noisy respiratory pattern called central neurogenic hyperventilation. Because respiration is affected by so many factors (e.g., fear, hysteria, chest injuries, spinal cord injuries, diabetes), it is not as useful an indicator as are the other vital signs in monitoring the course of head injury. Abnormal respiratory patterns may indicate a chest injury or other problem that could lead to hypoxia if untreated.

TABLE 8-1		Glasgow Coma Score.			
Eye Opening		**Verbal Response**		**Motor Response**	
	Points		**Points**		**Points**
Spontaneous	4	Oriented	5	Obeys commands	6
To voice	3	Confused	4	Localizes pain	5
To pain	2	Inappropriate words	3	Withdraws	4
None	1	Incomprehensible sounds	2	Abnormal flexion	3[*]
		Silent	1	Abnormal extension	2[**]
				No movement	1

[*]Decorticate posturing to pain
[**]Decerebrate posturing to pain

TABLE 8-2	Comparison of Vital Signs in Shock and Head Injury.	
	Shock	**Head Injury with Increased Intracranial Pressure**
Level of consciousness	Decreased	Decreased
Respiration	Increased	Varies but frequently decreased
Pulse	Increased	Decreased
Blood pressure	Decreased	Increased
Pulse pressure	Narrows	Widens

2. *Pulse*: Increasing ICP causes the pulse rate to decrease.

3. *Blood pressure*: Increasing ICP causes increased blood pressure. This hypertension is usually associated with a widening of the pulse pressure (systolic minus diastolic pressure). Other causes of hypertension include fear and pain. *Hypotension in the presence of a head injury is usually caused by hemorrhagic or neurogenic shock and should be treated as if caused by hemorrhage.* It is a rare (5%) finding in the patient with a severe TBI. The injured brain does not tolerate hypotension. A single instance of hypotension (BP ≤ 90 mm Hg systolic) in an adult with a brain injury may increase the mortality rate by 150%. The increase in mortality rate for hypotension and a severe TBI is even worse in children.

History: Begin obtaining the history before and during the exam. It is essential to obtain as thorough a history about the event as possible. The circumstances of the head injury may be extremely important for patient management and may be of prognostic importance to the ultimate outcome. Pay particular attention to reports of near drowning, electrocution, lightning strike, drug abuse, smoke inhalation, hypothermia, and seizures. Always inquire about the patient's behavior from the time of the head injury until the time of your arrival. Try to obtain the past medical history; nontraumatic events can also cause an alteration in the LOC.

Detailed Exam

Head trauma patients with altered mental status are load-and-go. The Detailed Exam (see Chapter 2) will be done during transport (or not at all, if a short transport).

Ongoing Exam

Each time you perform the Ongoing Exam, record the level of consciousness, the pupil size and reaction to light, the Glasgow Coma Score, and the development (or improvement) of focal weakness or paralysis. This, along with the vital signs, provides enough information to monitor the condition of the head-injured patient. Decisions on the management of the head trauma patient are based on the changes in all the parameters of the physical and neurologic examination. You are establishing the baseline from which later judgments must be made; record your observations.

MANAGEMENT OF THE HEAD TRAUMA PATIENT

Your job is to prevent secondary injury. It is extremely important to make a rapid assessment and then transport the patient to a facility capable of managing head trauma. Appropriate triage of the patient to facilities capable of managing TBI can have a signifi-

TABLE 8-3	Normal Ventilation Rates and Hyperventilation Rates.	
Age Group	Normal Ventilation Rate	Hyperventilation Rate
Adult	10–12 breaths/minute	20 breaths/minute
Children	20 breaths/minute	30 breaths/minute
Infants	25 breaths/minute	35 breaths/minute

cant impact on the outcome of the patient. The important points of management in the prehospital phase are listed below.

✋ PROCEDURE

1. Secure the airway and provide good oxygenation. The injured brain does not tolerate hypoxia, so good oxygenation is mandatory. If possible, monitor the oxygen saturation with a pulse oximeter. Maintain good ventilation (not hyperventilation) with high-flow oxygen at a rate of about one breath every 5-6 seconds (10–12 breaths per minute). Because head-injured patients are prone to vomiting, be prepared to log-roll the motion-restricted patient and to suction the oropharynx.

2. Stabilize the patient on a backboard. Restrict motion of the neck in a rigid collar and a padded head motion-restriction device.

3. Record baseline observations. Record vital signs (describe rate and pattern of breathing), the level of consciousness, the pupils (size and reaction to light), the Glasgow Coma Score, and the development (or improvement) of focal weakness or paralysis. If the patient develops hypotension, suspect hemorrhage or spinal injury.

4. Monitor the observations listed above continuously. Record them every five minutes.

CASE STUDY

Joyce, Dan, and Buddy have been dispatched to a private home where a man has fallen off of a ladder. As they respond they decide that Joyce will be team leader. When they arrive they find a small group of people huddled around a 40-year-old man who was taking down Christmas decorations and slipped off the ladder landing on his head. The scene is safe and he is the only patient. His fall was witnessed by his wife who, with tears in her eyes (she nagged him into removing the decorations that day), says that when his foot slipped it caught in the rung of the ladder and he swung like a pendulum, striking his head. He was unconscious for a few minutes and she was sure that he was dead, but he began to awaken. He is now awake but can't remember going up the ladder. She says he is in good health, takes no medications and has no allergies. She prepared him a hamburger at lunch about two hours ago. He complains of a headache and nausea and says his neck hurts.

PEARLS

1. *Cervical spine injury*: Always anticipate a cervical spine injury in the head-injured patient.

2. *Hypoxia*: Patients with serious head injuries can't tolerate hypoxia or hypotension. Give high-flow oxygen and monitor oxygenation with a pulse oximeter.

3. *Shock*: Any unexplained shock in a patient with head injury is hypovolemic until proven otherwise.

4. *Seizures*: Seizures in TBI patients are usually caused by hypoxia. Seizures should always cause you to recheck the airway, ventilation, and oxygenation of your patient.

5. *Vomiting*: Patients with head trauma frequently vomit. You must remain alert to prevent aspiration. Keep mechanical suction available and be prepared to log-roll the patient onto his side (maintaining motion restriction of the spine).

6. *Rapidly deteriorating condition*: A patient who *after correction of hypoxia and hypotension* shows rapid progression of brain injury (e.g., unresponsive with dilated pupil; decerebrate posturing; or drop in GCS of >2 with an initial GCS of <9) should be transported rapidly to a trauma center capable of managing severe TBI patients. This is the only situation in which hyperventilation is still indicated (see Table 8-3). Hyperventilation, while known to cause ischemia, may decrease brain swelling temporarily. Although a desperate measure, this might buy enough time to get the patient to surgery that might be lifesav-

(continued)

PEARLS
(continued)

ing. Radio ahead so that a neurosurgeon can be available and the operating room prepared by the time you arrive at the hospital.

7. *Nontraumatic causes of altered mental status*: Remember that hypoglycemia, hypoxia, cardiac dysrhythmias, and drugs can also cause altered mental status. Monitor the heart and oxygenation and check the blood glucose level on all patients with altered mental status.

8. *Pediatric patients*: Usually pediatric patients have a better recovery from TBI. If an adult and a child have the same injury, the child has a much better chance of recovery. However, hypoxia and hypotension appear to eliminate any neuroprotective mechanism normally afforded by age. If the child with a serious brain injury is allowed to become hypoxic or hypotensive, the chance of recovery is even worse than an adult with the same injury.

Joyce introduces the team and cautions him not to move while they are examining him. Her initial impression is cautiously good, but she is worried by the drainage from his nose. Dan stabilizes his neck while Joyce begins the exam and Buddy brings the backboard. The airway is open because the patient (Guido) can speak normally. He responds appropriately to questions but has amnesia for the event. He has a strong, regular pulse and his respiration is normal. Because of the mechanism she does a Rapid Trauma Survey. There is a hematoma on the right side of the head in the temporal area. The pupils are 5 mm and equal and there are ecchymoses of both upper eyelids. There is dried blood in both nostrils and a thin, serosanguineous drainage from the right nostril. The face feels stable. There is tenderness and spasm of the neck but no palpable deformity. The neck veins are flat and trachea is in the midline. The chest is normal to inspection with no tenderness, and breath sounds are present and equal. Heart sounds are easily heard. The abdomen is nontender. The pelvis is stable and nontender. The extremities are nontender with normal PMS. A cervical collar is placed on the patient and he is log-rolled onto the backboard (the back is normal) and packaged. Joyce decides to transport immediately, so he is transferred to the ambulance. Buddy drives.

While Dan obtains the vital signs, Joyce does a neurological exam. The patient is awake and oriented with a retrograde amnesia. He has a GCS of 15 (E-4, V-5, M-6). His pupils are still 5 mm and react equally. He has good sensation and movement in his fingers and toes bilaterally. The vital signs are: BP 140/80, pulse 95, Resp. 12, and pulse oximeter 100% on oxygen by nasal cannula at 3 liters per minute. Joyce notifies Medical Direction that they have a patient with a probable anterior basilar skull fracture with a spinal fluid leak and are taking him directly to the local trauma center. The patient begins to get restless and becomes more confused. He tries to pull out his IV and then vomits the hamburger he had for lunch. Joyce immediately does an Ongoing Exam. Exam of the head reveals no change in the temporal hematoma, but the right pupil is now 8 mm and poorly reactive. The left pupil is still 5 mm. The neck, chest, and abdomen are unchanged. There is now noted a slight difference in strength on the left side compared to the right. The vital signs are: BP 170/80, pulse 70, Resp 8, and pulse oximeter 95% on oxygen by nasal cannula at 3 liters per minute. Dan begins to assist respiration at a rate of 8-12 breaths/minute with 100% oxygen by bag-valve mask.

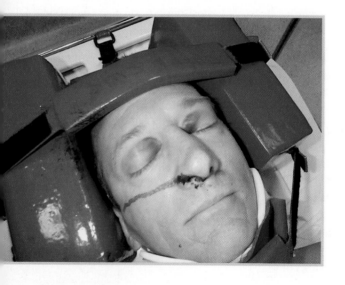

Guido is no longer restless but is now less reactive. He still localizes to pain. He opens his eyes to verbal stimuli but his speech is mostly unintelligible sounds and cursing. His GCS is now 11 (E-3, V-3, M-5). Joyce notifies Medical Direction of the change, and she has the trauma team meet them at the ambulance. Guido is taken straight to CAT scan, where a right epidural hematoma is revealed. He is then taken directly to surgery, where the bleeding right middle meningeal artery is ligated and the hematoma evacuated. After surgery, x-rays reveal a nondisplaced fracture of the fifth cervical vertebra. Guido recovers completely from his injuries and returns home.

CASE STUDY WRAP-UP

The mechanism of injury, coupled with the spinal fluid draining from the nose, alerted Joyce that the patient had an anterior basilar skull fracture. The mechanism was also suspicious for spinal injury. The patient was packaged for transport. As is common with an injury of this type, the patient initially looked good but began to deteriorate soon afterwards. He developed symptoms of an epidural hematoma with increased ICP but never deteriorated enough to require hyperventilation. Joyce was wise in bypassing lower levels of care to go to a trauma center where he would receive immediate evaluation and life-saving surgery before he reached the point of cerebral herniation. He was in danger of developing meningitis from the basilar skull fracture from which the spinal fluid was leaking. He was lucky that it sealed and healed without any infection developing. He could easily have had a spinal cord injury in this situation but his cervical spinal fracture was stable and healed without further surgery.

SUMMARY

Head injury is a serious complication of trauma. In order to give your patient the best chance of recovery, you should be familiar with the important anatomy of the head and central nervous system and understand how trauma to the various areas presents clinically. The most important steps in the management of the head-injured patient are rapid assessment, good airway management, prevention of hypotension, rapid transport to a trauma center, and frequent Ongoing Exams. In no other area of trauma care is the recording of repeated assessments so important to future management decisions.

BIBLIOGRAPHY

1. Chestnut, R. M., L. F. Marshall, M. R. Klauber, and others. "The Role of Secondary Brain Injury in Determining Outcome from Severe Head Injury." *Journal of Trauma*, Vol. 34 (1993), pp. 216–222.

2. LaHaye, P. A., G. F. Gade, and D. P. Becker. "Injury to the Cranium." In *Trauma*, eds. K. L. Mattox, E. E. Moore, and D. V. Feliciano, pp. 237–249. Norwalk, CT: Appleton & Lange, 1988.

3. Rimel, R. W., J. A. Jane, and R. F. Edlich. "An Injury Severity Scale for Comprehensive Management of Central Nervous System Trauma." *Annals of Emergency Medicine* (December 1979), pp. 64–67.

4. The Brain Trauma Foundation. *Guidelines for Prehospital Management of Traumatic Brain Injury*. New York: 2000.

Answer to Question on p. 126:
What is wrong with this picture? Someone has inserted a nasogastric tube into the nose of a child with raccoon eyes (anterior basilar skull fracture). This is contraindicated because of the danger of the tube going through the fractured cribriform plate and into the brain.

Chapter 9

Spinal Trauma

James J. Augustine, M.D., F.A.C.E.P.

Objectives

Upon completion of this chapter, you should be able to:

1. Explain the normal anatomy and physiology of the spinal column and spinal cord.

2. Define *spinal motion restriction* (SMR) and explain why this term is preferred to the term *spinal immobilization*.

3. Describe mechanisms of injury that indicate SMR may be required.

4. Describe the process of SMR from extrication through transportation, including airway maintenance.

5. Explain the difference between Emergency Rescue and Rapid Extrication techniques and give examples of when each would be appropriate.

6. Describe history and assessment criteria that identify patients who do not need SMR.

7. Give examples of special situations for which SMR techniques may need to be altered.

8. Using the clinical evaluation, differentiate neurogenic shock from hemorrhagic shock.

CASE STUDY

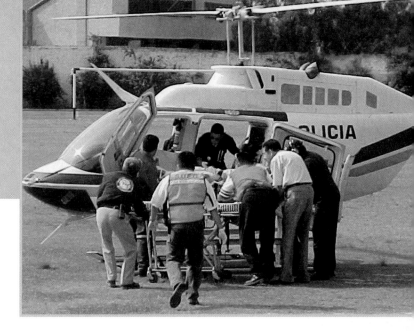

(Photo courtesy of Eduardo Romero Hicks, M.D.)

Dan, Joyce, and Buddy of the Emergency Transport System have been called to the local public swimming pool. They are told that there has been a diving injury. What injuries should they expect with a mechanism of this type? Is a spinal injury likely? What other emergency may be associated with a diving injury? Keep these questions in mind as you read the chapter. The case study will continue at the end of the chapter.

Spinal cord injury is a devastating and life-threatening result of modern trauma. If a patient with a spinal cord injury survives, it will cost an average of $1.5 million to support him for a lifetime. The management of trauma patients requires continuous vigilance for spinal injuries.

A variety of terms has been used through the years to describe the process by which emergency personnel attempt to prevent spinal cord injuries. It has been called traction, then immobilization, and now the preferred term is spinal motion restriction (SMR). This term is now used to most accurately define the process because in certain patients, especially in the prehospital environment, the spine cannot be completely immobilized. To prevent misunderstandings about what was done in the field, the more accurate term "spinal motion restriction" will replace the term "spinal immobilization."

Judgment must be used in determining which patients require SMR, as this procedure is also associated with complications. EMS providers must skillfully assess the mechanism of injury and the patient to provide safe and appropriate SMR to trauma patients. This chapter reviews the process of evaluating the mechanism of injury, providing a structured assessment, and packaging, treating, and transporting patients with known or potential spinal cord injuries.

THE NORMAL SPINAL COLUMN AND CORD
Spinal Column

It is important to differentiate the spinal column from the spinal cord. The spinal column is a bony tube composed of 33 vertebrae (see Figure 9-1). It supports the body in an upright position, allows the use of our extremities, and protects the delicate spinal cord. The column's 33 vertebrae are aligned in an S-shaped curve and are identified by their location: 7 cervical (the C-spine), 12 thoracic (the T-spine), 5 lumbar (the L-spine), and the remainder fused together as the posterior portion of the pelvis (5 sacral and 4 coccygeal). The vertebrae are numbered in each section, from the head down to the pelvis. The third cervical vertebra from the head is designated C-3, the sixth is called C-6, and so forth. The thoracic vertebrae are T1 through T12, and each attaches to one of the 12 pairs of ribs. The lumbar vertebrae are numbered L1 through L5, with L5 being the last vertebra above the pelvis.

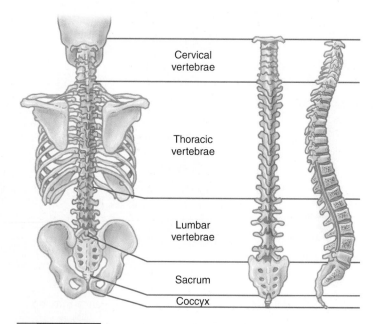

Figure 9-1 Anatomy of the spinal column.

The vertebrae are each separated by a fibrous disc that acts as a shock absorber. The alignment is maintained by strong ligaments between the vertebrae and by muscles that run along the length of the bony column from head to pelvis (these are the muscles strained when one lifts improperly). The spinal column is aligned in a gentle S-curve that is most prominent at the C5–C6 and T12–L1 levels in adults, making these areas the most susceptible to injury.

Spinal Cord

The spinal cord is an electrical conduit that serves as an extension of the brain stem. It continues down to the level of the first lumbar vertebra. The cord is 10 to 13 mm in diameter and is suspended in the middle of the vertebral foremen (see Figure 9-2). The cord is

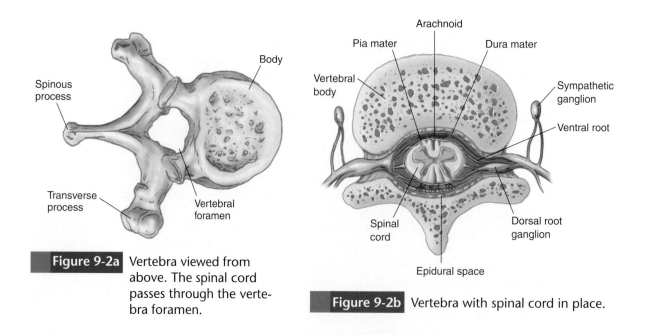

Figure 9-2a Vertebra viewed from above. The spinal cord passes through the vertebra foramen.

Figure 9-2b Vertebra with spinal cord in place.

soft and flexible like a cotton rope, and is surrounded and bathed by cerebrospinal fluid along its entire length. The fluid and the flexibility provide some protection to the cord from injury. The cord is composed of specific bundles of nerve tracts, much as a rope is composed of individual strands of fiber that are arranged in a predictable manner. The spinal cord passes down the vertebral canal and gives off pairs of nerve roots that exit at each vertebral level (see Figure 9-3). The roots lie next to the intervertebral discs and the lateral part of the vertebrae, making the nerve roots susceptible to injury when trauma occurs in these areas (see Figure 9-4). The nerve roots carry sensory signals from the body to the spinal cord and then to the brain. The roots also carry signals from the brain to specific muscles, causing them to move. These signals pass back and forth rapidly, and some are strong enough to cause actions on their own, called *reflexes*. This reflex system can be demonstrated by tapping the patella tendon below the knee causing the lower leg to jerk. If you accidentally put your finger on a hot burner, your reflex system causes your hand to move even before your brain receives the warning message. Strong signals also can overwhelm the spinal cord's ability to keep signals moving separately to the brain. This is why a trauma patient with a fractured hip may complain of knee pain or a patient with a ruptured spleen may complain of shoulder pain.

The integrity of spinal cord function is tested by motor, sensory, and reflex functions. The level of sensory loss is most accurate for

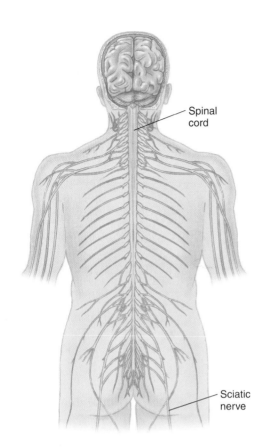

Spinal cord

Sciatic nerve

Figure 9-3 Spinal cord. The spinal cord is a continuation of the central nervous system outside the skull.

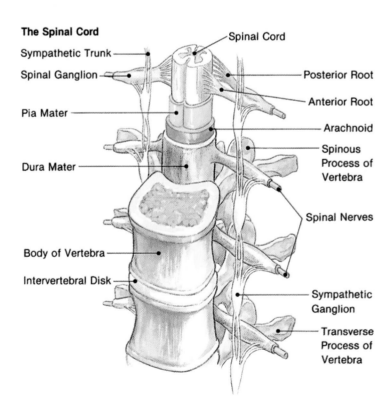

The Spinal Cord

Sympathetic Trunk

Spinal Ganglion

Pia Mater

Dura Mater

Body of Vertebra

Intervertebral Disk

Spinal Cord

Posterior Root

Anterior Root

Arachnoid

Spinous Process of Vertebra

Spinal Nerves

Sympathetic Ganglion

Transverse Process of Vertebra

Figure 9-4 Relationship of the spinal cord to the vertebra. Note how the nerve roots exit between the vertebra.

predicting the level of spinal cord injury. Muscle strength is another function that is easy to assess in the conscious patient. Reflexes are helpful for distinguishing complete from partial spinal cord injuries, but are best left for hospital assessment. The spinal cord is also an integrating center for the autonomic nervous system, which assists in controlling heart rate, blood vessel tone, and blood flow to the skin. Injury to this component of the spinal cord results in neurogenic shock (commonly called *spinal shock*), which is discussed later.

MECHANISMS OF BLUNT SPINAL INJURY

A normal healthy spinal column can be severely stressed and maintain its integrity without damage to the spinal cord. But certain mechanisms of trauma can overcome the protective defenses, injuring the spinal column and cord. The most common mechanisms are hyperextension, hyperflexion, compression, and rotation. Less commonly, lateral stress or distraction will injure the cord. These mechanisms and their subsequent injuries are illustrated in Table 9-1.

Spinal Column Injury

The head is a relatively large ball perched on top of the neck. Sudden movement of the head or trunk will produce flexion, extension, or lateral stresses that may damage the bony or connective tissue components of the spinal column. Injury to the spinal column is like injury to any other bone in the body. It requires a significant amount of force, unless there is a preexisting weakness or defect in the bone. For that reason, the elderly and those with severe arthritis are at higher risk for spinal injuries. Like other bone injuries, pain is the most common symptom, but it may be unnoticed by the patient. This is especially true if the patient has other painful injuries. At the site of a bone injury, local muscle spasm may occur. Injury to individual nerve roots can result from bony spinal column injury, with resulting localized pain, paralysis, or sensory loss. Therefore, signs that may indicate spinal injury include back pain, tenderness along the spinal column, pain with movement of the back, obvious deformity or wounds of the back, paralysis, weakness, or paresthesias (tingling or burning feeling to the skin).

Fortunately, spinal column injury can occur without injuring the spinal cord. Statistically, only 14% of all *column* injuries have evidence of spinal *cord* damage. In the cervical spine region it is much more common to have cord injury, with almost 40% of column injuries having cord damage. The converse is also possible, in that cord injuries can occur in the absence of obvious spinal column damage. This is particularly true in children. Only 63% of spinal *cord* injuries have evidence of spinal *column* damage. This means that almost half of the patients with some degree of paralysis will have no obvious bone or ligament injury to the spinal column (even by x-ray). The unconscious trauma patient carries a high risk (15–20%) of spinal column injury. The injuries are frequently in more than one place, and therefore SMR should be performed immediately on the unconscious trauma patient.

Spinal Cord Injury

Spinal cord injury is devastating. It is most common in patients aged 16 to 35, typically those who are active and productive. There are 15,000 to 20,000 spinal cord injuries in the United States each year—56% involve MVCs (including pedestrians), 19% falls, 12% penetrating wounds, 7% recreational activities, and the remaining 6% are from all other causes. Under age 16, falls are the most common cause of spinal injury. Under age 8, the relatively large size of the head makes the upper end of the cervical cord the most common site of injury, which can be extremely devastating.

Spinal cord injury results in a defective signal conducting function, presenting as a loss of motor function and reflexes, loss or change in sensation, and/or neurogenic shock. The delicate structure of the spinal cord's nerve tracts makes it very sensitive to any form

TABLE 9-1	Mechanisms of Blunt Spinal Injury

DESCRIPTION	DIAGRAM	EXAMPLES
Hyperextension Excessive posterior movement of head or neck	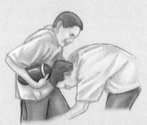	Face into windshield in MVC Elderly person falling to the floor Football tackler Dive into shallow water
Hyperflexion Excessive anterior movement of head onto chest	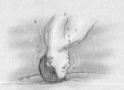	Rider thrown off of horse or motorcycle Dive into shallow water
Compression Weight of head or pelvis driven into stationary neck or torso		Dive into shallow water Fall of greater than 10 to 20 feet onto head or legs
Rotation Excessive rotation of the torso or head and neck, moving one side of the spinal column against the other		Rollover MVC Motorcycle accident
Lateral Stress Direct lateral force on spinal column, typically shearing one level of cord from another	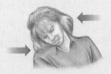	"T-bone" MVC Fall
Distraction Excessive stretching of column and cord	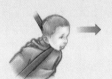	Hanging Child inappropriately wearing shoulder belt around neck Snowmobile or motorcycle under rope or wire

of trauma. What is termed *primary damage* occurs at the time of the trauma itself. Primary damage results from the cord being cut, torn, or crushed or by its blood supply being cut off. This damage is usually irreversible despite the best trauma care. *Secondary damage* occurs from hypotension, generalized hypoxia, injury to blood vessels, swelling, or compression of the cord from surrounding hemorrhage. Emergency efforts are directed at preventing secondary damage through attention to the ABCs and careful packaging of the patient.

NEUROGENIC SHOCK

Injury to the cervical or thoracic spinal cord can produce high-space shock (see Chapter 7). Neurogenic shock results from the malfunction of the autonomic nervous system in regulating blood vessel tone and cardiac output. Classically, this means the injured patient is hypotensive, with normal skin color and temperature and an inappropriately slow heart rate. In the healthy patient, blood pressure is maintained by the controlled release of catecholamines (epinephrine and norepinephrine) from the adrenal glands. Catecholamines cause constriction of the blood vessels, increase the heart rate and the strength of heart contraction, and stimulate sweat glands. Sensors in the aortic and carotid arteries monitor the blood pressure. The brain and spinal cord signal the adrenal glands to release catecholamines to keep the blood pressure in the normal range. In pure *hemorrhagic shock*, these sensors detect the hypovolemic state and compensate by constricting the blood vessels and speeding the heart rate. The high levels of catecholamines cause pale skin, tachycardia, and sweating. The mechanism of shock from spinal cord injury is just the opposite. There is no significant blood loss, but there is no signal going to the adrenals (the spinal cord cable is out), so no catecholamines are released. The blood vessels dilate; the blood pools, and the blood pressure cannot be maintained. The brain cannot correct this because it cannot get the message to the adrenal glands. The patient with neurogenic shock cannot show the signs of pale skin, tachycardia, and sweating because the cord injury prevents release of catecholamines. Intra-abdominal injury and bleeding can be difficult to determine because the patient with neurogenic shock usually has no sensation in the abdomen. The multiple-trauma patient may have both neurogenic shock and hemorrhagic shock. Neurogenic shock is a diagnosis of exclusion, after all other potential causes of shock have been ruled out. In the prehospital setting, neurogenic shock is treated in the same way as hemorrhagic shock (see Chapter 7).

PATIENT ASSESSMENT

All trauma patients are evaluated in the same manner using the assessment priority plan, of which evaluation of spinal cord function is a part. Clues to spinal cord injury are given in Table 9-2. Parts of the neurological exam are performed during the BTLS Primary Survey. The remainder of the neurological exam is performed during the Detailed Exam. This is frequently done after the patient is loaded into the ambulance. The patient that requires extrication is a special situation. Before beginning extrication you should check sensory and motor function in the hands and feet, and document these findings later in the written report. Not only does this pre-extrication neurological exam alert you to any spinal injury; it also provides documentation on whether there was loss of function before extrication was begun. Sadly, there are a few reports of patients who have claimed that their spinal injuries were caused by their rescuers. You will not have time to perform the pre-extrication neurological exam on the patient who requires *Emergency Rescue* and you may not have time on those requiring *Rapid Extrication*.

TABLE 9-2	Clues to Spinal Cord Injury on Patient Assessment.

The following are indicators that the spine may have been injured. These patients may require SMR (see Figure 9-8).

Mechanism of Injury

- Blunt trauma above the clavicle
- Diving accident
- Motor vehicle or bicycle accident
- Fall
- Stabbing or impalement anywhere near the spinal column
- Shooting or blast injury to the torso
- Any violent injury with forces that could act on the spinal column or cord

When the Patient Complains of

- Neck or back pain
- Numbness or tingling
- Loss of movement or weakness

When on Exam you Find

- Pain on movement of back or spinal column
- Obvious deformity of back or spinal column
- Guarding against movement of back
- Loss of sensation
- Weak or flaccid muscles
- Loss of control of bladder or bowels
- Erection of the penis (priapism)
- Neurogenic shock

The neurological exam is described in more detail in chapters 2 and 8, but we will review the exam of the peripheral nervous system here. This exam is kept brief and simple. If the conscious patient can move his fingers and toes, the motor nerves are intact. Anything less than normal sensation (tingling or decreased sensation) is suspicious for cord injury. The unconscious patient may withdraw if you pinch his fingers and toes. If so, you have demonstrated intact motor and sensory nerves and thus an intact cord. This does not mean you don't have to perform SMR. All unconscious trauma patients should have SMR. Flaccid paralysis, even in the unconscious head injury patient, usually means spinal cord injury. Document these important findings.

PATIENT MANAGEMENT

Based on the mechanism of injury, it is appropriate to place the head and neck in a neutral position as you first evaluate the patient. The spine is treated as a long bone, with its top being the head and its bottom being the pelvis. The motion of the spine is then restricted in this position until the patient is securely strapped to the long backboard. The purpose of SMR is to minimize spinal movement to avoid aggravating any spinal cord or column injury. Preparation for managing spinal column or cord injury can begin when you are dispatched to the scene of a motor vehicle collision, fall, explosion, head injury, or neck injury.

There are two types of situations that require modification of usual SMR. The patient who is in *immediate* danger of death may require *emergency rescue* from a vehicle or a structure. An example would be the patient who is in an MVC and when you arrive the auto is on fire. In cases where even a few seconds may mean the difference between life and death you are justified in saving the patient in any way possible. Anytime this manner of rescue is used you should document the reason and request a review of the chart by Medical Direction. Some examples of situations that might require *emergency rescue* are when Scene Size-up identifies a condition that may *immediately* endanger you or the patient:

1. Fire or immediate danger of fire
2. Immediate danger of explosion
3. Danger of being carried away by rapidly moving water
4. Structure in immediate danger of collapse
5. Continuing immediately-life-threatening toxic exposure

The second situation that requires modification of usual SMR is for patients whose Primary Survey indicates a critical degree of ongoing danger that requires an intervention within one or two minutes. Indications for *rapid extrication* are the following:

1. Airway obstruction that cannot be relieved by modified jaw thrust or finger sweep
2. Cardiac or respiratory arrest
3. Chest or airway injuries requiring ventilation or assisted ventilation
4. Deep shock or bleeding that cannot be controlled

Rapid extrication requires multiple rescuers who remove the patient along the long axis of the body, using their hands to minimize spinal movement (see skills in Chapter 10). When the rapid extrication technique is used, the written report should also be carefully reviewed to ensure appropriate documentation of the technique and its indication.

The most easily applied and readily available method of cervical motion restriction is with your hands or knees. Your hands should be placed to stabilize the neck in relation to the long axis of the spinal column (see Figure 9-5). "Pulling traction" is not a prehospital option, and the term *traction* is not an appropriate description for motion restriction of the spine. Traction will usually result in further instability of any spinal column injury. The correct approach is stabilization, without pulling on the neck. When packaging the body on a backboard, the neutral in-line position allows the most room for the spinal cord, so that is the optimal position for SMR.

You can place an appropriately sized cervical spinal extrication collar on the patient as airway assessment is being done. These one- or two-piece collars are not definitive devices for restricting cervical spine motion, but should be used only as a reminder that SMR is necessary and to prevent gross neck movement. The rescuer's hands can be removed only when the patient (head and body) has been strapped on a backboard with an attached head motion restriction device. For the conscious patient, positioning the head and neck in the position of patient comfort is a good guideline. Inadequate strapping will torque the neck against the body if the patient moves, rolls, is dropped, or is rotated.

Once the patient is secured to the board, a rescuer must be present and capable of rolling the board if the patient begins to vomit or loses his airway. Placing and strapping a patient on the board effectively eliminates the patient's ability to protect the airway, and therefore the rescuer is responsible. This rule continues in effect in the emergency department. An emergency department staff person must then assume responsibility for airway

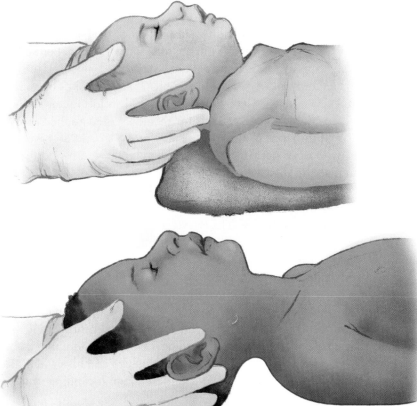

a. Due to the large heads of younger children, you may need to raise the shoulders with padding.

b. In older children, obtain neutral positioning with shoulders and head on a firm, flat surface.

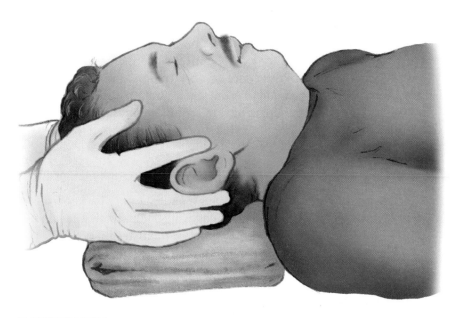

c. With adults, elevate the head 1 to 2 inches.

Figure 9-5 Neutral spinal positioning for adult, child, and infant patients. **a.** Due to the large heads of younger children, you may need to raise the shoulders with padding. **b.** In older children, obtain neutral positioning with shoulders and head on a flat surface. **c.** With adults, elevate the head one to two inches.

protection. Definitive SMR occurs when the body is strapped securely to the board with cushions, blanket, or towel rolls maintaining the head, cervical spine, torso, and pelvis in-line. In the past, sandbags have been used for motion restriction of the head and perform well when the patient is kept supine. However, if the board is tilted or the patient and the board are rotated (to prevent aspiration when the patient vomits), the weight of the sandbags may cause a dangerous amount of head movement. Therefore sandbags are an extremely poor option for prehospital SMR. Lighter-weight bulky objects, such as towel rolls, blanket rolls, or head cushions, are better tools for this job. When applied properly, these devices allow removal of the front portion of the cervical collar and observation of the neck, as in the patient with open neck wounds. Commercial cervical motion restriction devices may be left in place on the backboard.

There are some patients (frightened children and patients with altered mental status) who will struggle so violently that they defeat your attempts to eliminate spinal movement. There may be no good solution to this. The Reeves sleeve (see Figure 9-7a) may be the best device to restrict spinal motion in the combative adult patient. You should always carefully document those situations in which the patient refuses to cooperate with SMR.

Studies have suggested that a true neutral position for an adult is obtained with the use of one to two inches of occipital padding on a long backboard. This slightly elevates the head and brings the neck into a neutral position that tends to make the patient more comfortable. This is accomplished with the head pad on a cervical motion restriction device or the padding that is used with many backboard devices. Some padding is a necessity in elderly patients whose necks have a natural flexed posture and also in children, whose large heads will cause flexion of the neck unless there is some padding under the shoulders.

In certain situations, once the patient is packaged onto the backboard, the board and patient may have to be rolled up onto his or her side (see Figure 9-6). Careful strapping can prevent lateral movement of the spine in this situation but use of the vacuum backboard is far superior for this. Women who are more than 20 weeks pregnant should always be transported with the backboard tilted 20 to 30 degrees to the patient's left side to keep the uterus off the inferior vena cava. Patients with airway problems who are not intubated are better transported on their side. This is especially critical when there is uncontrolled bleeding into the airway or if there is massive face or neck trauma. In these situations gravity helps drain fluids out of the airway and may prevent aspiration if the patient vomits. Because of the danger of vomiting and aspiration, unconscious patients who are not intubated should be transported rolled to the side.

Log-Roll

This technique is used for moving a patient onto a backboard. It is commonly used because it is easy to perform with a minimum number of rescuers. As yet no movement technique has been devised that maintains complete spinal immobilization while moving a patient onto a backboard. Properly performed, the log-roll technique will minimize movement of the spinal column as well as any other technique.

The log-roll technique moves the spinal column as a single unit with the head and pelvis. It can be performed on patients lying prone or supine. Using three or more rescuers, controlled by the rescuer at the patient's head, the patient (with her arms at her side) is rolled onto the uninjured side, a board is slid underneath, and the patient is rolled face up onto the board. The log-roll technique is then completed when the patient's chest, pelvis, and head

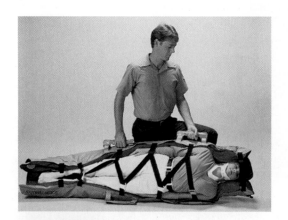

Figure 9-6 Patient in vaccum backboard turned on side. Notice that the body is maintained in a straight line.

are secured to the board. Log-roll may be modified for patients with painful arm, leg, and chest wounds who need to be rolled onto their uninjured side. The side to which you turn the patient during the log-roll procedure is not critical and can be changed in situations in which you can only place the backboard on one side of the patient. The log-roll technique is useful for most trauma patients, but for those patients with an unstable fractured pelvis it may aggravate the injury to roll their weight onto the pelvis. If the pelvic fracture appears stable, the log-roll should be carefully performed, turning the patient onto the uninjured side (if it can be identified). Patients with obviously unstable pelvic fractures should not be log-rolled but should be lifted carefully onto a board by four or more rescuers. The scoop stretcher could also be used to move patients with unstable pelvic fractures onto the backboard.

Spinal Motion Restriction Devices

There is a wide range of devices currently marketed to provide SMR for injured patients (Figure 9-7a through e). No device has yet been proven to excel over all others, and no device will ever be produced that can be used to provide SMR for all patients. No device is better than the crew that is using it; training with the available tools is the most critical factor in providing good patient care.

The Complications of SMR

There are complications of strapping a patient to a board. The patient will be uncomfortable and will often complain of head and low back pain that is directly related to being strapped onto the hard backboard. The head and airway are in a fixed position, which can produce airway compromise and aspiration if the patient vomits. Obese patients and those with congestive heart failure can suffer life-threatening hypoxia. On a rigid board there is uneven skin pressure that can result in pressure sores. Lifting the patient and the board can cause injuries to rescue personnel. SMR should be applied appropriately to those who will most likely benefit, and it should be avoided if not necessary.

Indications for SMR

It has always been accepted as fact that all patients with a risk of spinal trauma require careful SMR. However, there have never been any scientific studies confirming that view. Some countries do not perform SMR, and they report no difference in outcome. At least one study has been done comparing the EMS systems of a country that performs no SMR (Malaysia) and one that consistently performs SMR (the U.S.). The study concluded that prehospital SMR had little or no effect on neurologic outcome in patients with blunt spinal trauma. This is not to condemn SMR, but to remind us that what we are doing is based on logic and not actually based on scientific evidence. There is no doubt that some patients require SMR. Recent studies have documented circumstances under which spinal column or cord injury is very unlikely, and therefore the patient can be managed without SMR. These studies have resulted in a clinical pathway referred to as the Maine Protocol for Spinal Motion Restriction, written by Peter Goth, M.D. (see Figure 9-8). This protocol is supported by the National Association of EMS Physicians (see Table 9-3 for NAEMSP's position paper on spinal motion restriction). You must assess the mechanism of injury, interview and examine the patient, then use this information to determine which patients need SMR. From the Scene Size-up, history, and assessment come the clues that identify those patients who do not need SMR.

Under the Maine pathway, the rescuer first assesses the mechanism of injury. SMR is not required if there is no mechanism of injury that would damage the spine (foot crushed by a car). If the mechanism is a high-risk event, SMR is performed regardless of other clinical findings. These high-risk situations include high-speed MVCs, falls of greater than three times the patient's height, penetrating wounds into or near the spinal

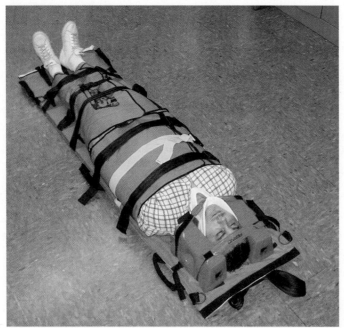

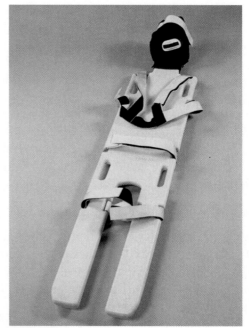

a.   b.

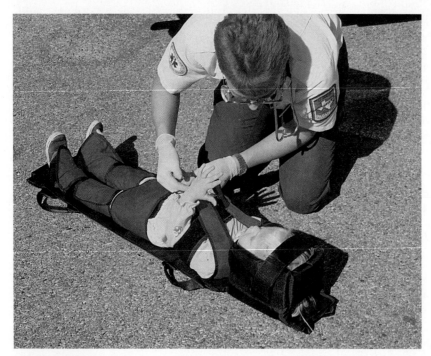

c.

Figure 9-7 **a.** Reeves sleeve. **b.** Miller body splint. **c.** Pediatric SMR device. **d.** Kendrick extrication device.
e1. Short backboard **e2.** Short backboard.

column, sports injuries to the head or neck, diving accidents, and any trauma situation in which the patient is still unconscious. If the danger of spinal injury is uncertain (ground-level fall, low-speed "fender bender"), the rescuer will manually stabilize the spine and then assess the patient for signs of spinal injury. The patient must be reliable enough to understand the EMS provider and answer the questions accurately, so children and patients with altered mental status or acute stress reactions are excluded. The patient is assessed for evidence of intoxication or distracting injuries that may not allow the patient to clearly feel the pain associated with a spinal injury. The patient is asked if he has pain in

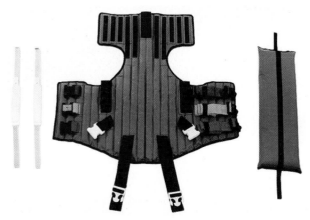

d.

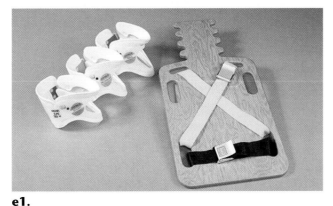

e1.   **e2.**

 Figure 9-7 (continued)

the area of the spinal column. If no pain is present in the neck or back, and no other injuries are so painful as to distract the patient from comprehending back or neck pain, the rescuer then carefully examines the spinal column and performs a neurological exam. If there is any tenderness on palpation of the spinal column area or if the patient complains of midline pain when asked to move his back, SMR is performed. SMR is also performed if there are alterations in the motor or sensory exam.

If the patient has no high-risk mechanism of injury, no alteration of mental status, no distracting injuries, is not intoxicated, has no pain or tenderness along the spine, and has no neurological deficits, the patient may be treated and transported without SMR. This

TABLE 9-3	Position Paper on Spinal Motion Restriction by the National Association of EMS Physicians

Spinal motion restriction is indicated in prehospital trauma patients who sustain an injury with a mechanism having the potential for causing spinal injury and who have at least one of the following clinical criteria:

1. Altered mental status

2. Evidence of intoxication

3. A distracting painful injury (e.g., long bone extremity fracture)

4. Neurologic deficit

5. Spinal pain or tenderness

Initial Assessment of Spinal Injury
Clinical Criteria

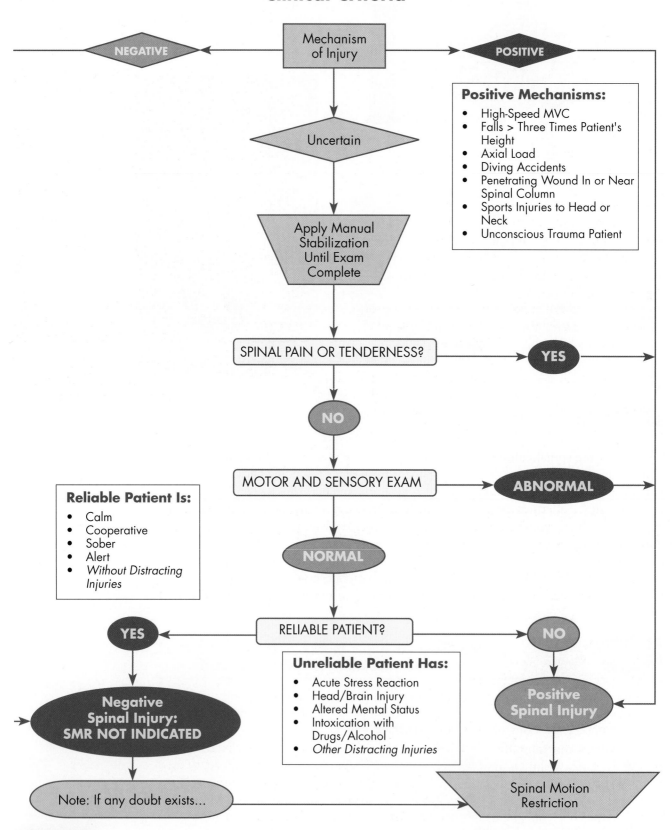

Figure 9-8 Decision tree for spinal immobilization. *(Reprinted by permission of Peter Goth, M.D.)*

protocol has proven effective in research studies but, like all protocols, must be approved for local use by Medical Direction and followed up with a quality assurance program.

AIRWAY INTERVENTION

When the rescuer performs SMR in any manner, the patient loses some of her ability to maintain her own airway. As mentioned earlier, the rescuer must then assume this responsibility until the patient has a controlled airway or has the spinal column cleared in the emergency department and is released from the motion-restricting equipment (see Figure 9-9). This is particularly critical in children, who have a greater potential for vomiting and aspiration after a traumatic injury.

Airway manipulations in the trauma patient require careful application. Current research indicates that any airway intervention will cause some movement of the spinal column. In-line manual stabilization is the most effective manner for minimizing this movement. Cervical collars are only partially helpful in preventing movement. Nasotracheal, orotracheal, or cricothyroid intubations all induce some bony movement. Your priority plan should include manual stabilization, then the use of the airway control method that you are most skilled at performing. When weighing the risks and benefits of each airway procedure, recall that the risk of dying with an uncontrolled airway is greater than the risk of inducing spinal cord damage using a careful approach to airway intervention.

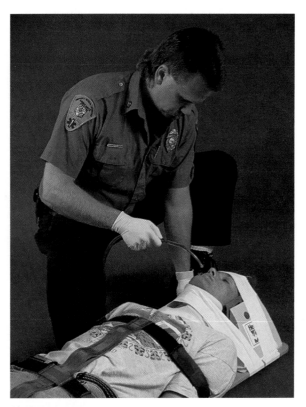

Figure 9-9 You are responsible for the patient's airway once the patient is strapped to a backboard.

SPECIAL SMR SITUATIONS

You must be prepared to stabilize the spinal column of all patients who sustain major trauma. In some patients (see below), traditional techniques must be modified to provide safe and effective SMR:

1. Patients in closed spaces
2. Patients in water
3. Patients in a prone or standing position
4. Pediatric patients
5. Elderly patients
6. Patients in protective helmets
7. Very large or obese patients
8. Patients with disfiguring or penetrating neck wounds

Closed-space rescues are performed in a manner appropriate for the clinical condition of the patient. The only general rules that can be applied to these rescues are to prevent gross cervical spine movement and to move patients in-line with the long axis of the body (see Figure 9-10). Safety of the rescuer is of prime importance in all closed-space rescues. Asphyxia, toxic gases, and structure collapse are dangers of closed-space rescue. Never enter a closed space unless you are properly trained, equipped (air pack, safety line, etc.), and sure of scene safety.

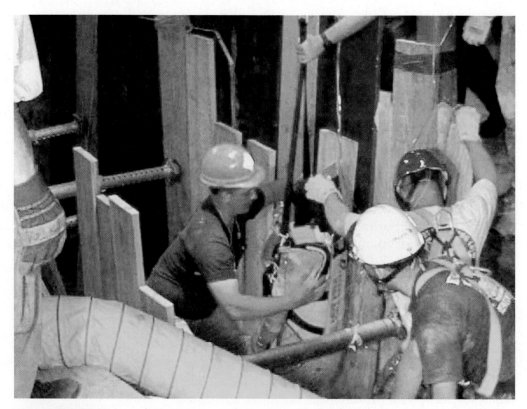

Figure 9-10 Patient entrapped in trench cave-in being lifted out along the long axis of the body. *(Photo courtesy of Roy Alson, M.D.)*

You can perform water rescues by moving the patient in-line, preventing gross cervical movement. When the rescuers are in a stable position for performing SMR, the backboard is floated under the patient, and the patient is then secured and removed from the water (see Figure 9-11). Safety of both rescuers and patients is of paramount importance. If you are not trained in water rescue, do not attempt to rescue victims in hazardous situations such as deep or swift water.

Prone and standing patients are stabilized in a manner that minimizes spinal column movement, ending with the patient in the conventional supine position. Prone patients are log-rolled onto a backboard, with the careful coordination of head and chest rescuers. Seated patients may be stabilized using short backboards or their commercial adaptations. Used appropriately, these provide initial stabilization of the cervical and thoracic spine and then facilitate the movement of the patient onto a long backboard. Standing patients may be placed against the long board while upright and then strapped in place. The board is then gently lowered to the supine position.

It is best to provide initial SMR of the pediatric patient with your hands, and then use cushions or towel rolls to help secure the child on an appropriate board or device. Some pediatric trauma specialists suggest padding beneath the *back and shoulders* on the board in a child under the age of 3 (see Figures 9-5 and 9-12). These children normally have a relatively large head that flexes the neck when placed on a straight board. Padding under the back and shoulders will prevent this flexion and also make the child more comfortable. Children who are involved in an MVC while restrained in a child safety seat but have no apparent injuries may be packaged in the safety seat for transport to the hospital (see Pediatric BTLS textbook). Using towel or blanket rolls, cloth tape, and a little reassurance, you can secure the child in the safety seat and then belt the seat into the ambulance (see

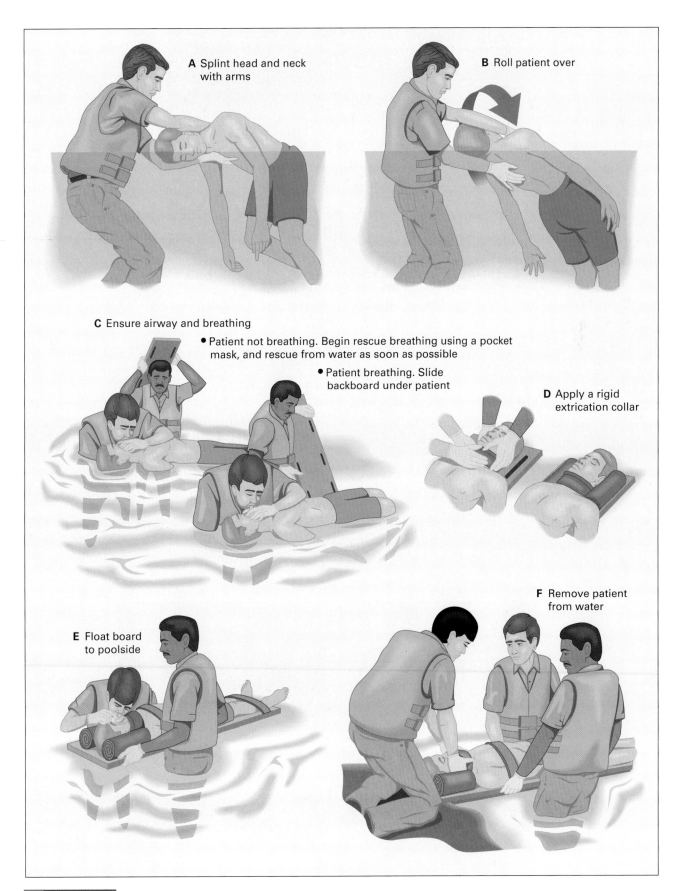

A Splint head and neck with arms

B Roll patient over

C Ensure airway and breathing
- Patient not breathing. Begin rescue breathing using a pocket mask, and rescue from water as soon as possible
  - Patient breathing. Slide backboard under patient

D Apply a rigid extrication collar

E Float board to poolside

F Remove patient from water

Figure 9-11 Water rescue, possible spinal injury.

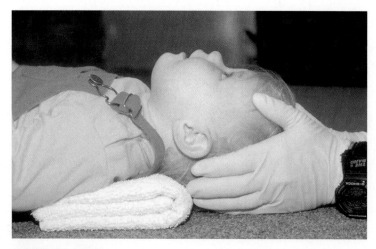

Figure 9-12 Most children require padding under back and shoulders to keep the cervical spine in a neutral position. *(Courtesy of Bob Page, NREMT-P)*

Figure 9-13). This technique minimizes movement of the child and provides a secure method for child transport in the ambulance. Some autos come with built-in child-restraint seats that cannot be removed. Children in such seats will have to be extricated onto a backboard or another pediatric SMR device. For the child who is frightened and struggling, there may be no good way to obtain SMR. Careful reassurance, the presence of a comforting family member, and gentle management will help prevent more complications and further struggling.

Elderly patients require flexibility in packaging techniques. Many elderly patients have arthritic changes of the spine and very thin skin. Such patients will be very uncomfortable when placed on a backboard. Some arthritic spines are so rigid that the patient cannot be laid straight on the board, and some elderly patients have rigid flexion of the neck that will result in a large gap between the head and the board. You can make use of towels, blankets, and pillows to pad the elderly patient and prevent movement and dis-

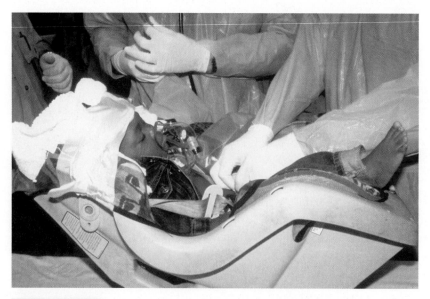

Figure 9-13 Infant secured in car seat. *(Courtesy of David Effron, M.D., FACEP)*

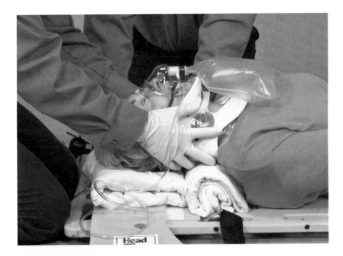

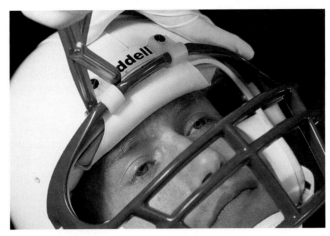

Figure 9-14 Additional padding, such as rolled blankets or towels behind the head, may be needed to keep the head in a neutral, in-line position.

Figure 9-15 The face guard of football helmets can be removed with rescue scissors or a screwdriver.

comfort on the backboard (see Figure 9-14). This is a situation in which the vacuum backboard (which conforms to the shape of the patient) works very well (see Figure 9-6).

Athletes and cyclists wearing helmets are another special set of patients. Large helmets used in these sports must be removed at some point to permit complete assessment and care. Helmets used in different sports present different management problems for rescuers. Football and ice hockey helmets are custom fitted to the individual. Unless special circumstances exist, such as respiratory distress coupled with an inability to access the airway, the helmet should not be removed in the prehospital setting. Athletic helmet design will generally allow easy airway access once the face guard is removed. The face guard can easily be removed with a screwdriver or cut off using rescue scissors (see Figure 9-15). The athlete wearing shoulder pads has his neck in a neutral position when on the backboard with the helmet in place. If the helmet is removed, padding must be inserted under the head to keep the neck from extending (see Figure 9-16a and b). After arrival at the emergency facility the cervical spine can be x-rayed with the helmet in place. Once the spine is evaluated, the helmet can be removed by stabilizing the head and neck, removing the

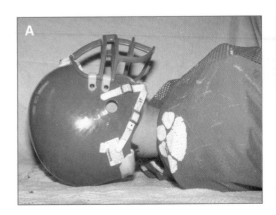

Figure 9-16 **a.** Patients with shoulder pads and helmets are usually best immobilized with the helmet in place. The spine is maintained in a neutral position with a minimum of movement. *(Photo courtesy of Bob Page, NREMT-P)* **b.** Patients with shoulder pads must have padding under the head to maintain a neutral position if the helmet is removed.

PEARLS

1. Spinal clearance is not a priority in the patient suffering from multiple trauma; spinal motion restriction is.

2. Restriction of motion of the cervical spine is different for the adult, child, and in the elderly patient.

3. Injury to the spinal cord can produce high-space shock, with the patient experiencing hypotension, normal skin color and temperature, and an inappropriately slow heart rate.

4. *Emergency Rescue* is reserved for those situations where there is immediate (within seconds) environmental threat to the life of the victim and/or rescuer. Patients should be moved to a safe area in a manner that places the rescuer at the least risk.

5. *Rapid Extrication* should be considered for patients whose medical conditions or situations require fast intervention (one or two minutes—but not seconds) to prevent death.

6. Perform brief motor and sensory checks in the upper and lower extremities before and after moving any patient.

7. Do not apply traction to the head and neck. Maintain in-line stabilization of the head, neck, and spine.

8. Sandbags are not used for prehospital spine management. Consider spinal motion restriction devices, light bulky items such as towel rolls, blankets, and head cushions.

9. A patient in spinal motion restriction is at risk for aspiration and other problems. You are responsible for checking and maintaining the airway.

10. Infants and small children involved in MVCs can be transported in their car seats as long as they have no apparent injury and the device is not damaged.

cheek pads, releasing the air inflation system, and then sliding the helmet off in the usual manner.

In contrast, motorcycle helmets often must be removed in the prehospital setting. The removal technique is modified to accommodate the different design. Motorcycle helmets are often designed with a continuous solid face guard that limits airway access. These helmets are not custom designed and frequently are poorly fitted to the patient. Their large size will usually produce significant neck flexion if left in place when the patient is placed on a backboard (see Figure 9-17). Motorcycle accidents are usually associated with much more violent force than are athletic injuries. The motorcycle helmet will make it difficult to stabilize the neck in a neutral position, may obstruct access to the airway, and may hide injuries to the head or neck; it should be removed in the prehospital setting using the techniques described in Chapter 10.

Very large or obese patients may not fit appropriately in standard equipment. You must be flexible, even using sheets of plywood and head cushions or towel rolls to stabilize. In cold-weather climates, patients in bulky warm clothing will need to be snugly secured to prevent excessive movement.

Patients with penetrating or disfiguring wounds of the neck or lower face must be continually observed. Cervical collars will prevent continued examination of the wound site and may compromise the airway in wounds with expanding hematomas or subcutaneous air. If the mandible is fractured, the collar may again cause airway compromise. Therefore, for patients with these injuries, it may be wise to avoid collars, using manual stabilization and then head cushion devices or blanket rolls for cervical motion restriction.

Trauma patients with paralysis or neurogenic shock have lost vascular control and thus cannot control blood flow to the skin. They may lose heat rapidly, so it is important for you to prevent hypothermia.

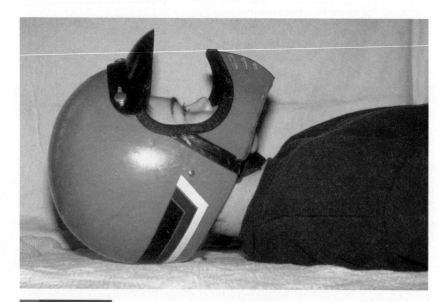

Figure 9-17 Full-face helmets obstruct access to the patient's airway. Notice that the helmet flexes the neck in a patient who is not wearing shoulder pads. *(Courtesy of Bob Page, NREMT-P)*

CASE STUDY

Dan, Joyce, and Buddy of the Emergency Transport System have been called to the local public swimming pool. They are told that there has been a diving injury. They decide that Dan will be the team leader on this case. When they arrive they see that the fire department is already on-scene but bystanders had pulled the patient from the water with no spinal stabilization. The firemedic states that the patient was chasing some friends and dived into the shallow end of the pool, striking his head on the bottom. He was briefly dazed but not unconscious and did not suffer near-drowning because his friends immediately pulled him from the shallow water.

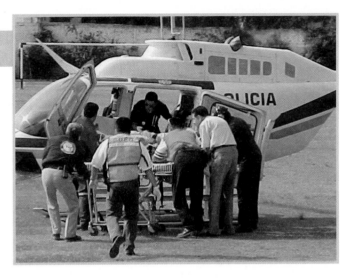

(Photo courtesy of Eduardo Romero Hicks, M.D.)

The patient complains of severe pain in his neck with weakness in both arms and legs. Rapid Trauma Survey reveals tenderness along the cervical spine with spasm of the cervical spinal muscles and weakness, but no total paralysis below the neck. He is breathing with his diaphragm only. The patient is carefully packaged on a long backboard, given 100% oxygen to breathe, and transported to the level I trauma center by helicopter. Vital signs just before lift-off are normal. On arrival he is found to be able to flex his arms at the elbow but cannot move his trunk or legs. His blood pressure has dropped to 80/50 with a pulse of 72. A CT scan reveals a compression fracture of the fifth cervical vertebra, causing cord compression. The patient requires spinal decompression and stabilization surgery and months of physical therapy in order to regain some use of his arms and legs. He eventually is able to walk with a cane and is able to return to school.

CASE STUDY WRAP-UP

Diving injuries or falls in which the victim lands on his head cause axial loading of the spinal column and can cause compression fractures of the cervical spine and cervical spinal cord injury. Falls or jumps in which the victim lands on his feet are more likely to cause lumbar compression fractures as well as lower extremity fractures. Gentle handling and 100% oxygen can help prevent secondary spinal cord injury. Obviously, patients who sustain diving injuries often drown before anyone recognizes that they are in trouble.

SUMMARY

Spinal cord injury is a devastating consequence of modern-day trauma. Unstable or incomplete damage to the spinal column or cord is not completely predictable; therefore, trauma patients who are unconscious or have any dangerous mechanism of injury affecting the head, neck, or trunk should have SMR. Those trauma patients with uncertain mechanisms may not require SMR if they meet the physical exam criteria. Special trauma cases may require special SMR techniques. Once SMR is performed, the patient loses some ability to control his airway; you must be prepared at all times to intervene should the patient vomit or have evidence of airway compromise.

BIBLIOGRAPHY

1. Aprahamian, L. "Experimental Cervical Spine Injury Model: Evaluation of Airway Management and Splinting Techniques." *Annals of Emergency Medicine*, Vol. 13 (1994), p. 584.

2. Domeier, R. M. The National Association of EMS Physicians Standards and Clinical Practice Committee. *Prehospital Emergency Care*, Vol. 3 (1999), pp. 251–253.

3. Goth, P. C. *Spine Injury, Clinical Criteria for Assessment and Management*, pp. 1–36. Augusta, ME: Medical Care Development, 1994.

4. Hauswald, M., G. Ong., D. Tandberg, and X. Omar. "Out-of-hospital spinal immobilization: Its effect on neurologic injury. *Academic Emg Med*, Vol. 5 (1998) pp. 214–219.

5. Henry, G. L., and N. Little. *Neurologic Emergencies*. New York: McGraw-Hill, 1985.

6. Illinois State Medical Association. *Guidelines for Helmet Fitting and Removal in Athletes*. Chicago: The Association, 1990.

7. Jacobs, L. M. "Prospective Analysis of Acute Cervical Spine Injury." *Annals of Emergency Medicine*, Vol. 15 (1986), p. 44.

8. Podolsky, S. "Efficacy of Cervical Spine Immobilization Methods." *Journal of Trauma*, Vol. 23 (1983), p. 461.

9. Seaman, P. J. "Log-Roll Technique." *Emergency*, Vol. 24 (1992), p. 18.

Spine Management Skills

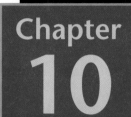

Chapter 10

Donna Hastings, EMT-P

Objectives

Upon completion of this chapter, you should be able to:

1. Describe the essential components of a spinal motion restriction (SMR) system.

2. Explain when to use SMR.

3. Perform SMR with a short backboard.

4. Perform log-rolling of a patient onto a long backboard.

5. Properly secure a patient to a long backboard.

6. Perform SMR on a patient from a standing position.

7. Stabilize the head and neck when a neutral position cannot be safely attained.

8. Perform rapid extrication.

9. Explain when helmets should and should not be removed from injured patients.

10. Properly remove a motorcycle helmet.

11. Demonstrate proper stabilization of the neck in patients who are wearing shoulder pads and helmets.

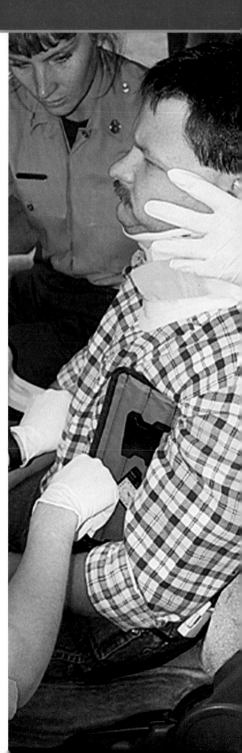

ESSENTIAL COMPONENTS OF A SPINAL MOTION RESTRICTION SYSTEM

There are four components of a full spinal motion restriction system:

1. *Backboard*: This may be of several different types; its purpose is to keep the spinal column from moving.

2. *Cervical collar*: There are also several different types of these devices. They do not completely immobilize the neck but remind the patient not to move his neck, and provide some support.

3. *Head motion restriction device*: There are also several different types of these devices. These attach to the backboard and are used to restrict movement of the patient's head after the patient's body has been strapped to the backboard. After this has been applied, the cervical collar can be removed if necessary.

4. *Straps*: As above, there are several different types of strapping systems that are used to bind the patient's body to the backboard to restrict movement of the spinal column. The straps should be positioned to decrease patient movement from side to side and from sliding up and down on the backboard.

PATIENTS REQUIRING SPINAL MOTION RESTRICTION

The goal of SMR is to limit movement of the spine and thus prevent further harm. See Figure 10-1 for indications for SMR. Patients requiring SMR must have it done before they are moved at all. In the case of an automobile collision, you must stabilize the patient's spine before removing him from the wreckage. More patient movement is involved in extrication than at any other time, so you must carefully stabilize the neck and spine before beginning extrication. *Remember*: Traction can cause permanent paralysis. You are stabilizing the spine, not pulling on it. Except in situations requiring Emergency Rescue and sometimes Rapid Extrication, always try to document sensation and motor function in the extremities before you move the patient.

SMR USING THE SHORT BACKBOARD

The short backboard is used for patients who are in a position (such as in a motor vehicle) that does not permit use of the long backboard. There are several different devices of this type: Some of them have strapping mechanisms different from the one explained here. You must be familiar with your equipment (practice, practice, practice . . .) before employing it in an emergency.

✋ PROCEDURE

✳ Technique

(These steps are illustrated in Figures 10-2 through 10-14.)

1. Remember that the priorities of evaluation and management are done before the SMR devices go on.

2. One rescuer must, if possible, station himself behind the patient, place his hands on either side of the patient's head, and stabilize the neck in a neutral position. This step is part of the ABCs of evaluation. It is done at the same time that you begin evaluation of the airway.

3. When you have finished the Primary Survey and have checked extremities for movement (document later), you must apply a semirigid extrication collar. If you have

Initial Assessment of Spinal Injury
Clinical Criteria

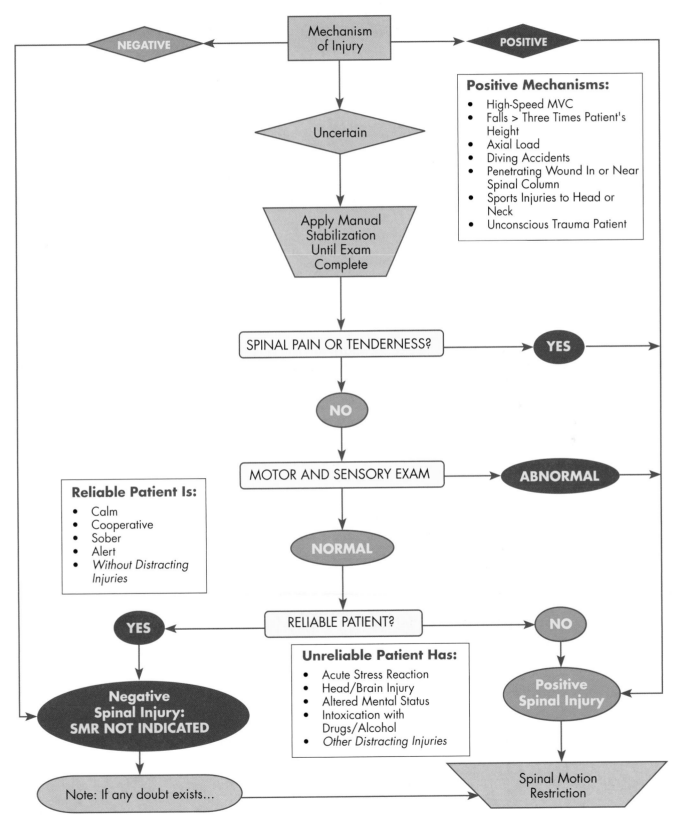

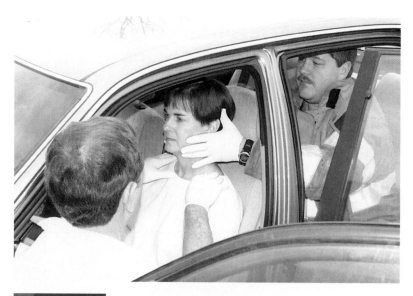

Figure 10-2 Stabilize neck and perform primary survey.

enough people, this can be done while someone else is doing the ABCs of evaluation and management. If you have limited help, apply the collar after finishing the Rapid Trauma Survey, but before transferring the patient to the backboard.

4. Position the short backboard behind the patient. The first rescuer continues to stabilize the neck while the short backboard is being maneuvered into place. The patient may have to be moved forward to get the backboard into place; great care must be taken so that moves are coordinated to support the neck and back.

5. Secure the patient to the board: There are usually three straps for this. Place the short strap under the armpits and across the upper chest as an anchor. Bring each long strap over a leg, down between both legs, back around the outside of the same leg, across the chest, and then attach them to the upper strap opposite that which was brought across the shoulders.

6. Tighten the straps until the patient is held securely.

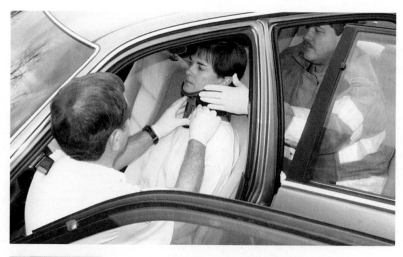

Figure 10-3 Apply a semirigid extrication collar.

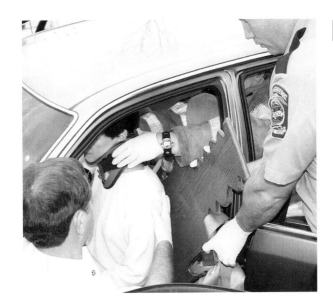

7. Secure the patient's head to the board by wide tape or elastic wraps around the forehead. Apply padding under the neck and head as needed to maintain a neutral position.

8. Transfer the patient to a long backboard. Turn the patient so that her back is to the opening through which she is to be removed. Someone must support her legs so that the upper legs remain at a 90-degree angle to her torso. Position the long backboard through the opening until it is under the patient. Lower the patient back onto the long backboard and slide the patient and the short backboard up into position on the long backboard. Loosen the straps on the short board and allow the patient's legs to extend out flat, then retighten the straps. Now secure her to the long backboard with straps, and secure her head with a padded motion-restriction device. When she is secured in this way, it is possible to turn the whole board up on its side if the patient has to vomit. The patient should remain securely strapped, with little or no movement.

EMERGENCY RESCUE AND RAPID EXTRICATION

Patients left inside vehicles following a collision are usually stabilized on a short backboard (or extrication device) and then transferred onto a long backboard. Although this is the best way to extricate anyone with a possible spinal injury, there are certain situations in which a more rapid method must be used. *Note*: BTLS International offers a one-day course (BTLS Access) on basic extrication from automobiles. Call 1-800-495-2857 for information.

Situations Requiring Emergency Rescue

This procedure is used only in situations in which the patient's life is in *immediate* danger. In some of these situations you may not have time to use any technique other than pulling the patient to safety. This is an example of "desperate situations may demand desperate measures." Use good judgment; do not sacrifice your life in a dangerous situation. Whenever you use this procedure, it should be noted in the written report, and you should be prepared

PEARLS

1. When placing the straps around the legs on a male, do not catch the genitals in the straps.

2. Do not use the short backboard as a "handle" to move the patient. Move patient and board as a unit. Many short backboard devices come with built-in handles. These are not to be used ALONE to move a patient.

3. When you are applying the horizontal strap (long backboard) around a woman, place the upper strap above her breasts and under her arms, not across the breasts.

4. When you are applying the lower horizontal strap on a pregnant woman, place it across the pelvis and not across the uterus.

5. You may need to modify your strapping techniques, depending on injuries.

6. Secure the patient well enough so that little or no motion of the spine will occur if the board is turned on its side. Do not make straps so tight that they interfere with breathing.

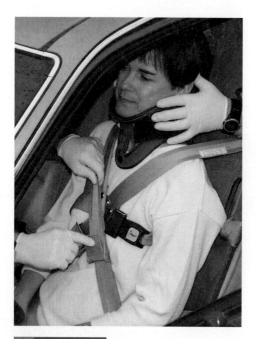

Figure 10-5 Apply straps and tighten securely.

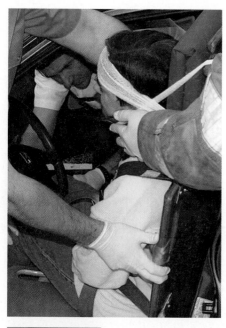

Figure 10-6 Turn the patient carefully; then lower onto the backboard.

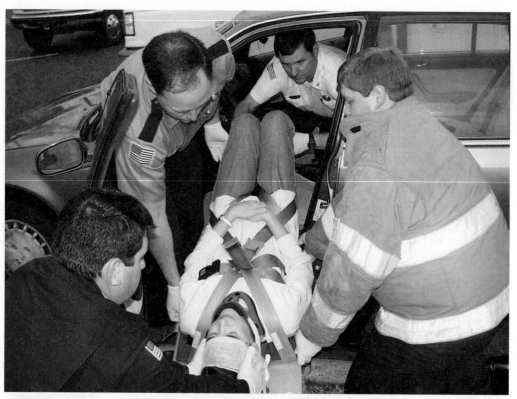

Figure 10-7 Slide the patient on the short backboard up into position on the long backboard. Loosen the straps and allow the legs to extend out flat; then retighten the straps. Secure the patient and the short backboard to the long backboard. Apply a padded SMR device to secure the patient's head and neck.

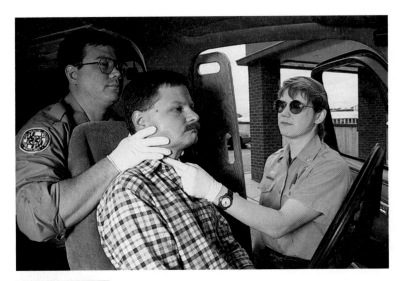

Figure 10-8 Kendrick extrication device; stabilize the neck and perform the Primary Survey.

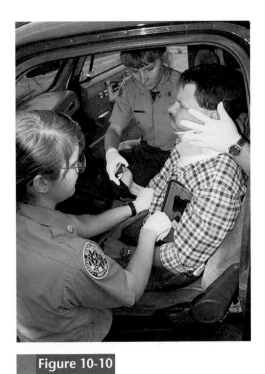

Figure 10-10

Position the device behind the patient. Coordinate all movements to restrict spinal motion. Position the chest panels up well into the armpits.

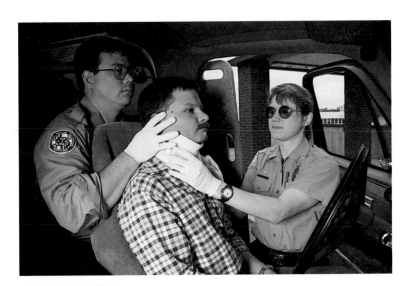

Figure 10-9 Apply semirigid extrication collar.

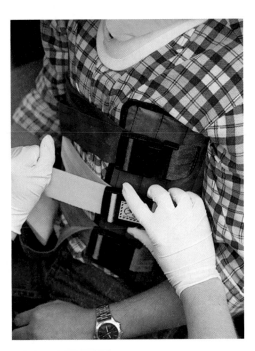

Figure 10-11 Tighten the chest straps.

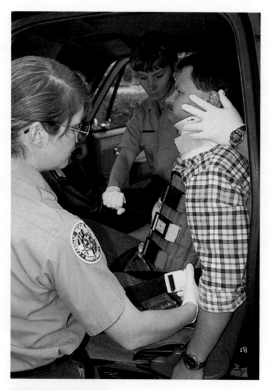

Figure 10-12

Loosen each leg strap around the ipsilateral (same side) leg and back to the buckle on the same side. Fasten snugly.

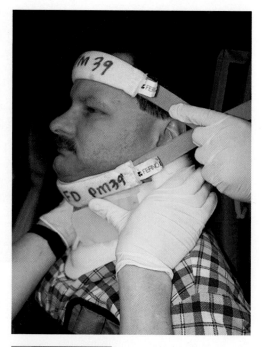

Figure 10-13

Apply firm padding as needed between the head and the headpiece to keep the head in a neutral position. Bring the head flaps around to the side of the head and secure firmly with straps, tape, or elastic wrap.

to defend your actions at a review by your Medical Director. You should perform Emergency Rescue if the Scene Size-up identifies a condition that may immediately (within seconds) endanger you and/or the patient (see Figure 10-23 on p. 160).

Examples

1. Fire or immediate danger of fire
2. Immediate danger of explosion
3. Danger of being carried away or drowned by rapidly moving water
4. Structure in immediate danger of collapse
5. Continuing immediately-life-threatening toxic exposure

Situations Requiring Rapid Extrication

You should perform Rapid Extrication if your BTLS Primary Survey of the patient identifies a critical degree of ongoing danger that requires an intervention within one to two minutes. You must act immediately and rapidly, but you have time to stabilize the patient to some degree as you extricate them.

Examples

1. Airway obstruction that you cannot relieve by jaw thrust or finger sweep
2. Cardiac or respiratory arrest
3. Chest or airway injuries requiring ventilation or assisted ventilation
4. Deep shock or bleeding that you cannot control

PROCEDURE

Technique

(These steps are illustrated in Figures 10-15 through 10-22.)

1. One rescuer must, if possible, station himself behind the patient, place his hands on either side of the patient's head, and stabilize the neck in a neutral position. This step is part of the ABCs. It is done at the same time that you begin evaluation of the airway.

2. Do a Rapid Survey; then quickly apply a cervical collar. You should have the collar with you when you begin.

3. If your BTLS Primary Survey of the patient reveals one of the situations above, go to the Rapid Extrication technique. This requires at least four, and preferably five or six, persons to perform well.

4. Immediately slide the long backboard onto the seat and, if possible, at least slightly under the patient's buttocks.

5. A second rescuer stands close beside the open door of the vehicle and takes over control of the cervical spine.

6. Rescuer 1 or another rescuer is positioned on the other side of the front seat ready to rotate the patient's legs around.

7. Another rescuer is also positioned at the open door by the patient. By holding the upper torso, he works together with the rescuer holding the legs to turn the patient carefully.

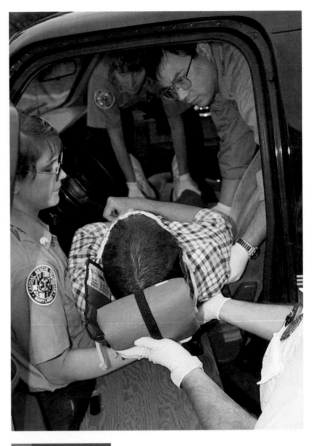

Figure 10-14

Turn the patient and the device as a unit; then lower onto a long backboard. Slide the patient and the device up into position on the board. Loosen the leg straps and allow the legs to extend out flat; then retighten the straps. Secure the patient and the device to the backboard.

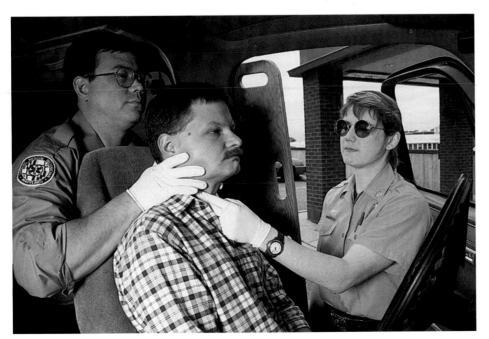

Figure 10-15

Stabilize the neck and perform the Primary Survey.

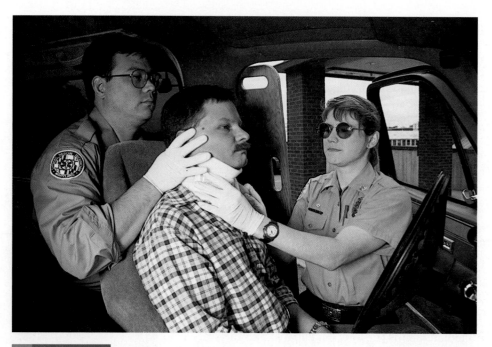

Figure 10-16 Apply a semirigid extrication collar.

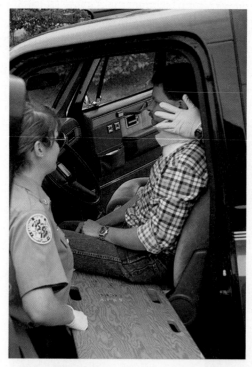

Figure 10-17 Slide the longboard onto the seat and slightly under the patient.

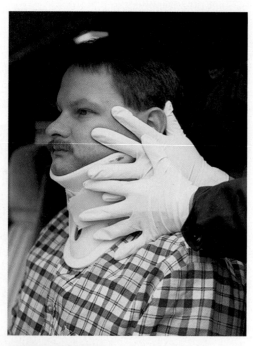

Figure 10-18 A second rescuer stands beside the open door of the vehicle and takes over control of the cervical spine.

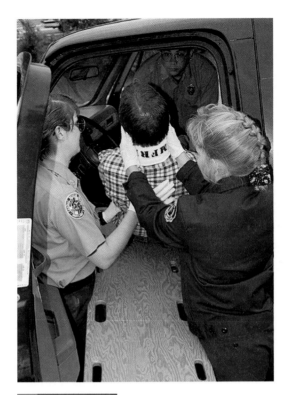

Figure 10-19 Carefully supporting the neck, torso, and legs, the rescuers turn the patient.

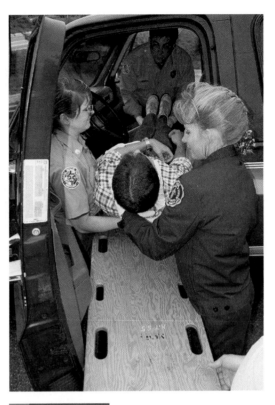

Figure 10-20 The legs are lifted and the back is lowered to the backboard.

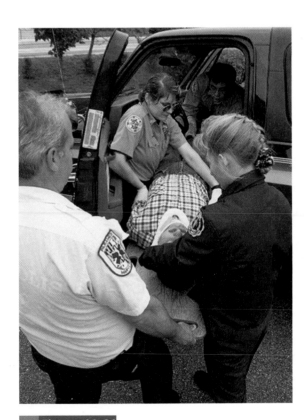

Figure 10-21

Carefully slide the patient to the full length of the backboard.

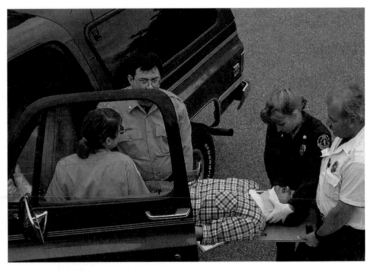

Figure 10-22 The patient is immediately moved away from the vehicle and into the ambulance, if available. Secure the patient to the backboard as soon as possible.

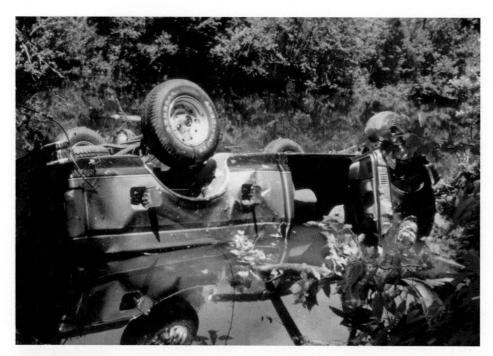

Figure 10-23 Example of a situation in which you may have to perform emergency rescue. *(Courtesy of Bonnie Meneely, EMT-P)*

8. The patient is turned so that his back is toward the backboard. His legs are lifted and his back is lowered to the backboard. The neck and back are not allowed to bend during this maneuver.

9. Using teamwork, the patient is carefully slid to the full length of the backboard and his legs are carefully straightened.

10. The patient is then moved immediately away from the vehicle (to the ambulance if available), and resuscitation is begun. He is secured to the backboard as soon as possible.

✋ PROCEDURE—SMR USING THE LONG BACKBOARD

✳ Log-Rolling the Supine Patient

(These steps are illustrated in Figures 10-24 through 10-32.)

1. Rescuer 1 stabilizes the neck in a neutral position. Do not apply traction. Grasp the patient's shoulders at the neck and gently position the patient's head between the rescuer's forearms. A semirigid extrication collar is applied. Even with the collar in place, Rescuer 1 maintains the head and neck in a neutral position until the log-rolling maneuver is completed.

2. The patient is placed with her legs extended in the normal manner and her arms (palms inward) extended by her sides. The patient will be rolled up

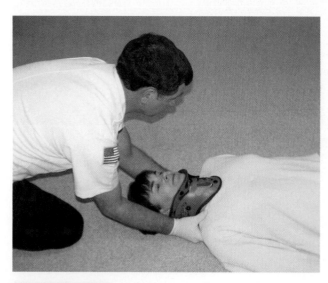

Figure 10-24 Rescuer 1 maintains the neck stabilized in a neutral position.

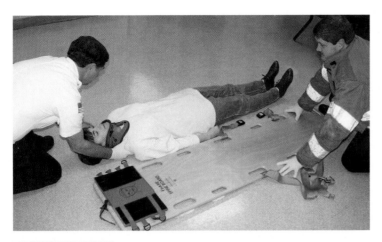

Figure 10-25 The long board is positioned beside the patient.

on one arm with that arm providing proper spacing and acting as a splint for the body.

3. The long backboard is positioned next to the body. If one arm is injured, place the backboard on the injured side so that the patient will roll upon the uninjured arm.

4. Rescuers 2 and 3 kneel at the patient's side opposite the board.

5. Rescuer 2 is positioned at the midchest area and Rescuer 3 is by the upper legs.

6. With his knees, Rescuer 2 holds the patient's near arm in place. He then reaches across the patient and grasps the shoulder and the hip, holding the patient's far arm in place. Usually, it is possible to grasp the patient's clothing to help with the roll.

7. With one hand, Rescuer 3 reaches across the patient and grasps the hip. With his other hand, he holds the feet together at the lower legs.

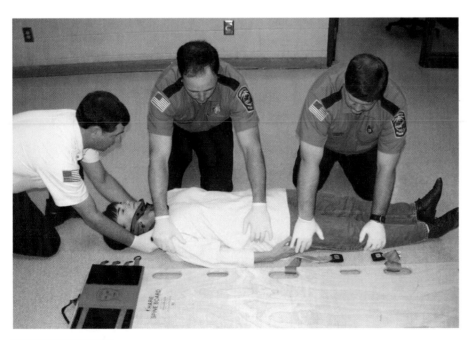

Figure 10-26 Rescuer 2 and Rescuer 3 assume their positions at the patient's side opposite the board.

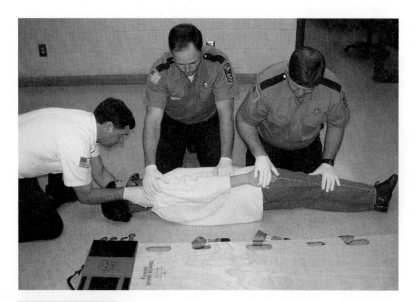

Figure 10-27 The patient is carefully rolled upon her side.

8. When everyone is ready, Rescuer 1 gives the order to log-roll the patient.

9. Rescuer 1 carefully keeps the head and neck in a neutral position (anteroposterior as well as laterally) during the roll.

10. Rescuers 2 and 3 roll the patient up on her side toward them. The patient's arms are kept locked to her side to maintain a splinting effect. The head, shoulders, and pelvis are kept in line during the log-roll.

11. When the patient is on her side, Rescuer 2 (or Rescuer 4, if available) quickly examines the back for injuries.

12. The backboard is now positioned next to the patient and held at a 30- to 45-degree angle by Rescuer 4. If there are only three rescuers, the board is pulled into place by Rescuer 2 or 3. The board is left flat in this case.

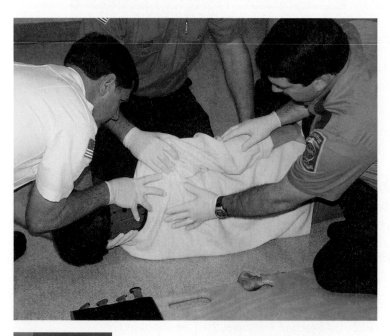

Figure 10-28 Quickly examine the back for injuries.

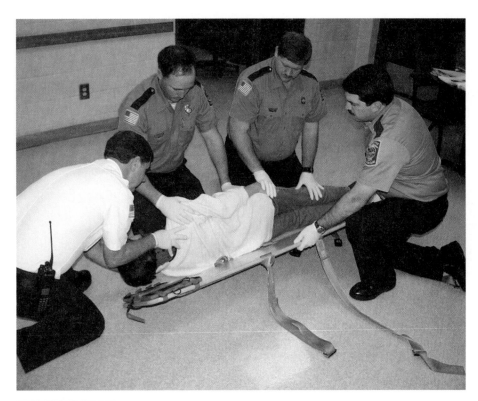

Figure 10-29 If another person is available, he positions the backboard next to the patient at a 30- to 45-degree angle.

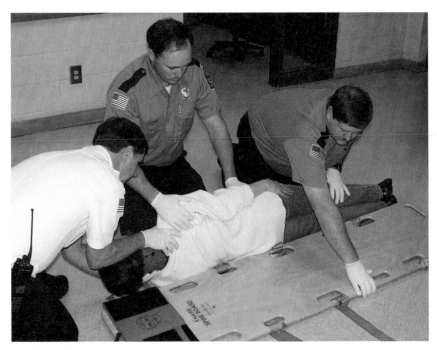

Figure 10-30 If no other help is available, Rescuer 2 or 3 positions the backboard and leaves it flat.

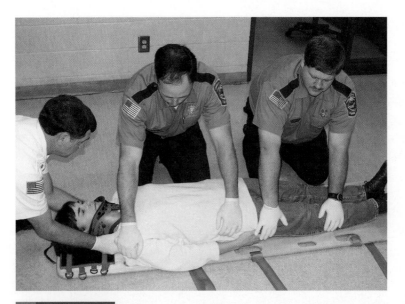

Figure 10-31 At Rescuer 1's order, the patient is rolled onto the backboard. All movements are coordinated so that the spine is kept straight at all times.

13. When everybody is ready, Rescuer 1 gives the order to log-roll the patient onto the backboard. This is accomplished by keeping head, shoulders, and pelvis in line.

Log-Rolling the Prone Patient with Airway Considerations

The status of the airway is critical for decisions on the order in which the log-rolling procedure is done. There are three clinical situations that dictate how you should proceed.

1. The patient who is not breathing or who is in severe respiratory difficulty must be log-rolled immediately to manage the airway. Unless the backboard is already positioned, you must log-roll the patient, manage the airway, and then transfer the patient to the backboard (in a second log-rolling step) when ready to transport.

2. The patient with profuse bleeding of the mouth or nose must not be turned to the supine position. Profuse upper airway bleeding in a supine patient is a guarantee of aspiration. This patient will have to have careful SMR and be transported prone or on his side, allowing gravity to help keep the airway clear. The vacuum backboard could be very useful in this situation (see Chapter 9, Figure 9-6).

3. The patient with an adequate airway and respiration should be log-rolled directly onto a backboard.

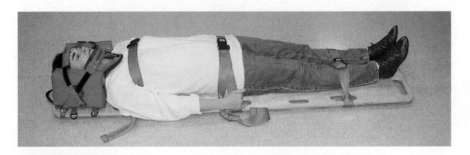

Figure 10-32 Log roll completed.

✋ PROCEDURE

❇ Log-Rolling the Prone Patient Who Has an Adequate Airway (See Figure 10-33.)

1. Rescuer 1 stabilizes the neck in a neutral position. When placing the hands on the head and neck, the rescuer's thumbs always point toward the patient's face. This prevents having the rescuer's arms crossed when the patient is log-rolled. A semirigid extrication collar is applied.

2. A BTLS Rapid Trauma Survey is done (including the back), and the patient is placed with his legs extended in the normal manner and his arms (palms inward) extended by his sides. The patient will be rolled up on one arm, with that arm acting as a splint for the body.

3. The long backboard is positioned next to the body. The backboard is placed on the side of first rescuer's lower hand (if the first rescuer's lower hand is on the patient's right side, the backboard is placed on the patient's right side). If the arm next to the backboard is injured, carefully raise the arm above the patient's head so he does not roll on the injured arm.

4. Rescuers 2 and 3 kneel at the patient's side opposite the board.

5. Rescuer 2 is positioned at the midchest area, and Rescuer 3 is by the upper legs.

6. Rescuer 2 grasps the shoulder and the hip. Usually, it is possible to grasp the patient's clothing to help with the roll.

7. Rescuer 3 grasps the hip (holding the near arm in place) and the lower legs (holding them together).

8. When everyone is ready, Rescuer 1 gives the order to log-roll the patient.

9. Rescuer 1 carefully keeps the head and neck in a neutral position (anteroposterior as well as laterally) during the roll.

10. Rescuers 2 and 3 roll the patient up on his side away from them. The patient's arms are kept locked to his side to maintain a splinting effect. The head, shoulders, and pelvis are kept in line during the roll.

11. The backboard is now positioned next to the patient and held at a 30- to 45-degree angle by Rescuer 4. If there are only three rescuers, the board is pulled into place by Rescuer 2 or 3. The board is left flat in this case.

12. When everyone is ready, Rescuer 1 gives the order to roll the patient onto the backboard. This is accomplished by keeping the head, shoulders, and pelvis in line.

When log-rolling the patient with chest or abdominal injuries, try to roll onto the uninjured side. The roll should be executed quickly enough to not compromise lung expansion. When log-rolling a patient with injures to the lower extremities, position Rescuer 2 at the feet of the patient to provide in-line support to the injured leg(s) during the log-roll. Again try to roll onto the uninjured side. The side to which you turn the patient during the log-roll procedure is not critical and can be changed in situations where you can only place the backboard on one side of the patient. The log-roll technique is useful for most trauma

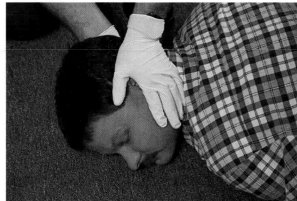

Figure 10-33

When stabilizing the neck of the prone (or supine) patient, your thumbs always point toward the face (not the occiput). This prevents having your arms crossed when the patient is rolled over.

patients, but for those patients with a fractured pelvis it may aggravate the injury to roll their weight onto the pelvis. If the pelvic fracture appears stable, the log-roll should be carefully performed, turning the patient onto the uninjured side (if it can be identified). Patients with obviously unstable pelvic fractures should not be log-rolled but rather should be lifted carefully onto a board using four or more rescuers. The scoop stretcher (see Chapter 2, Figure 2-4) is a supplemental device that may help move the patient onto the backboard when specific injuries complicate log-rolling.

Securing the Patient to the Backboard

There are several different methods of securing the patient using straps. Two examples of commercial devices for full body immobilization are the Reeves sleeve and the Miller body splint. The Reeves sleeve is a heavy-duty sleeve into which a standard backboard will slide. Attached to this sleeve are the following:

1. A head motion restriction device
2. Heavy vinyl-coated nylon panels that go over the chest and abdomen and are secured with seat belt-type straps and quick-release connectors
3. Two full-length leg panels to secure the lower extremities
4. Straps to hold the arms in place
5. Six handles for carrying the patient
6. Metal rings (2,500-lb strength) for lifting the patient by rope

When the patient is in this device, he remains immobilized when lifted horizontally, vertically, or even carried on his side (like a suitcase). This device is excellent for the confused, combative patient who must be restrained for his safety (see Figure 10-34).

The Miller body splint is a combination backboard, head immobilizer, and body immobilizer (see Chapter 9, Figure 9-7b). Like the Reeves sleeve, it does an excellent job of SMR with a minimum of time and effort.

There are several different commercial strapping systems available. As with all equipment, you should become familiar with your strapping system before using it in an emergency situation.

Figure 10-34

Patient restrained in a Reeves sleeve. Combative patients can have their arms enclosed within the panels and the straps.

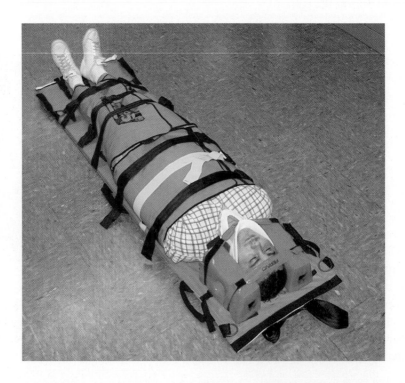

👆 PROCEDURE

✳️ Applying and Securing a Long Backboard to a Standing Patient

1. Rescuer 1 stands in front of the patient and stabilizes the head and neck in a neutral position. Rescuer 2 applies a semirigid cervical collar while Rescuer 1 continues to maintain the neck in a neutral position.

2. Rescuer 2 places a long backboard against the patient's back.

3. Rescuer 3 secures the patient to the board using nylon straps. These must include an anchor strap high on the chest as well as ones that cross over the shoulders and the pelvis and legs to prevent movement when the board is tilted down.

4. Rescuer 3 places padding behind the patient's head to maintain a neutral position, and applies and secures a blanket roll or commercial head motion restriction device using elastic wraps or wide tape.

5. Rescuers 2 and 3 carefully tilt the board back onto a stretcher and secure the legs.

Stabilizing the Head and Neck When a Neutral Position Cannot Be Attained Safely

If the head or neck is held in an angulated position and the patient complains of pain on any attempt to straighten it, you should stabilize it in the position found. The same is true of the unconscious patient whose neck is held to one side and does not easily straighten with a gentle attempt. You cannot use a cervical collar or commercial head motion restriction device in this situation. You must use pads or a blanket roll and careful taping to stabilize the head and neck in the position found.

HELMET MANAGEMENT

👆 PROCEDURE

✳️ Removing a Motorcycle Helmet from a Patient with a Possible Cervical Spine Injury (See Figure 10-35a to g.)

1. Position yourself above or behind the patient. Place your hands on each side of the helmet and stabilize the head and neck by holding the helmet and the patient's neck.

2. Your partner positions himself to the side of the patient and removes the chin strap. Chin straps can usually be removed easily without cutting them.

3. Your partner then assumes the stabilization by placing one hand under the neck and the occiput and the other hand on the anterior neck with the thumb pressing on one angle of the mandible and the index and middle fingers pressing on the other angle of the mandible.

4. You now remove the helmet by pulling out laterally on each side to clear the ears and then up to remove. Tilt full-face helmets back to clear the nose (tilt the helmet, not the head).

PEARLS

1. Patients wearing both helmets and shoulder pads usually can have their spines maintained in a more neutral position by leaving the helmet in place and padding and taping the helmet to the backboard.

2. Patients wearing helmets but no shoulder pads usually can have their spines maintained in a more neutral position by removing the helmet.

3. Face masks on helmets can be removed with screwdrivers or rescue scissors.

4. Full-face motorcycle-type helmets must be removed to evaluate and manage the airway.

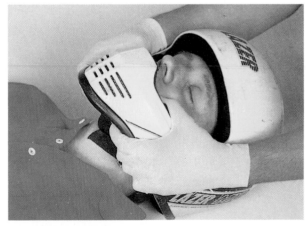

Figure 10-35a

One rescuer applies stabilization by placing hands on each side of the helmet with fingers on the patient's mandible. This prevents slippage if the strap is loose.

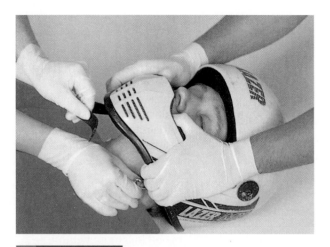

Figure 10-35b A second rescuer loosens the strap at the D-rings while stabilization is maintained.

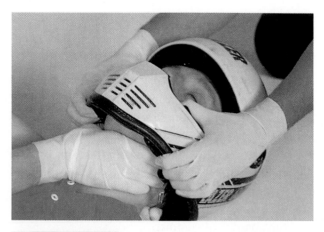

Figure 10-35c The second rescuer places one hand on the mandible at the angle, thumb on one side, long and index fingers on the other.

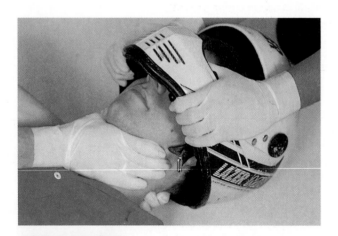

Figure 10-35d

With the other hand, the second rescuer holds the occipital region. This maneuver transfers the stabilization responsibility to the second rescuer. The rescuer at the top removes the helmet in two steps, allowing the second rescuer to readjust his hand position under the occipital region. Three factors should be kept in mind: (a) The helmet is egg-shaped and therefore must be expanded laterally to clear the head. (b) If the helmet provides full facial coverage, glasses must be removed first. (c) If the helmet provides full facial coverage, the nose will prevent removal. To clear the nose, the helmet must be tilted backward and raised over it.

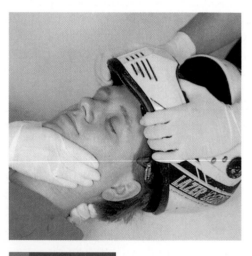

Figure 10-35e

Throughout the removal process, the second rescuer maintains in-line stabilization from below in order to prevent head tilt.

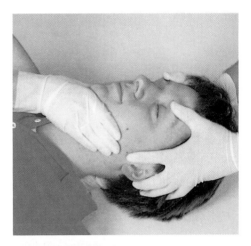

Figure 10-35f

After the helmet has been removed, the rescuer at the top replaces his hands on either side of the patient's head with his palms over the ears, taking over stabilization.

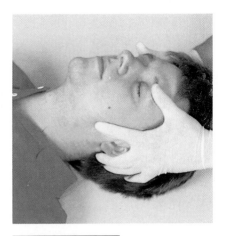

Figure 10-35g

Stabilization is maintained from above until SMR is completed.

5. If the patient is wearing glasses, remove them through the visual opening before removing the full-face helmet. Your partner maintains stabilization of the neck during this procedure.

6. After removal of the helmet, you again assume stabilization of the neck by grasping the head on either side, with your fingers holding one angle of the jaw and the occiput.

7. Your partner now applies a suitable cervical collar.

✋ PROCEDURE

✳ Alternate Procedure for Removing a Helmet (See Figure 10-36a to d.)

This has the advantage of one person maintaining stabilization of the neck throughout the whole procedure. This procedure does not work well with full-face helmets.

1. Position yourself above or behind the patient and place your hands on each side of the neck at the base of the skull. Stabilize the neck in a neutral position. If necessary, you may use your thumbs to perform a modified jaw thrust while doing this.

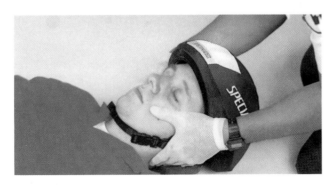

Figure 10-36a Apply steady stabilization in neutral position.

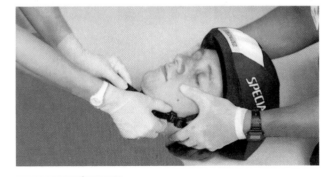

Figure 10-36b Remove the chin strap.

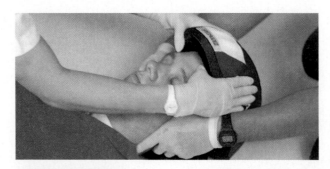

Figure 10-36c Remove the helmet by pulling gently on each side.

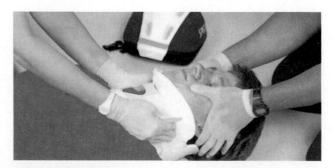

Figure 10-36d Apply a suitable cervical spine extrication collar and secure the patient to a long backboard.

2. Your partner positions himself over to the side of the patient and removes the chin strap.

3. Your partner now removes the helmet by pulling out laterally on each side to clear the ears and then up to remove. You maintain stabilization of the neck during the procedure.

4. Your partner now applies a suitable cervical collar.

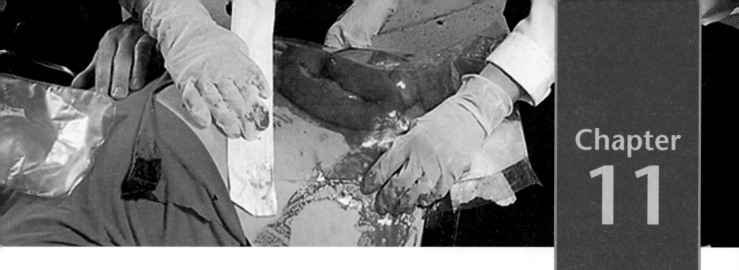

Abdominal Trauma

Arthur H. Yancey II, M.D., M.P.H., F.A.C.E.P.

Objectives

Upon completion of this chapter, you should be able to:

1. Identify the basic anatomy of the abdomen and explain how abdominal and chest injuries may be related.

2. Relate how injuries apparent on the exterior of the abdomen can damage underlying structures.

3. Differentiate between blunt and penetrating injuries and identify complications associated with each.

4. Describe possible intra-abdominal injuries based on findings of history, physical examination, and mechanism of injury.

5. Describe the treatment required for the patient with protruding viscera.

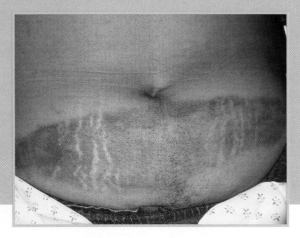

Dan, Joyce, and Buddy of the Emergency Transport System have been called to the scene of a single auto collision in which the auto ran into a tree. The single victim is still in the auto. He is restrained. What injuries would you expect from a mechanism of this type? Keep this question in mind as you read the chapter. The case study will continue at the end of the chapter.

Injury to the abdomen can be a difficult condition to evaluate even in the hospital. In the field it is usually more so. Nevertheless, since *intra-abdominal injury is the second leading cause of preventable traumatic death,* even the possibility of intra-abdominal injury must be recognized, documented, and addressed immediately. Penetrating abdominal injuries obviously need immediate surgical attention; blunt injuries may be more subtle, but potentially are just as deadly. Whether the result of blunt or penetrating trauma, abdominal injury presents two life-threatening dangers: hemorrhage and infection. Hemorrhage has immediate consequences, and thus you must be alert to the danger of early shock in all abdominal injury patients. Infection may be just as deadly, but does not require field intervention because its onset is slower.

The role of prehospital providers in the management of abdominal trauma has been the subject of some controversy. Studies in the mid-1980s demonstrated that appropriate and timely intervention by well-trained paramedics could improve the hemodynamic status of critically injured patients with wounds to the abdomen. More recent studies have suggested that pneumatic antishock garment (PASG) application and vigorous IV fluid resuscitation in the prehospital setting may do more harm than good for patients with penetrating abdominal trauma (see Chapter 7 and the bibliography for this chapter). The effects in blunt trauma are less well studied.

In the field, you need to remember rapid patient assessment and treatment of shock in order to manage the patient with abdominal trauma. These tools are important, because blood loss from an abdominal injury can be fatal if appropriate care is not rendered in a rapid and efficient fashion.

ANATOMY

The abdomen is traditionally divided into three regions: the thoracic abdomen, the true abdomen, and the retroperitoneal abdomen. The thoracic portion of the abdomen is located underneath the thin sheet muscle, the diaphragm, and is enclosed by the lower ribs (see Figure 11-1). It contains the liver, gallbladder, spleen, stomach, and transverse colon. Injury to the liver and spleen can result in life-threatening hemorrhage.

The true abdomen contains the small intestines and the bladder (see Figure 11-2). Damage to the intestines can result in infection, peritonitis, and shock. In the female, the uterus, fallopian tubes, and ovaries are considered to be part of the pelvic portion of the true abdomen.

The retroperitoneal abdomen lies behind the thoracic and true portions of the abdomen (see Figure 11-3). This area includes the kidneys, ureters, pancreas, posterior duodenum, ascending and descending colon, abdominal aorta, and the inferior vena cava. Because of its location away from the body surface, injuries here are difficult to evaluate. While hemorrhage in the true abdomen may cause the anterior abdominal wall to become distended, hemorrhage severe enough to cause shock may occur in the retroperitoneal space without this dramatic sign. In the pelvic part of the retroperitoneal abdomen are the iliac vessels. These vessels may be damaged by abdominal trauma or pelvic fracture. Injury to them can cause exsanguinating hemorrhage with few early symptoms.

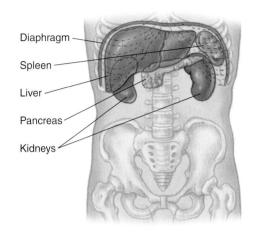

Figure 11-1 Intrathoracic abdomen.

TYPES OF INJURIES

Injuries to the abdomen are usually described as being blunt or penetrating. The penetrating group is subdivided into gunshot and stab wound categories. Blunt trauma is the most common mechanism of abdominal injury. Blunt abdominal injuries have relatively high mortality rates of 10 to 30%, usually because of the frequency of accompanying injuries to the head, chest, or an extremity(s) in as many as 70% of MVC victims. Blunt abdominal injury may be from direct compression of the abdomen, with fracture of solid organs and blowout of hollow organs, or from deceleration, with tearing of organs or their blood vessels. The patient who has suffered blunt trauma may have no pain and little external evidence of injury, which may give you a false sense of security. *Patients with multiple lower rib fractures are notorious for having severe intra-abdominal injuries without significant abdominal pain.* In this case the less noticeable abdominal pain is completely overshadowed by the severe rib pain. This patient may bleed to death because the abdomen is overlooked.

Gunshot wounds to the abdomen, as a rule, will be treated in the operating room. These patients have mortality rates of between 5 and 15%. These rates are much higher than those of stab wounds because of greater incidence of injury to abdominal viscera from the higher energy imparted to the intra-abdominal organs (see Chapter 1).

The mortality rate from abdominal stab wounds is relatively low (1–2%). Unless the knife penetrates a major vessel or organ, such as the liver or spleen, the patient may not initially appear to be in shock at the scene. However, some of these patients can develop life-threatening peritonitis over the next few hours. These wounds need to be carefully evaluated in the hospital because approximately one-third of these patients require surgery.

You should remember that the path of the penetrating object might not be readily apparent from the wound location. A stab to the chest may penetrate the abdomen, and vice versa. The course of a bullet may pass through numerous structures in different body locations. It is important to look at the patient's entire posterior surface because *penetrating trauma in the gluteal area (iliac crests to the gluteal folds, including the rectum) is associated with up to a 50% incidence of significant intra-abdominal injuries.*

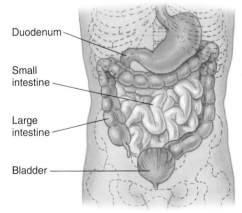

Figure 11-2 True abdomen.

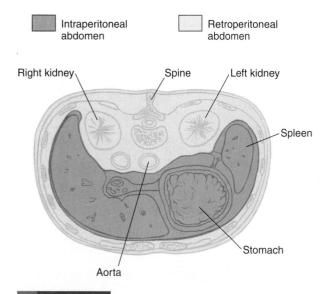

Intraperitoneal abdomen

Retroperitoneal abdomen

Right kidney   Spine   Left kidney

Spleen

Stomach

Aorta

Figure 11-3 Retroperitoneal abdomen.

In the prehospital phase, with both blunt and penetrating trauma, you must be most concerned about intra-abdominal bleeding with hemorrhagic shock.

EVALUATION AND STABILIZATION
Scene Size-Up

You can glean much important information from the scene by noting the circumstances surrounding the patient's injury. An accurate but rapid assessment of the scene will usually tip you off to the possibility of abdominal trauma. Do circumstances on the scene suggest that the victim has fallen from a height or been hit by a passing vehicle? Has there been an explosion that could have hurled the victim against immobile objects or transmitted blast pressure to organs inside the abdomen? Has the passenger of an automobile crash had the shoulder strap under the arm rather than over the shoulder? Or was the lap belt worn too high over the soft true abdomen instead of correctly across the pelvis? Any of these mechanisms can lead to penetrating or blunt abdominal injury.

If the patient was involved in a motor vehicle crash, as you do your Scene Size-up, quickly observe the damage to the vehicle, such as passenger compartment intrusion, broken windows, bent steering wheel/steering column, and location of occupants. If the patient needs to be extricated, note the location of the safety belts; although they certainly save lives, incorrectly worn safety belts can cause blunt abdominal injuries by compressing the intra-abdominal organs against the spine.

The person who is stabbed or shot may be able to give you some idea as to the size of the instrument or trajectory of the bullet. With gunshot wounds, it is also important to know the caliber, the range from which it was fired, and the number of times it was fired. A bystander or the police may be able to provide such information. When you arrive at the hospital (optimally a trauma center), be sure to report any mechanism that suggests abdominal injury. However, while at the scene, it is important not to spend a great deal of time attempting to obtain a history. *The major cause of preventable mortality in abdominal trauma is delayed diagnosis and treatment.*

Evaluation

As in treating any other traumatic condition, the patient should first undergo the BTLS Primary Survey. If shock is discovered (Chapter 7) and is not accounted for by injuries elsewhere, intra-abdominal injury must be assumed to be the cause. The essence of the prehospital abdominal examination in the Primary Survey is rapid visual evaluation and palpation. Observe the torso for deformities, contusions, abrasions, and punctures (DCAP), evisceration, and distention. Note any tenderness or tenseness. The chest is only one thin muscle sheet (the diaphragm) away from the abdominal cavity, so injury to both is not uncommon. Be mindful that splenic injury may present with left posterior shoulder pain, and liver injury may present with right posterior shoulder pain. *Distention of the abdomen should be interpreted as a sign of severe hemorrhage as should tenderness or tenseness over the abdominal wall.* Gentle palpation of the iliac crests (pelvic wings) and pubis of the pelvis may reveal the tenderness or the bony crepitus associated with fractures. Pelvic fractures frequently result in hemorrhagic shock. Signs of intra-abdominal injury usually don't appear early, so if signs of intra-abdominal injury are present in the prehospital phase, there is usually significant injury. Shock may be imminent (see Chapter 7). Abdominal tenderness or distention is an indication for immediate transport to the hospital. But remember that tenderness is an unreliable indicator of injury in a patient with an altered mental status and/or spinal injury at or above the level of the abdomen. Auscultation or percussion in the field loses critical time and little useful information is gained. Abdominal wounds should never be probed with your finger or with an instrument.

If clothing must be removed to visualize injury, try to preserve important potential legal evidence by cutting around (rather than through) areas that have signs of possible penetration.

Stabilization

Interventions should follow the protocol outlined in Chapter 2. They should proceed in the same order in which evaluation occurred: airway (**A**), breathing (**B**), and circulation (**C**). In critically injured patients, evaluation and treatment should occur simultaneously in the foregoing order. This means that even if a patient has only an abdominal injury, supplemental oxygen by mask should be delivered through a confirmed open airway. Breathing should be verified to be adequate or the patient treated to ensure adequate ven-

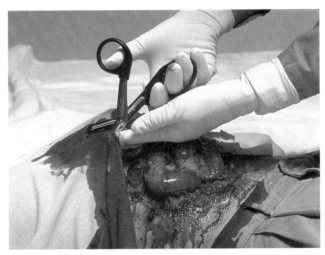

a. Remove clothing from around the abdominal wound.

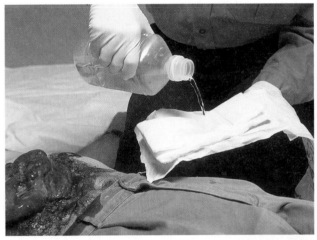

b. Cover the wound with a sterile dressing soaked with normal saline.

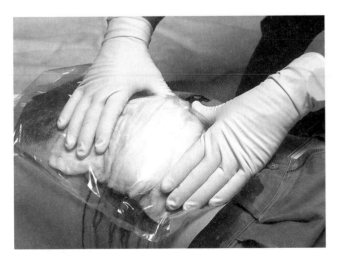

c. Cover the moistened dressing with a sterile occlusive dressing to prevent evaporative drying.

Figure 11-4   Evisceration care.

tilation. Then, and only then, should the consequences of any abdominal injury be addressed as part of the circulation assessment.

Apply oxygen at 12 to 15 L/min by mask or at 5 L/min by nasal cannula (see Chapter 4). The patient should be readied for rapid transport.

If the system in which you practice allows the use of the PASG, these may be placed on the patient but inflated only after consultation with on-line Medical Direction. The more critically ill the patient, the more important it is to transport the patient early and apply the PASG en route. Gently cover any organ or viscera protruding from a wound with gauze moistened with saline or water. If you have a long transport time, you can apply a nonadherent material, such as plastic wrap or aluminum foil, to prevent drying of the gauze and intestines (see Figure 11-4). If the intestines are allowed to dry, they may become irreversibly damaged. Do not ever push any abdominal contents protruding from a wound back into the abdomen. Similarly, if a foreign body (e.g., knife, glass shard) is impaled in the abdomen, do not attempt removal or manipulation. Carefully stabilize the object in place without moving it. Pregnant patients deserve the special considerations addressed in Chapter 17.

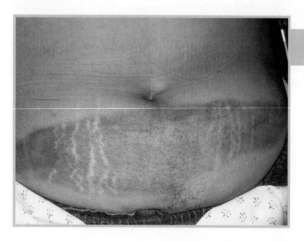

CASE STUDY

Dan, Joyce, and Buddy of the Emergency Transport System have been called to the scene of a single auto collision in which the auto ran into a tree. As they respond they decide that Joyce will act as team leader. They prepare for a patient with chest, abdomen, extremity, or spinal injuries. Upon their arrival they find the police and a local rescue squad already on-scene. The scene is safe. There is only one victim. The victim was driving an old truck without shoulder straps or airbags. He did have his lap belt on when he lost control on a curve and ran out of the road, striking a tree. There was significant impact, with the truck engine being pushed back almost to the passenger compartment. The ETS team helps the rescue squad extricate the patient from the vehicle.

The patient is awake but has the odor of an alcoholic beverage on his breath and is obviously confused. He does follow commands and is able to move his hands and feet before they begin extrication. They use a short backboard device and they extricate him onto a long backboard, where he is secured. As they are extricating him, they note that there are no obvious injuries to the back. Initial Assessment reveals an obese young white male who is awake but confused. He is talking and has an open airway. His breathing is somewhat labored and he complains of pain when he breathes. He has a strong but rapid pulse at the wrist. Joyce identifies him as a load-and-go patient because of the mechanism along with altered mental status and tachycardia. She performs a Rapid Trauma Assessment while Buddy applies a non-rebreathing oxygen mask and has suction ready in case the patient vomits. The airway is clear with no obvious trauma to the head or neck. Breath sounds are present but decreased on the left side. There is no obvious chest trauma. The abdomen has a large bruise from the seat belt and is diffusely tender. There are no obvious extremity injuries.

After transferring the patient to the ambulance, Joyce performs a brief neurological exam (patient awake but confused, eyes open spontaneously, and he obeys commands = GCS 14). She also performs vital signs. Blood pressure 140/90, pulse 130, respiration 30, and pulse oximeter reading is 93% on 100% oxygen. The patient complains of abdominal and chest pain and states he thinks a deer ran in front of his truck and he lost control trying to miss it. He has no allergies, takes no medications, has no past history of serious illness, and he ate two hamburgers and drank "three" beers just before the collision.

Joyce reports to Medical Direction and is instructed to take the patient to the local level II trauma center. Detailed exam reveals no other injuries but Joyce thinks she can hear bowel sounds in the left chest. Before arrival (20 minute transport time) the patient becomes pale and diaphoretic and his blood pressure drops to 70/40. Upon arrival at the trauma center he is taken directly to surgery where he is found to have a diaphragmatic hernia on the left as well as a ruptured spleen and a contusion of the liver. After a stormy course complicated by delirium tremens, he eventually survives to drink and drive again.

CASE STUDY WRAP-UP

A deceleration motor vehicle collision can cause injuries to almost any system, but patients wearing only a lap belt are prone to compression fractures of the lumber spine (clasp-knife effect). The lap belt is prone to cause intra-abdominal injuries if it is worn across the abdomen rather than across the pelvis. Sudden compression of the abdomen can cause rupture of the diaphragm and herniation of abdominal contents into the chest. This usually occurs on the left because the large mass of the liver protects the right side. Anyone with significant abdominal trauma is subject to develop hemorrhagic shock, so always be prepared.

SUMMARY

Effective prehospital management of the patient with abdominal trauma entails:

1. Scene size-up for mechanisms and pertinent history from the patient and/or witnesses
2. Rapid patient assessment
3. Rapid transport to the appropriate hospital (optimally, a trauma center)
4. Other interventions as needed (usually performed en route)

The enemies of the abdominal trauma patient are bleeding and time elapsed from injury until optimal care. If you can minimize on-scene delays, you will help to maximize the patient's chance for survival.

BIBLIOGRAPHY

1. Aprahamian, C., B. M. Thompson, J. B. Towne, and others. "The Effect of a Paramedic System on Mortality of Major Open Intra-Abdominal Vascular Trauma." *Journal of Trauma,* Vol. 23 (1983), pp. 687–690.

2. Bickell, W. H., M. J. Wall, P. E. Pepe, and others. "Immediate Versus Delayed Fluid Resuscitation for Hypotensive Patients with Penetrating Torso Injury." *New England Journal of Medicine,* Vol. 331 (October 1994), pp. 1105–1109.

3. Mattox, K. L., W. H. Bickell, P. E. Pepe, and others. "Prospective MAST Study in 911 Patients." *Journal of Trauma,* Vol. 29 (1989), pp. 1104–1112.

4. Pons, P. T., B. Honigman, C. E. Moore, and others. "Prehospital Advanced Trauma Life Support for Critical Penetrating Wounds to the Thorax and Abdomen." *Journal of Trauma,* Vol. 25 (1985), pp. 828–832.

Extremity Trauma

John E. Campbell, M.D., F.A.C.E.P.

Chapter

12

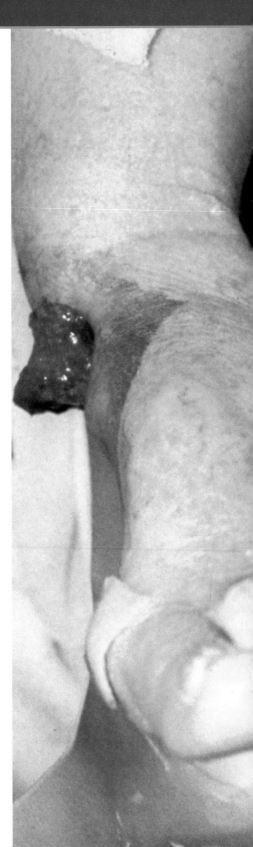

Objectives

Upon completion of this chapter, you should be able to:

1. Prioritize extremity trauma in the assessment and management of life-threatening injuries.

2. Discuss the major complications and treatment of the following extremity injuries:
   a. Fractures
   b. Dislocations
   c. Amputations
   d. Open wounds
   e. Neurovascular injuries
   f. Sprains and strains
   g. Impaled objects
   h. Compartment syndrome

3. Estimate blood loss from pelvic and extremity fractures.

4. Discuss major mechanisms of injury, associated trauma, potential complications, and management of injury to the following areas:
   a. Pelvis
   b. Femur
   c. Hip
   d. Knee
   e. Tibia/fibula
   f. Clavicle and shoulder
   g. Elbow
   h. Forearm and wrist
   i. Hand or foot

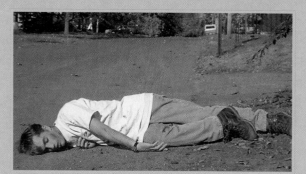

D an, Joyce, and Buddy of the Emergency Transport System have been called to the scene of an auto–pedestrian collision. They are told that the pedestrian is unconscious. What injuries should they expect with a mechanism of this type? Are head and spinal injuries likely? Keep these questions in mind as you read. The case study will continue at the end of the chapter.

You must never let distorted or wounded extremities occupy your attention when there may be more life-threatening injuries present. These dramatic injuries are easy to identify when you first encounter the patient and may be disabling, but are rarely immediately life-threatening. It is important to remember that the movement of air through the airway, the mechanics of breathing, the maintenance of circulating blood volume, and the appropriate treatment of shock always come before the splinting of any fracture.

Hemorrhagic shock is a potential danger of very few musculoskeletal injuries. Only direct lacerations of arteries or fractures of the pelvis or femur are commonly associated with enough bleeding to cause shock. Injuries to the nerves or vessels that serve the hands and feet are the most common complications of fractures and dislocations. Such injuries cause the loss of function that we lump under the term *neurovascular compromise*. Thus, evaluation of sensation and circulation (PMS: pulse, motor, and sensation) distal to fractures is very important.

INJURIES TO EXTREMITIES
Fractures

Fractures may be open (compound) with the broken end of the bone still protruding or having once protruded through the skin (see lead photo in chapter), or they may be closed (simple) with no communication to the outside (see Figure 12-1). Fractured bone ends are extremely sharp and are quite dangerous to all the tissues that surround the bone. Since nerves and arteries frequently travel near the bone, across the flexor side of joints, or very near the skin (hands and feet), they are frequently injured. Such neurovascular injuries may be due to lacerations from bone fragments or from pressure due to swelling or hematomas.

Closed fractures can be just as dangerous as open fractures because injured soft tissues often bleed profusely. It is important to remember that any break in the skin near a fractured bone may be considered to be an opening for contamination.

A closed fracture of one femur can cause the loss of up to a liter of blood; thus, two fractured femurs can cause life-threatening hemorrhage (see Figure 12-2). A fractured pelvis can cause extensive bleeding into the abdomen or the retroperitoneal space. The pelvis usually fractures in several places and may have 500 cc of blood loss for each fracture. Pelvic fractures may lacerate the bladder or the large pelvic blood vessels. Either of these structures can cause fatal hemorrhage into the abdomen. Remember, multiple fractures can cause life-threatening hemorrhage without any *external* blood loss.

Open fractures add the dangers of contamination as well as loss of blood outside the body. If protruding bone ends are pulled back into the skin when the limb is aligned, bacteria-contaminated debris will be pulled into the wound. Infection from such debris may prevent healing of the bone and may even cause death from septic complications.

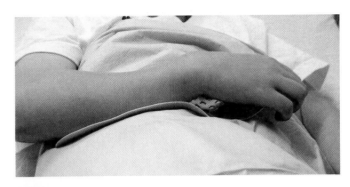

Figure 12-1 Closed forearm fracture. *(Photo courtesy of Roy Alson, M.D.)*

Dislocations

Joint dislocations are extremely painful injuries. They are almost always easy to identify because normal anatomy is distorted (see Figure 12-3). Major joint dislocations, though not life-threatening, are often true emergencies because of the neurovascular compromise that can, if not treated quickly, lead to amputation. It is impossible to know whether a fracture exists in combination with a dislocation. It is very important to check for PMS distal to major joint dislocations. Ordinarily, you splint injuries in the position you find them. There are certain exceptions to this rule. It is universally true, however, that one can apply only *gentle* traction to any distorted extremity in an effort to straighten it. In the few instances that you would use traction to straighten, use no more than 10 pounds of force. Most often the best treatment for the patient is padding and splinting the extremity in the most comfortable position and rapidly transporting to a facility that has orthopedic care available.

Amputations

These are disabling and sometimes life-threatening injuries. They have the potential for massive hemorrhage, but most often, the bleeding will control itself quite readily with ordinary pressure applied to the stump. The stump should be covered with a damp sterile dressing and an elastic wrap that will apply uniform, reasonable pressure across the entire stump. If bleeding absolutely cannot be controlled with pressure, a tourniquet may be used. In general, a tourniquet is to be avoided whenever possible.

You should make an effort to find the amputated part and bring it with you. This sometimes neglected detail can have serious future implications for the patient, since parts can frequently be used for graft material. Reimplantation is attempted only in very

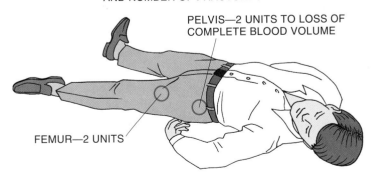

ESTIMATING BLOOD LOSS BY SITE
AND NUMBER OF FRACTURES

PELVIS—2 UNITS TO LOSS OF
COMPLETE BLOOD VOLUME

FEMUR—2 UNITS

THE MOST SEVERE BLOOD LOSS OCCURS IN
FRACTURE OF THE PELVIS

Figure 12-2 Internal blood loss from fractures.

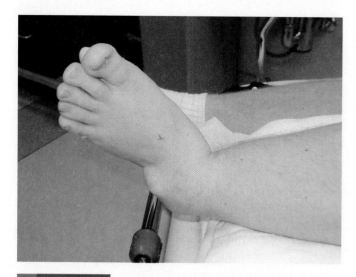

Figure 12-3 Ankle dislocation. *(Photo courtesy of Roy Alson, M.D.)*

limited situations. For this reason, you should not suggest to the patient that reimplantation will be done. Small amputated parts should be placed in a plastic bag (see Figure 12-4). If ice is available, place the bag in a larger bag or container containing ice and water. *Do not use ice alone and never use dry ice.* Cooling the part slows the chemical processes and will increase the viability from 4 hours to up to 18 hours. It is important to bring amputated parts even if reimplantation appears to be impossible.

Open Wounds

Cover wounds with a sterile dressing and bandage carefully. Gross contamination such as leaves or gravel should be removed from the wound, and smaller pieces of contamination can be irrigated from the wound with a normal saline drip in the same manner that you would irrigate a chemically contaminated eye. Bleeding can almost always be stopped with pressure dressings or pneumatic splints. Tourniquets should almost never be used to stop bleeding from a wound if amputation is not present. If necessary, a blood pressure cuff or pressure on a larger artery proximal to the injury may be appropriate.

Neurovascular Injuries

The nerves and major blood vessels generally run beside each other, usually in the flexor area of the major joints. They may be injured together, and loss of circulation and/or sensation can be due to disruption, swelling, or compression by bone fragments or hematomas. Foreign bodies or broken bone ends may well impinge on delicate structures and cause them to malfunction. Always check for PMS before and after any extremity manipulation, application of splint, or traction.

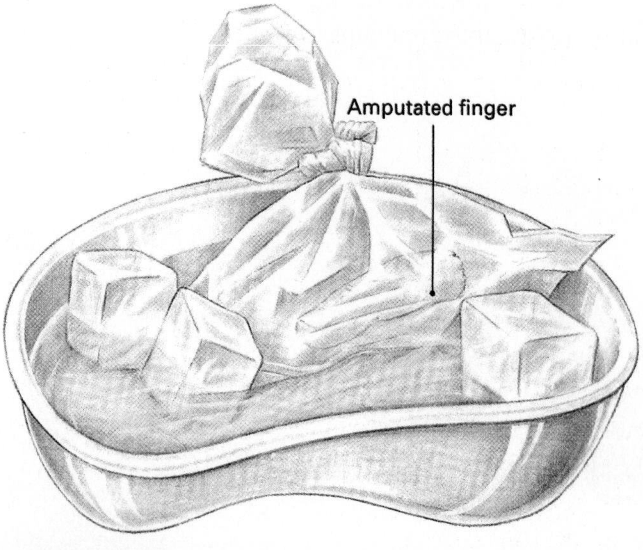

Amputated finger

Figure 12-4 Amputated parts should be put in a dry bag, sealed, and placed in water that contains a few ice cubes.

Sprains and Strains

These injuries cannot be differentiated from fractures in the field. Treat them as though they were fractures.

Impaled Objects

Do not remove impaled objects. Apply a very bulky type of padding to hold the object in place and transport the patient with the object in place. The skin is a pivot point in these cases, and any motion outside the body is translated or magnified within the tissues, where the end of the object may lacerate or harm sensitive structures. The cheek of the face is the exception to this rule because you can reach inside the mouth to put pressure on the bleeding.

Compartment Syndrome

The extremities contain muscle tissue in closed spaces that are surrounded by tough membranes that will not stretch. Trauma (crush injuries, closed or open fracture, or sustained compression) to these areas (forearm and lower leg most commonly) may cause bleeding and swelling within the closed spaces. As the area swells, pressure is transmitted to the blood vessels and nerves. This pressure may compress the blood vessels in such a manner that circulation is impossible. The nerves may also be compromised. These injuries usually develop over a period of hours. Late symptoms are the five Ps: pain, pallor, pulselessness, paresthesia, and paralysis. *The early symptoms are usually pain and paresthesia.* As with shock, you should think of this diagnosis before the later symptoms develop.

ASSESSMENT AND MANAGEMENT

Scene Size-Up and History

In extremity trauma, it is especially important to get a history because the apparent mechanism of injury and the condition of the extremity when you first arrive may give you important information on the severity of the injury. If you have enough rescuers, one rescuer can obtain the history while you are performing the BTLS Primary Survey. If not, you should not attempt to elicit a detailed verbal history until you have assessed the status of the airway, breathing, and circulation. In the conscious patient, you should obtain most of the history at the end of the Primary Survey.

Foot injuries from long jumps (falls landing on the feet) often have lumbar spine injuries associated with them. Any injury to the knee when the patient is in the sitting position may have associated injuries to the hip. In a like manner, hip injuries may refer pain to the knee, so the knee and the hip are intimately connected and must be evaluated together rather than separately. Falls onto the wrist frequently injure the elbow, and so the wrist and elbow must be evaluated together. The same is true of the ankle and the proximal fibula of the outside of the lower leg.

Any injury that appears to be in the shoulder must be carefully examined because it may easily involve either the neck, chest, or shoulder. Fractures of the pelvis are usually associated with very large amounts of blood loss. Whenever a fracture in the pelvis is identified, shock must be suspected and proper treatment begun.

ASSESSMENT

During the BTLS Primary Survey, you are concerned with obvious fractures to the pelvis and large bones of the extremities. You should also find and control major bleeding from the extremities.

During the Detailed Exam, you should quickly assess the full length of each extremity, looking for deformity, contusions, abrasions, penetrations, burns, tenderness, lacerations, and swelling (DCAP-BTLS). Feel for instability and crepitation (see chapters 2 and 3). Check the joints for pain and movement. Check and record distal PMS. Pulses may be marked with ballpoint pen to identify the area in which the pulse is best felt (see Figure 12-5). *Crepitation or grating of bone ends is a definite sign of fracture, and once identified, the bone ends should be immediately immobilized to prevent further soft tissue injury.* Checking for crepitation should be done *very gently*, especially when checking the pelvis. Crepitation means bone ends are grating on one another, and this means you are causing further tissue injury.

Management of Extremity Injuries

Proper management of fractures and dislocations will decrease the incidence of pain, disability, and serious complications. Treatment in the prehospital setting is directed at proper immobilization of the injured part by the use of an appropriate splint.

Purpose of Splinting: The objective is to prevent motion in the broken bone ends. The nerves that cause the most pain in a fractured extremity lie in the membrane surrounding

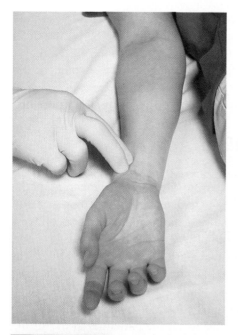

Figure 12-5a Palpate the radial artery. *(Photo courtesy of Michael Heron)*

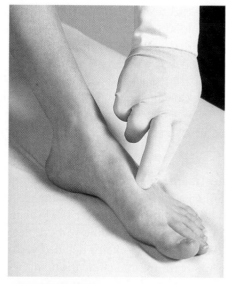

Figure 12-5b Palpate the dorsalis pedis pulse. *(Photo courtesy of Michael Heron)*

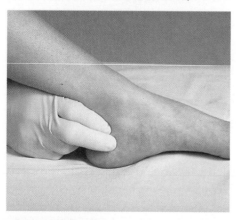

Figure 12-5c Palpate the posterior tibial pulse. *(Photo courtesy of Michael Heron)*

the bone. The broken bone ends irritate these nerves, causing a very deep and distressing type of pain. Splinting not only decreases pain, but also eliminates further damage to muscles, nerves, and blood vessels by preventing further motion of the broken bone ends.

When to Splint: There is no simple rule that determines the precise sequence to follow in every trauma patient. In general, the seriously injured patient will be better off if only splinting of the spine (long backboard) is done before transport. The patient who requires a load-and-go approach can have extremity fractures temporarily immobilized by careful packaging on the long backboard. This does not mean that you have no responsibility for identifying and protecting extremity fractures, but implies that it is better to do some splinting in the vehicle en route to the hospital. It is never appropriate to sacrifice time immobilizing a limb to prevent *disability*, when that time may be needed to save the patient's *life*. Conversely, if the patient appears to be stable, extremity fractures should be splinted before moving the patient.

✋ PROCEDURE

❊ Rules of Splinting

1. You must adequately visualize the injured part. Clothes should be cut off, not pulled off, unless there is only an isolated injury that presents no problem with maintaining immobilization.

2. Check and record distal sensation and circulation before and after splinting. Check movement distal to the fracture if possible (e.g., ask the conscious patient to wiggle his fingers or observe the motion of the unconscious patient when a painful stimulus is applied). Pulses may be marked with a pen to identify where they were last palpated.

3. If the extremity is severely angulated and pulses are absent, you should apply gentle traction in an attempt to straighten it (see Figure 12-6). This traction should never exceed 10 pounds of pressure. If resistance is encountered, splint the extremity in the angulated position. When you are attempting to straighten an extremity, it is very important to be honest with yourself with regard to resistance. It takes very little force to lacerate the wall of a vessel or to interrupt the blood supply to a large nerve. If the trauma center is near, always splint in the position found.

4. Open wounds should be covered with a sterile dressing before you apply the splint. Splints should always be applied on the side of the extremity away from open wounds to prevent pressure necrosis.

5. Use the splint that will immobilize one joint above and below the injury.

6. Pad the splint well. This is particularly true if there is any skin defect or if bony prominences might press against a hard splint.

7. Do not attempt to push bone ends back under the skin. If you apply traction and the bone end retracts back into the wound, do not increase the amount of traction. You should not use your hands or any tools to try to pull the bone ends back out, but be sure to notify the receiving physician. Carefully pad bone ends with bandages before applying pneumatic splints to the lower extremities. The healing of bone is improved if the bone ends are kept moist when transport time is prolonged.

8. In a life-threatening situation, injuries may be splinted while the patient is being transported. When the patient appears stable, splint all injuries before moving the patient.

9. If in doubt, splint a possible injury.

Types of Splints

Rigid Splint: This type of splint can be made from many different materials and includes all cardboard, hard plastic, metal, or wooden types of splints. The type of splint that is made rigid by evacuating air from a moldable splint (vacuum splint) is also classified as a rigid splint. Rigid splints should be padded well and should always extend one joint above and below the fracture.

Soft Splint: This type includes air splints, pillows, and sling- and swathe-type splints. Air splints are good for fractures of the lower arm and lower leg. The pneumatic antishock garment (PASG or MAST) is an excellent air splint (blow up only to air-splint pressures). Air splints have the advantage of compression, which helps to slow bleeding, but they have the disadvantage of increasing pressure as the temperature rises or the altitude increases. *They should not be put on angulated fractures* since they will automatically apply straightening pressure.

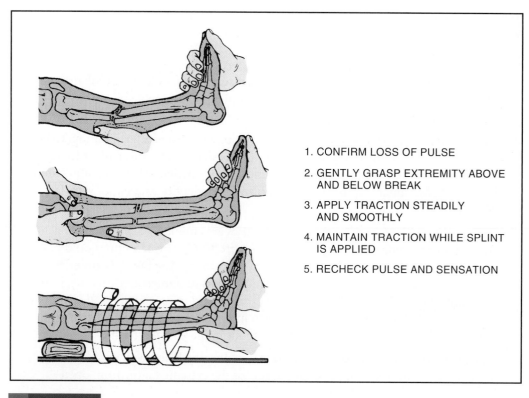

1. CONFIRM LOSS OF PULSE

2. GENTLY GRASP EXTREMITY ABOVE AND BELOW BREAK

3. APPLY TRACTION STEADILY AND SMOOTHLY

4. MAINTAIN TRACTION WHILE SPLINT IS APPLIED

5. RECHECK PULSE AND SENSATION

Figure 12-6 Straightening angulated fractures to restore pulses.

Other major disadvantages of air splints include the fact that the extremity pulses cannot be monitored while the splint is in place; the splints also often stick to the skin and are painful to remove.

Inflating the splints requires you to blow the splints up by mouth or by hand or foot pump (never by compressed air) until they give good support and yet *can easily be dented with slight pressure from a fingertip.* When using air splints, you must constantly check the pressure to be sure that the splint is not getting too tight or too loose (they often leak).

Remember that if air splints are applied in a cold environment and the patient is moved into the warm environment of the ambulance, the pressure will increase as the splints warm up. Where air ambulances are available, it must be remembered that the pressure in air splints increases if they are applied on the ground and then subsequently the patient is airlifted to the hospital. Also remember that if pressure is released during the flight, the pressure will be too low when the patient is returned to the ground.

Pillows make good splints for injuries to the ankle or foot. They are also helpful, along with a sling and a swathe, to stabilize a dislocated shoulder.

Slings and swathes are excellent for injuries to the clavicle, shoulder, upper arm, elbow, and sometimes the forearm. They utilize the chest wall as a solid foundation and splint the arm against the chest wall. Some shoulder injuries cannot be brought close to the chest wall without significant force being applied. In these instances, pillows are used to bridge the gap between the chest wall and the upper arm.

Traction Splint: This device is designed for fractures of the femur. It holds the fracture immobile by the application of a steady pull on the ankle while applying countertraction to the ischium and the groin. This steady traction overcomes the tendency of the very strong thigh muscles to spasm. If traction is not applied, the pain worsens because the bone ends tend to impact or override. Traction also prevents free motion of the ends of the femur, which could lacerate the femoral nerve, artery, or vein. There are many designs and types of splints available to apply traction to the lower extremity (see Figure 12-7a–c), but each must be carefully padded and applied with care to prevent excessive pressure on the soft tissues around the pelvis. It is also necessary to use a great deal of care in applying the ankle hitch so as not to interfere with the circulation of the foot. Many of these devices can be used with a buck's boot as an alternative to the ankle hitch.

Management of Specific Injuries

Spine: This is covered elsewhere in the book but included here to remind you that if there is any chance of spinal injury, proper SMR must be done to prevent lifelong paralysis or even death from a spinal cord injury. In the most urgent cases, careful packaging of the patient on the long backboard may be adequate splinting for a number of different extremity injuries. Remember that certain mechanisms of injury, such as a fall from a height in which the patient lands on both feet, may cause lumbar spine fracture because forces are transmitted all the way up the body.

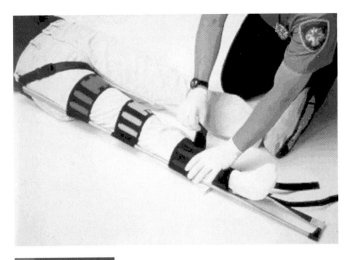

Figure 12-7a Kendrick traction device. *(Photo courtesy of Eduardo Romero Hicks, M.D.)*

Pelvis: It is practical to include injuries to the pelvis with extremities because they are frequently associated. Pelvic injuries are usually caused by motor vehicle accidents or by severe trauma such as falls from heights. *They are identified by gentle pressure being placed on the iliac crests, hips, and pubis during the patient survey.* There is always the potential for serious hemorrhage in pelvic fractures, so shock should be expected and the patient rapidly transported (load-and-go). Internal bleeding from unstable pelvic fractures can be decreased by circumferential stabilization of the pelvis. The PASG or slings made from sheets have been used in the past but there is now a commercially available pelvic sling that, when tightened, signals when the correct stabilizing pressure is reached (see Figure 12-8). The patient with a pelvic injury should always be transported on a backboard. The

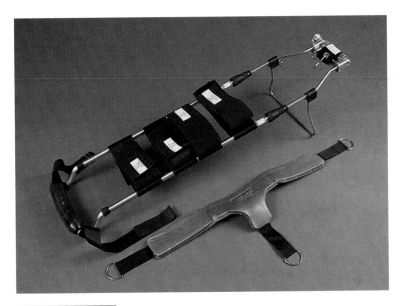

Figure 12-7b Hare traction splint.

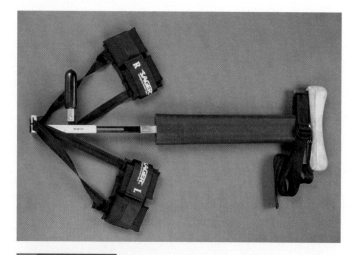

Figure 12-7c Sager traction splint.

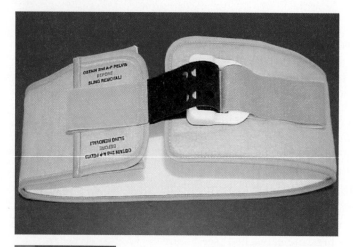

Figure 12-8a Commercial pelvic sling device. *(Photo courtesy of Sam Splints)*

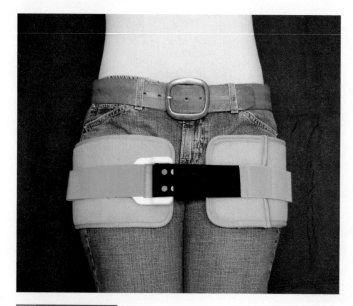

Figure 12-8b Pelvic sling applied. *(Photo courtesy of Sam Splints)*

vacuum backboard is especially useful here because it is much more comfortable than the hard backboard. Log-rolling a patient with an unstable pelvic fracture can aggravate the injury. Scoop stretchers (see Figure 2-4 on page 33) or adequate manpower is needed to move these patients to the backboard.

Femur: The femur usually fractures at the midshaft, although hip fractures are quite common. These fractures may have open wounds associated with them and, if so, they must be presumed to be open fractures. There is a lot of muscle tissue surrounding the femur, and when spasm develops after a femur fracture the bone ends tend to override, causing more muscle damage. Because of this, tractions splints are usually used to stabilize the fracture and prevent shortening. Because of the large muscle mass, a great deal of bleeding can occur into the tissue of the thigh. Bilateral femur fractures can be associated with a loss of up to 50% of the circulating blood volume. The PASG can be used with a traction splint with the air pressure of the PASG decreasing the internal bleeding around the femur fracture (see procedure for applying traction splint and PASG in Chapter 13).

Hip: Hip fractures are most often in the narrow "neck" of the femur, where strong ligaments may occasionally allow this type of fracture to bear weight. The ligaments are very strong, and there is very little movement of the bone ends in the most frequent type of hip fracture.

You must consider hip fractures in any elderly person who has fallen and has pain in the knee, hip, or pelvic region. This type of presentation and pain should be considered a fracture until an x-ray proves otherwise. In this age group, pain is frequently well tolerated and sometimes even ignored or denied. In general, the tissues in the elderly patient are more delicate, and less force is required to disrupt a given structure. Always remember that in the child and in the elderly patient, isolated knee pain may well be coming from damage to the hip. Do not use a traction splint for a hip fracture.

Hip dislocation is a different story. Most hip dislocations are a result of the knees being struck by the dashboard, forcing the relatively loose, relaxed hip out of the posterior side of its cup in the pelvis (see Figure 12-9). Thus, any patient in a severe automobile accident with a knee injury must have the hip examined very carefully. Hip dislocation is an orthopedic emergency and requires reduction as soon as possible to prevent sciatic nerve injury or necrosis of the femoral head due to interrupted blood supply. This is a very difficult reduction to perform because the amount of force required is very great and the movement must be quite precise.

The dislocated hip will usually be flexed, and the patient will not be able to tolerate having the leg straightened. The leg will almost invariably be rotated toward the midline. A posterior hip dislocation should be supported in the most comfortable position by the use of pillows and by splinting to the uninjured leg (see Figure 12-10). This patient requires rapid transport.

Knee: Fractures or dislocation of the knee (see Figure 12-11a and b) are quite serious because the arteries are bound down above and below the knee joint and are often bruised or lacerated if the joint is in an abnormal position. There is no way to know whether a fracture exists in an abnormally positioned knee and, in either case, the decision must be based on the circulation and neurological function below the knee in the foot. Some authorities state that about 50% of knee dislocations have associated injuries to the vessels, and many knee injuries later require amputation. It is important to restore the circulation below the knee whenever possible.

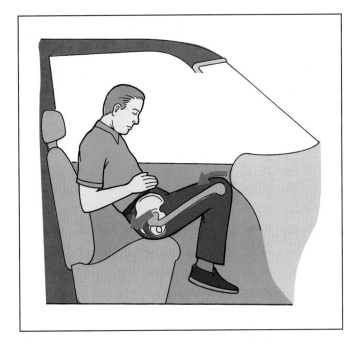

Figure 12-9 Mechanism of posterior dislocation of the hip, "down and under."

Prompt reduction of knee dislocation is very important. If there is loss of pulse or sensation, you should apply gentle traction that may be by hand or by a traction splint. You must be careful to apply *no more than 10 pounds of force.* This force must be applied along the long axis of the leg. If there is resistance to straightening the knee, splint it in the most comfortable position and transport the patient rapidly. This may be considered to be a true orthopedic emergency.

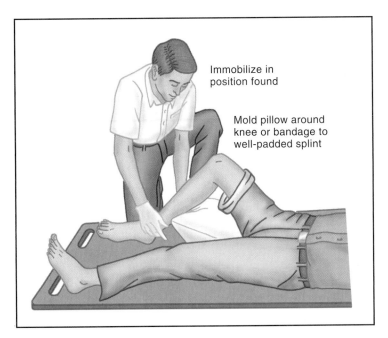

Immobilize in position found

Mold pillow around knee or bandage to well-padded splint

Figure 12-10 Splinting posterior dislocation of the hip.

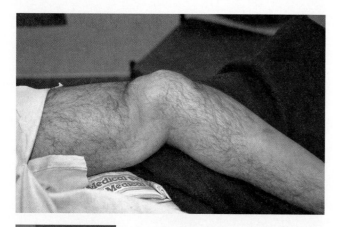
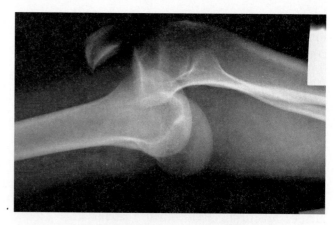

Figure 12-11 Knee dislocation: (a) presentation of a knee dislocation; (b) x-ray of the dislocation.

Tibia/Fibula: Fractures of the lower leg are often open due to thin skin over the front of the tibia and often have significant internal and/or external blood loss. Internal blood loss can interrupt the circulation to the foot if a compartment syndrome develops. It is rarely possible for patients to bear weight on fractures of the tibia, but fractures of the distal fibula are frequently mistaken for sprains. Fractures of the lower tibia/fibula may be splinted with a rigid splint, an air splint, or a pillow (see Figure 12-12). Pneumatic splints will adequately splint upper tibia fractures. Here again it is important to dress any wound and pad any bone ends that may be put under an air splint or PASG.

Clavicle: This, the most frequently fractured bone in the body, rarely causes problems (see Figure 12-13). It is best immobilized with a sling and swathe. Rarely, there may be injuries to the subclavian vein and artery or to the nerves of the arm when this area is injured. It is also very important that the ribs and chest be very carefully evaluated whenever an injury to the shoulder or clavicle is discovered.

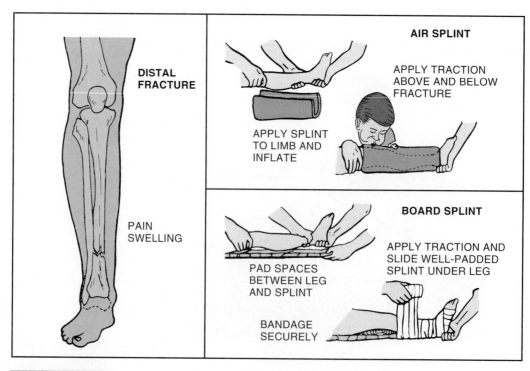

Figure 12-12 Splinting lower leg fractures with splint or board splint.

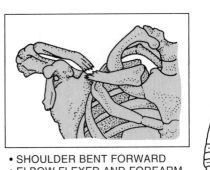

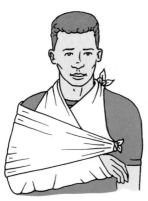

- SHOULDER BENT FORWARD
- ELBOW FLEXED AND FOREARM
  HELD ACROSS CHEST
- PAIN IN SHOULDER AREA
- SWELLING OR LUMP

FOLD ARM OF INJURED SIDE
ACROSS CHEST

PLACE ARM IN SLING AND
SECURE IT TO BODY WITH
SWATHE

Figure 12-13 Fractured clavicle.

Shoulder: Most shoulder injuries are not life-threatening, but they may be associated with severe injuries of the chest or neck. Many shoulder injuries are dislocations or separations of joint spaces and may show up as a defect at the upper outer portion of the shoulder. The upper humerus is fractured with some degree of frequency, however. The radial nerve travels quite close around the humerus and may be injured in humeral fractures. Injury to the radial nerve results in an inability of the patient to lift the hand (wrist drop). Dislocated shoulders are very painful and quite often require a pillow between the arm and body to hold the upper arm in the most comfortable position. Shoulders that are held in abnormal positions should never be forced into a more anatomic alignment (see Figure 12-14).

Elbow: It is often difficult to tell whether there is a fracture or dislocation; both can be serious because of the danger of damage to the vessels and nerves that run across the flexor surface of the elbow. Elbow injuries should always be splinted in the most comfortable position and the distal function clearly evaluated (see Figure 12-15). Never attempt to straighten or apply traction to an elbow injury because the tissues are quite delicate and the structure is very complicated.

Forearm and Wrist: This a very common fracture (see Figure 12-16), usually as a result of a fall on the outstretched arm. Usually it is best immobilized with a rigid splint or an air splint (see Figure 12-17). If a rigid splint is used, a roll of gauze in the hand will hold the arm in the most comfortable position of function. The forearm is also subject to internal bleeding that can interrupt the blood supply to the fingers and the hand (compartment syndrome).

Hand or Foot: Many industrial accidents involving the hand or the foot produce multiple open fractures and

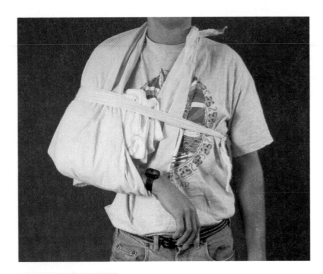

Figure 12-14 Dislocated shoulder.

Figure 12-15

Fractures or disloca-
tions of the elbow.

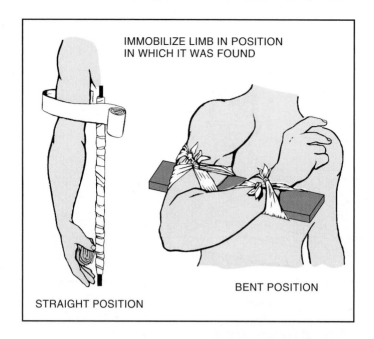

IMMOBILIZE LIMB IN POSITION
IN WHICH IT WAS FOUND

BENT POSITION

STRAIGHT POSITION

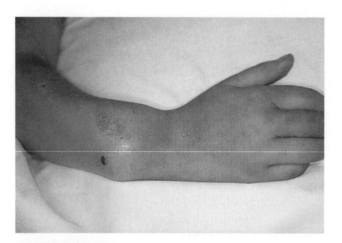

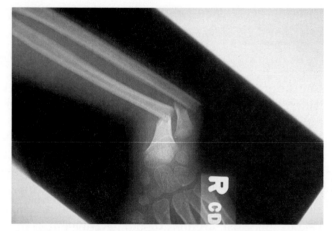

Figure 12-16 Presentation of a forearm fracture: (a) a fracture will often present with deformity; (b) an x-ray
of the fracture.

Figure 12-17

Fractures of the fore-
arm and wrist.

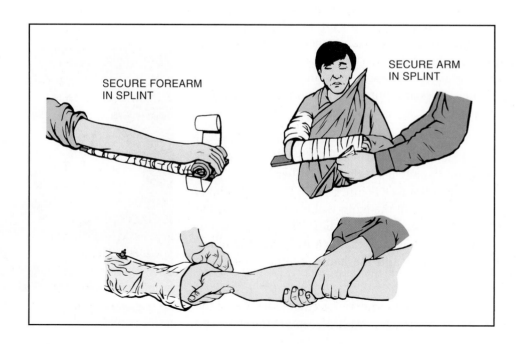

SECURE ARM
IN SPLINT

SECURE FOREARM
IN SPLINT

avulsions. These injuries are often gruesome in appearance but are seldom associated with life-threatening bleeding. A pillow may be used to support these injuries very effectively (see Figure 12-18). An alternative method of dressing the hand is to insert a roll of gauze in the palm, then arrange the fingers and thumb in their normal position. The entire hand is then wrapped as though it were a ball inside a very large and bulky dressing. Elevating the isolated hand or foot injury above the level of the heart will almost always reduce bleeding dramatically during transport.

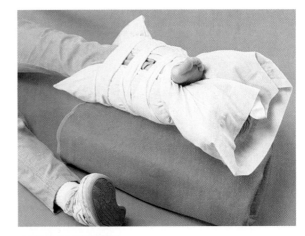

Figure 12-18 Pillow splinting an injured foot.

CASE STUDY

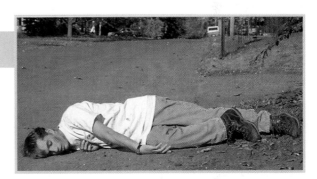

Dan, Joyce, and Buddy of the Emergency Transport System have been called to the scene of an auto–pedestrian collision. They are told that the pedestrian is unconscious. During travel to the scene they decide that Buddy will be team leader and they prepare to care for a patient with serious multisystem injuries. They arrive on the local college campus where a male student stepped out in front of a car and was hit. He was thrown about 15 feet, and has been unconscious since the injury. Nothing is known about him, as no bystanders know him. The scene is safe. He is the only victim.

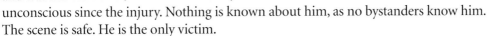

As they approach, their general impression is bad: The patient is lying on his right side with his right leg at an abnormal angle. He is not moving. He does not respond when Buddy speaks to him. Initial assessment reveals that his airway is open, but his respiration is shallow and slow. He has a weak, rapid pulse at the wrist. The ETS team checks his back (no apparent injuries) as they log-roll him onto a backboard. Joyce begins assisted ventilation with 100% oxygen while Buddy does the BTLS Rapid Trauma Survey. The patient has a hematoma of the right temporal area and only moans when his fingers and toes are pinched. There is no deformity of the neck and the neck veins are flat. The chest has no apparent injuries and breath sounds are present and equal. Heart sounds are easily heard. The abdomen is soft and the patient does not seem to have pain when the abdomen is palpated. The pelvis is stable but seems to be tender, as the patient moans when the pelvis is palpated. There is an obvious deformity of the right thigh but PMS of all extremities is present (the patient withdraws his fingers and toes to pinching).

Buddy gets the team to move him immediately to the ambulance and they begin transport. A brief neurological done in the ambulance reveals that the patient opens his eyes to pain (pupils 3 mm and react equally to light), moans to pain, and withdraws to pain. His GCS is calculated to be 8 (severe brain injury). He has no gag reflex so Joyce inserts an oral airway and keeps suction immediately available. Vital signs are: BP 90/60, pulse 130, respiration assisted at 10 per minute. His pulse oximeter saturation is 100%. While Joyce ventilates the patient, Buddy and Dan apply a Hare traction splint to the right leg. By the time they contact Medical Direction they are almost at the hospital, as the transport time was only five minutes. The patient was found to have an epidural hematoma and this was immediately evacuated with good results. The patient also had a fractured pelvis and right femur, but no other injuries. He responded well to treatment and was back in school by the next semester. He had no residual neurological symptoms.

CASE STUDY WRAP-UP

This patient had multiple system trauma that is the usual case with auto–pedestrian collisions. His shock was secondary to the fractured femur and pelvis and not to any other internal injuries. The patient's coma was due to the epidural hematoma that is one of the few head injuries that usually respond immediately to decompression. The outcome might have been different had he been allowed to remain hypotensive.

SUMMARY

While usually not life-threatening, extremity injuries are often disabling. These injuries may be more obvious than more serious internal injuries, but do not let extremity injuries distract you from following the usual steps of the BTLS Primary Survey. Pelvic and femur fractures can be associated with life-threatening internal bleeding, so patients with these injuries are in the load-and-go category. Proper splinting is important to protect the injured extremity from further injury. Dislocations of elbows, hips, and knees require careful splinting and rapid reduction to prevent severe disability to the affected extremity.

BIBLIOGRAPHY

1. Committee on Trauma, American College of Surgeons. "Musculoskeletal Trauma." In *Advanced Trauma Life Support Program*, pp. 301–320. Chicago: The College, 1997.

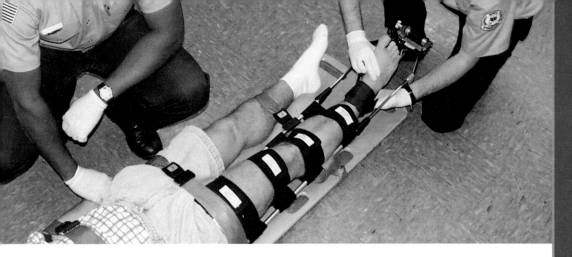

Extremity Trauma Skills

Donna Hastings, EMT-P

Upon completion of this chapter, you should be able to:

1. Explain when to use a traction splint.

2. Describe the complications of using a traction splint.

3. Apply the most common traction splints:

    a. Thomas splint

    b. Hare splint

    c. Sager splint

USE OF TRACTION SPLINTS

Traction splints are designed to immobilize fractures of the femur. They are not useful for fractures of the hip, knee, or lower leg. Applying firm traction to a fractured or dislocated knee may tear the blood vessels behind the knee. If there appears to be a pelvic fracture, you cannot use a traction splint because it may cause further damage to the pelvis. Fractures below the midthigh that are not angulated or are severely shortened may just as well be immobilized by air splints or the antishock garment. Traction splints work by applying a padded device to the back of the pelvis (ischium) or to the groin. A hitching device is then applied to the ankle, and countertraction is applied until the limb is straight and well immobilized. Apply the splints to the pelvis and groin very carefully to prevent excessive pressure on the genitalia. Also use care when attaching the hitching device to the foot and ankle so as not to interfere with circulation. To prevent any unnecessary movement, do not apply traction splints until the patient is on a long backboard. If the splint extends beyond the end of the backboard, be very careful when moving the patient and when closing the ambulance door. You must check the circulation in the injured leg, so remove the shoe before attaching the hitching device. In every case at least two people are needed. One must hold steady, *gentle* traction on the foot and leg while the other applies the splint. When dealing with load-and-go situations, do not apply the splint until the patient is in the ambulance (unless the ambulance has not arrived).

✋ PROCEDURE

✳ Applying a Thomas Traction Splint (Half-Ring Splint)

The Thomas splint was used exclusively prior to the advent of modern traction devices. During World War I its use decreased the mortality rate for battlefield femur fractures from 80 to 40%. At that time it was considered one of the greatest advancements in medical care. It is still used in some countries, and in the absence of other options (see Figure 13-1).

1. Support the leg and maintain gentle traction while your partner cuts away the clothing and removes the shoe and sock to check the pulse and sensation at the foot.
2. Position the splint under the injured leg. The ring goes down and the short side goes to the inside of the leg. Slide the ring snugly up under the hip, where it will be pressed against the ischial tuberosity.
3. Position two support straps above the knee and two below the knee.
4. Attach the top ring strap.
5. Apply padding to the foot and ankle.
6. Apply the traction hitch around the foot and ankle (see Figure 13-2).
7. Maintain gentle traction by hand.
8. Attach the traction hitch to the end of the splint.
9. Increase traction by Spanish windlass action using a stick or tongue depressors.
10. Release manual traction and reassess circulation and sensation.
11. Support the end of the splint so that there is no pressure on the heel.

✳ Applying a Hare Traction Splint

This is the modern version of the Thomas splint (see Scan 13-1).

1. Position the patient on the backboard or stretcher.
2. Support the leg and maintain gentle traction, while your partner cuts away the clothing and removes the shoe and sock to check pulse and sensation at the foot.
3. Using the uninjured leg as a guide, pull the splint out to the correct length.
4. Position the splint under the injured leg. The ring goes down and the short side goes to the inside of the leg. Slide the ring up snugly under the hip against the ischial tuberosity.
5. Attach the ischial strap.
6. Apply the padded traction hitch to the ankle and foot.
7. Position and attach two support straps above the knee and two below the knee.
8. Maintain gentle manual traction.

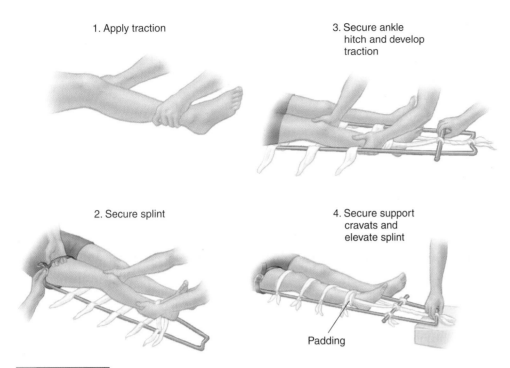

1. Apply traction

3. Secure ankle hitch and develop traction

2. Secure splint

4. Secure support cravats and elevate splint

Padding

Figure 13-1 Applying a Thomas traction splint.

9. Attach the traction hitch to the windlass by way of the S-hook.
10. Turn the ratchet until the correct tension is applied.
11. Reassess PMS of leg.
12. Release manual traction and recheck circulation and sensation.
13. To release traction, pull the ratchet knob outward and then slowly turn to loosen.

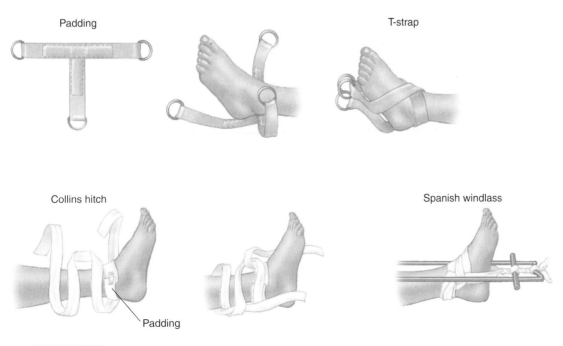

Padding

T-strap

Collins hitch

Padding

Spanish windlass

Figure 13-2 Applying a traction hitch to the ankle.

Applying a Hare Traction Splint

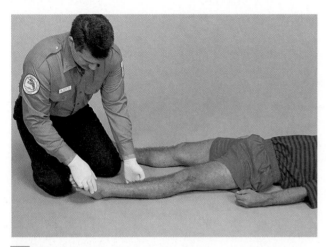

1. Assess distal pulses and a motor and sensory function.

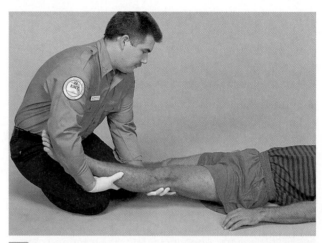

2. Stabilize the injured leg by applying manual traction.

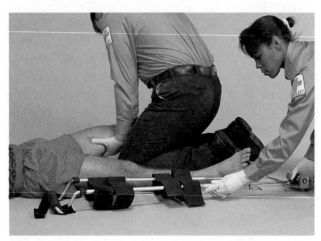

3. Adjust the splint for proper length.

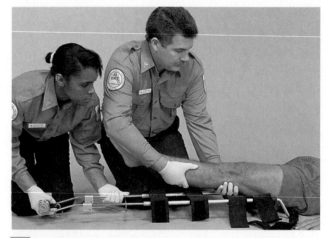

4. Position the splint under the injured leg until the ischial pad rests against the bony prominence of the buttocks. Once the splint is in position, raise the heel stand.

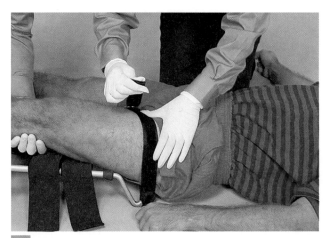

5. Attach the ischial strap over the groin and thigh.

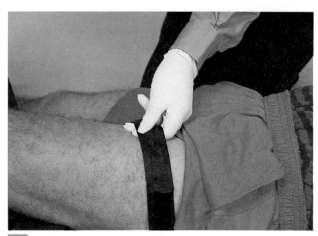

6. Make sure the ischial strap is snug but not tight enough to reduce distal circulation.

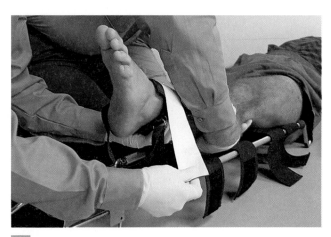

7. With the patient's foot in an upright position, secure the ankle hitch.

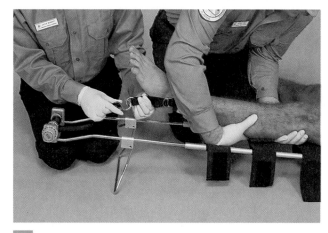

8. Attach the S hook to the D ring and apply mechanical traction. Full traction is achieved when the mechanical traction is equal to the manual traction and the pain and muscle spasms are reduced. In an unresponsive patient, adjust the traction until the injured leg is the same length as the uninjured leg.

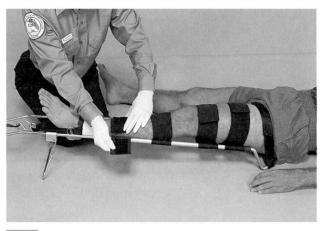

9. Fasten the leg support straps.

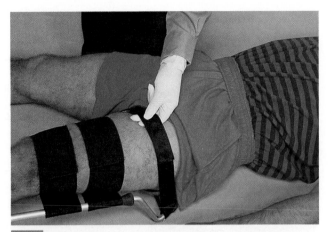

10. Reevaluate the ischial strap and ankle hitch to ensure that both are securely fastened.

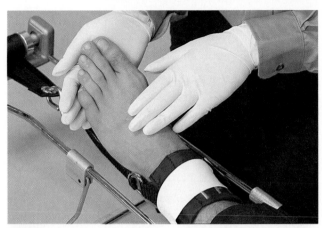

11. Reassess distal pulses and motor and sensory function.

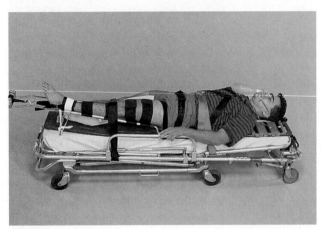

12. Place the patient on a longboard and secure with straps. Pad between the splint and uninjured leg. Secure the splint to the backboard. Except in cases of isolated injury, the patient should be on the backboard before applying the splint.

✳ Applying a Sager Traction Splint

This splint is different in several ways. It works by providing countertraction against the pubic ramus and the ischial tuberosity medial to the shaft of the femur; thus it does not go under the leg. The hip does not have to be slightly flexed, as with the Hare. The Sager splint is also lighter and more compact than other traction splints. You can also splint both legs with one splint if needed. The current Sager splints are significantly improved over older models and may represent the state of the art in traction splints (see Scan 13-2).

1. Position the patient on a long backboard or stretcher.
2. Support the leg and maintain gentle traction while your partner cuts away the clothing and removes the shoe and sock to check the pulse and sensation at the foot.
3. Using the uninjured leg as a guide, pull the splint out to the correct length.

Applying a Sager Traction Splint

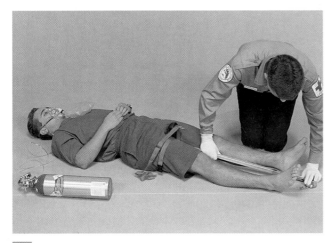

1. Place the splint along the medial aspect of the injured leg. Adjust it so that it extends about four inches beyond the heel.

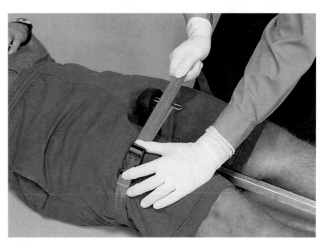

2. Secure the strap to the thigh.

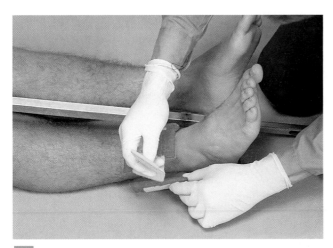

3. Apply the ankle hitch and attach it to the splint.

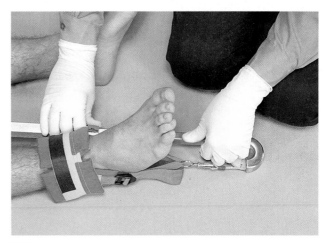

4. Apply traction by extending the splint. Adjust the splint to 10% of the patient's body weight.

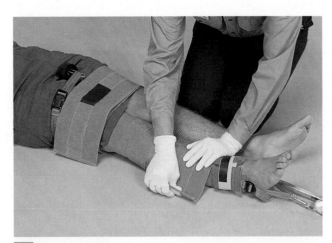

5. Apply the straps to secure leg to splint. Reassess distal pulses and motor and sensory function.

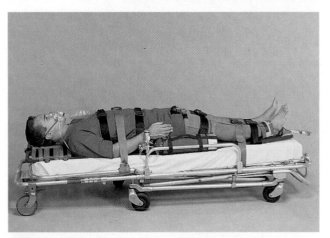

6. Place the patient onto a long backboard. Strap the ankles together and secure to the board. Except in cases of isolated injury, the patient should be on the backboard before applying the splint.

4. Position the splint to the inside of the injured leg with the padded bar fitted snugly against the pelvis in the groin. Attach the strap to the thigh. The splint can be used on the outside of the leg, using the strap to maintain traction against the pubic ramus. Be very careful not to catch the genitals under the bar (or strap).

5. While maintaining gentle manual traction, attach the padded hitch to the foot and ankle.

6. Extend the splint until the correct tension is obtained.

7. Apply the elastic straps to secure the leg to the splint.

8. Release manual traction and recheck circulation and sensation.

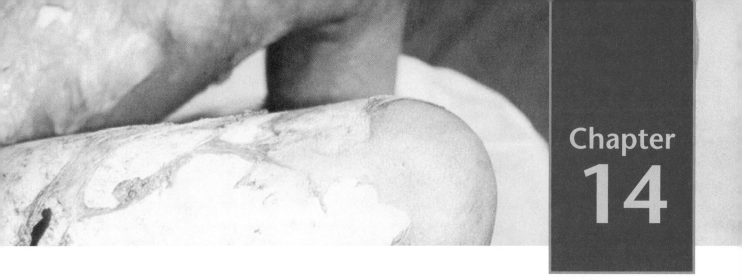

Chapter 14

Burns

Roy L. Alson, Ph.D., M.D., F.A.C.E.P.

Objectives

Upon completion of this chapter, you should be able to:

1. Identify the basic anatomy of the skin including:
   a. Epidermal and dermal layers
   b. Structures found within
2. List the basic functions of the skin.
3. Identify the descriptive categories of burns.
4. Identify complications and describe the management of:
   a. Thermal burns
   b. Chemical burns
   c. Electrical burns
5. List situations and physical signs that may indicate:
   a. Upper airway injury
   b. Inhalation injury
6. List signs and symptoms of carbon monoxide poisoning.
7. Discuss how carbon monoxide causes hypoxia.
8. Describe the treatment for carbon monoxide poisoning.
9. Estimate depth of burn based on skin appearance.
10. Estimate extent of burn using the rule of nines.
11. Identify which patients may require transport to a burn center.

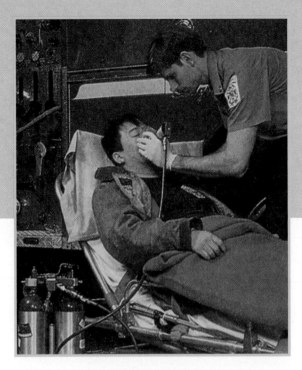

CASE STUDY

Dan, Joyce, and Buddy of the Emergency Transport System have been called to the scene of a warehouse fire. They are told that the watchman has just been rescued after being trapped in an upstairs bathroom. What injuries should they expect with a mechanism of this type? Is carbon monoxide poisoning possible? Are there medical problems that can be precipitated or aggravated by this mechanism? Keep these questions in mind as you read. The case study will continue at the end of the chapter.

According to the American Burn Association, there are over 1 million burn injuries per year in the United States, resulting in more than 4,500 deaths. Thousands more are injured. Many who survive their burns are left severely disabled and/or disfigured. While the number of those killed or injured has decreased in the last 30 years, particularly with the use of smoke detectors and the improvements in burn care, burn injury is still a major problem for our society. Applying the basic principles taught here can help decrease death, disability, and disfigurement from burn injuries. As the rescue of burn patients can be extremely dangerous, following the rules of scene safety is extremely important. Multiple agents (see below) can cause burn injuries, but in general, pathologic damage to the skin is similar. Specific differences among the types of burns will be discussed in later sections.

TYPES OF BURN INJURIES

1. Thermal
   a. Flame
   b. Scald
   c. Steam

2. Electrical
3. Chemical
4. Radiation

ANATOMY AND PATHOLOGY

The largest organ of the body, the skin, is made up of two layers. The outer layer that we can see on the surface is called the *epidermis*. It serves as a barrier between the environment and our body. Underneath the thin epidermis is a thick layer of collagen connective

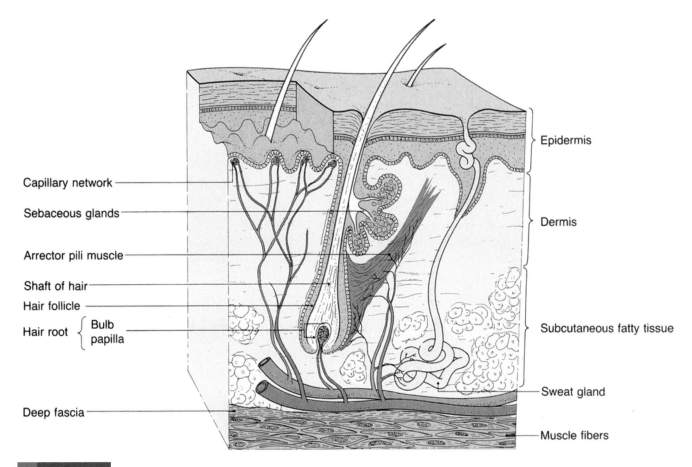

Capillary network
Sebaceous glands
Arrector pili muscle
Shaft of hair
Hair follicle
Hair root { Bulb
            papilla
Deep fascia

Epidermis
Dermis
Subcutaneous fatty tissue
Sweat gland
Muscle fibers

Figure 14-1 The Skin.

tissue called the *dermis*. This layer contains the important sensory nerves and also the support structures such as the hair follicles, sweat glands, and oil glands (see Figure 14-1). The skin has many important functions, which include acting as a mechanical and protective barrier between the body and the outside world, sealing fluids inside and preventing bacteria and other microorganisms from readily entering the body. The skin is also a vital sensory organ that provides input to the brain on general and specific environmental data and serves a primary role in temperature regulation. Damage to the skin renders it unable to carry out these functions and puts the body at risk for serious problems.

Burn damage to the skin occurs when heat or caustic chemicals come in contact with the skin and damage its chemical and cellular components. In addition to actual tissue injury, the body's inflammatory response to the skin damage may also result in additional injury or increase the severity of the burn. Burns are characterized, based on the depth of tissue damage and skin response, as superficial (first degree), partial-thickness (second degree), or full-thickness (third degree). Superficial burns result in minor tissue damage to the outer epidermal layer only, but do cause an intense and painful inflammatory response. The most common injury of this type is "sunburn." Although no medical treatment is usually required, various medications can be prescribed that significantly speed healing and reduce the painful inflammatory response. Partial-thickness burns cause damage through the epidermis and into a variable depth of the dermis. These injuries will heal (usually without scarring) because the cells lining the deeper portions of the hair follicles and sweat glands will multiply and grow new skin for healing. Antibiotic creams or various specialized types of dressings are routinely used to treat these burns and, therefore, appropriate medical evaluation and care should be provided for patients with these

TABLE 14-1	Characteristics of Various Depths of Burns.		
	Superficial (first degree)	**Partial-Thickness (second degree)**	**Full-Thickness (third degree)**
Cause	Sun or minor flash	Hot liquids, flashes, or flame	Chemicals, electricity, flame, hot metals
Skin color	Red	Mottled red	Pearly white and/or charred, translucent and parchmentlike
Skin surface	Dry with no blisters	Blisters with weeping	Dry with thrombosed blood vessels
Sensation	Painful	Painful	Anesthetic
Healing	3–6 days	2–4 weeks, depending on depth	Requires skin grafting

injuries. Emergency care of partial-thickness burns involves cooling the burn and covering with a dry sterile dressing.

Flash burns are virtually always superficial or partial-thickness burns. A flash burn occurs when there is some type of explosion, but no sustained fire. The single heat wave traveling out from these explosions results in such short patient–heat contact that full-thickness burns almost never occur. Only areas directly exposed to the true heat wave will be injured. Typically, face and hands are involved. An example of this type of burn is seen when someone pours gasoline on a charcoal fire in order to get it to heat up faster. *In situations of possible flash explosion risk, you should ALWAYS wear proper protective clothing and avoid entry into explosive environments.* Other injuries (fractures, internal injuries, blast chest injuries, etc.) may occur as a result of explosion.

Full-thickness burns cause damage to all layers of the epidermis and dermis. No more skin cell layers are left, so healing by regrowth of epidermal cells is impossible. All full-thickness burns leave scars which later may contract and limit motion of the extremity (or restrict movement of the chest wall). Deeper full-thickness burns usually result in skin protein becoming denatured and hard, forming a firm, leatherlike covering that is referred to as *eschar*. Characteristics of these burns are listed in Table 14-1, and the depth levels and examples are shown in Figures 14-2, 14-3, and 14-4.

The body's normal inflammatory response to the burn injury can result in progressive tissue damage for a day or two following burn injury, which may well result in an increase in burn depth. Any condition that either

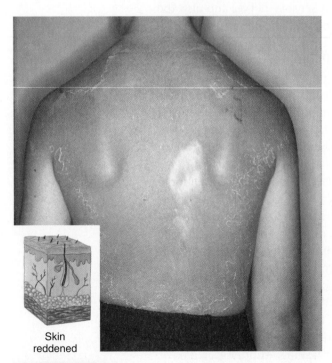

Skin reddened

Figure 14-2 Superficial (first degree) burn.

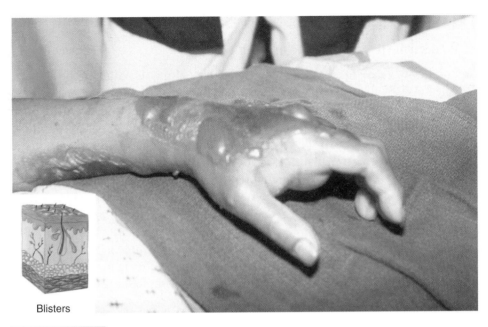

Blisters

Figure 14-3 Partial-thickness (second degree) burn. *(Courtesy of Roy Alson, M.D.)*

reduces circulation (shock) to this damaged tissue or by itself causes further tissue damage will lead to burn progression with increasing burn depth. Because of this process of burn progression, it is not essential to determine exactly the burn depth in the field. You should, however, be able to clearly discern between superficial and deep burns. Because transport to a burn center depends on both depth and extent of the burn, you should be able to estimate the amount of body surface involved in the burn.

Initial care that is directed specifically toward the burn should concentrate on limiting any progression of the burn depth and extent.

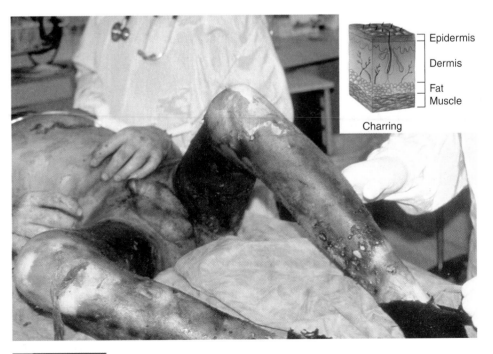

Epidermis
Dermis
Fat
Muscle

Charring

Figure 14-4 Full-thickness (third degree) burn. *(Courtesy of Roy Alson, M.D.)*

INITIAL FIELD CARE
Patient Assessment and Management

Evaluation of the burn patient is often complicated by the dramatic nature of the injuries. You can easily be overwhelmed by the extent of the injury. You must remember that even patients with major burns rarely expire in the initial postburn period from the burn injury. Death in the immediate postburn period is a consequence of associated trauma or conditions such as airway compromise or smoke inhalation. A careful, systematic approach to patient evaluation will allow you to identify and manage critical life-threatening problems and to improve patient outcome.

The steps for assessing a major burn patient are the same as for any other major trauma patient. Begin by performing a Scene Size-up as outlined in Chapter 1, with an emphasis on your safety. After this size-up is completed, your next priority is to remove the patient from the source of the burn. Removing the burn source is the first step in treating a burn patient, and the most important concept in removing the burn source is the maintenance of safety. This involves both maintaining your safety *and* maintaining patient safety. There are specific and significant dangers in removing the burn source in all types of burn injuries. As a structure fire progresses, there is a point at which flashover occurs. Flashover is the *sudden* explosion into flame of everything in the room, with the temperature rising instantaneously to over 2,000 degrees centigrade. There is often little warning before this happens; *thus removal of patients from burning buildings takes priority over all other treatment*. Remember also that fire consumes oxygen and produces large quantities of toxic products and smoke. Thus, personnel making entry to carry out rescue should wear breathing apparatus or risk becoming victims themselves.

Chemicals are not always easy to detect, either on patients or on other objects in the environment. Severe chemical burns to rescuers have occurred because of the failure to note sources of toxic and caustic chemicals and use appropriate personal protective equipment. Special training in hazardous materials management is recommended for all rescuers. Electricity is exceptionally dangerous, and handling of high voltage wires is extremely hazardous. Specialized training and knowledge are required to appropriately deal with these situations, and you should not attempt to remove wires unless specifically trained and equipped to do so. Even objects commonly felt to be safe, such as wooden sticks, manila rope, and firefighter's gloves, may not be protective and may result in electrocution. If at all possible, the source of electricity should be turned off before any attempt at rescue is made.

People do not actually die rapidly from burn injuries. Early burn deaths are usually the result of airway or trauma. Death from shock due to fluid loss from the burn will not be seen for many hours (or days) and sepsis takes days to develop. Even though the burn is highly visible and makes an intense impression at the scene, care of the burn itself has a lower priority than airway management. You should manage burn patients the same as any other *trauma* patients and perform a BTLS Primary Survey as soon as the burn victim is in a safe area. The BTLS Primary Survey should follow the standard format described in Chapter 2.

Begin by assessing and, if necessary, securing the airway, while simultaneously checking the initial level of consciousness and protecting the cervical spine. Assessment of breathing, circulation, and control of major hemorrhage is then carried out. Based upon the findings from the Scene Size-up and the Initial Assessment, a Rapid Trauma Survey is then performed, a baseline set of vital signs is obtained, and if possible, a SAMPLE history obtained. At this point a determination is made on the need for immediate transport and critical interventions. Critical problems in the burn patient that require immediate intervention include airway compromise, altered level of consciousness, or the presence of major injuries in addition to the burn. Clues from the mechanism of injury that point to critical problems include a history of being confined in a closed space with the fire or smoke, electrical burns, chemical exposure, falls from a height, or other major blunt force trauma. Supplemental oxygen should be initiated as soon as possible for all major burn patients.

The Rapid Trauma Survey of the burn patient is directed toward identification of airway and circulatory compromise. Besides clues from the mechanism of injury, other findings that should alert the responder to potential airway problems are the presence of facial and scalp burns, sooty sputum, and singed nasal hair and eyebrows. Remember that a history of smoke exposure in a closed space is the best predictor of smoke inhalation or other airway injury! Examine the oral cavity and look for soot, swelling, or erythema (redness). Ask the patient to speak. A hoarse voice or persistent cough suggests involvement of deeper airway structures. Auscultate the chest. Wheezing or rales should alert you to the presence of lower airway injury from inhalation. Examine burned areas and check for distal pulses. Circumferential full-thickness burns may lead to neurovascular compromise. While this is rarely a problem on the fire scene, this may become significant during an interfacility transfer. Full-thickness burns of the chest wall, with eschar formation, may compromise chest expansion and ventilation. Escharotomy (by qualified personnel) is necessary. Be sure to alert the receiving facility to the presence of full-thickness circumferential burns.

Once the immediate life-threats have been addressed, you should attend to the burn wound itself. You should try to limit burn wound progression as much as possible. Rapid cooling early in the course of a surface burn injury can help limit this progression. Following removal from the source of the burn, the skin and clothing are still hot and this heat continues to injure the tissues, causing an increase in burn depth and seriousness of the injury. Cooling halts this process and, if done appropriately, is beneficial. Cooling should be done with any source of clean water, but this should be undertaken for no more than a minute or two. Cooling for longer periods of time can induce hypothermia and subsequent shock.

Following the brief period of cooling, manage the burn by covering the patient with clean, dry sheets and blankets to keep the patient warm and to prevent hypothermia. *It is not necessary to have sterile sheets*. The patient should be covered even when the environment is not cold because damaged skin loses temperature regulation capacity. Patients should never be transported on wet sheets, wet towels, or wet clothing and *ice is absolutely contraindicated*. Ice will worsen the injury as it causes vasoconstriction and thus reduces the blood supply to already damaged tissue. Cooling the burn wound improperly can cause hypothermia and additional tissue damage and could be worse than not cooling the burn at all. Initial management of chemical and electrical burn injuries will be described in the sections on those injuries.

In your assessment of the burn patient, note and record the type of burn mechanism and the particular circumstances such as entrapment, explosion, mechanisms for other possible injuries, smoke exposure, chemical/electrical details, and so forth. An appropriate past medical history should also be documented in writing. If the patient is unable to speak, ask other witnesses and/or fire personnel about the circumstances of the injury.

Perform a standard Detailed Exam on stable patients. This survey should include an evaluation of the burn, estimating the depth based on appearance and also estimating the burn size. These findings are important in determining the level of medical care that is appropriate for the burn victim. The burn size is best estimated in the field using the rule of nines (see Figure 14-5). The body is divided into areas that are either 9 or 18% of the total body surface and by roughly drawing in the burned areas, the extent can be estimated. Only partial-thickness and full-thickness burns are used for this calculation. In small children there are some differences in body size proportions and a Lund and Browder chart is helpful (see Table 14-2). For smaller or irregular burns, the size can be

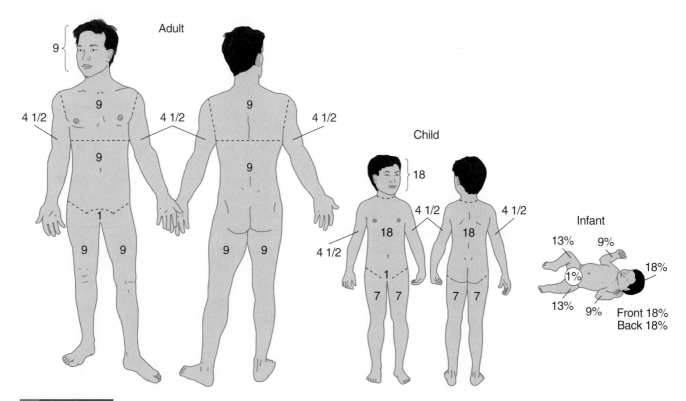

Figure 14-5 The rule of nines.

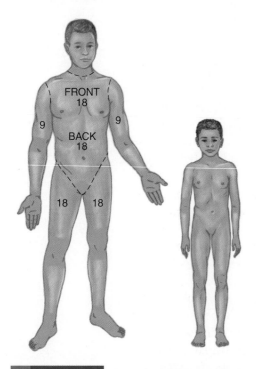

Figure 14-6 Areas in which small burns are more serious. Second- or third-degree burns in these areas (shaded portions) should be treated in the hospital.

estimated using the palmar surface of the patient's hand, which is about 1% of the total body surface area. Even small burns can be serious if they involve certain parts of the body which affect function or appearance (see Figure 14-6).

During the evaluation of the extent of the burn injury, you should remove the patient's loose clothing and jewelry. Cut around burned clothing that is adherent, but do not try to pull the clothing off of the skin.

It is appropriate that a physician see burn injuries. There are now available specialized forms of therapy that offer specific advantages to the treatment of superficial, partial-thickness, and full-thickness burns. We have all seen partial-thickness burns become infected and progress to full-thickness burns because of poor care. The sooner that specialized burn therapy can be initiated, the more rapid and satisfactory the results will be. Table 14-3 lists conditions that would benefit from care at a burn center. Based upon available local resources and protocols, it may be appropriate to bypass a local facility and transport these patients directly to the burn center.

SPECIAL PROBLEMS IN BURN MANAGEMENT

The following sections review management of specific types of burns, based upon the injury mechanism. Be aware that more than one type of burn can be present in a patient. For example, a high-voltage electrical burn injury may also produce flame burns due to ignition of the patient's clothing.

| TABLE 14-2 | Lund and Browder Chart | | | | | | | |

Area	Age (Years) 0–1	1–4	5–9	10–15	Adults	% 2°	% 3°	% Total
Head	19	17	13	10	7			
Neck	2	2	2	2	2			
Ant. Trunk	13	17	13	13	13			
Post. Trunk	13	13	13	13	13			
R. Buttock	$2\frac{1}{2}$	$2\frac{1}{2}$	$2\frac{1}{2}$	$2\frac{1}{2}$	$2\frac{1}{2}$			
L. Buttock	$2\frac{1}{2}$	$2\frac{1}{2}$	$2\frac{1}{2}$	$2\frac{1}{2}$	$2\frac{1}{2}$			
Genitalia	1	1	1	1	1			
R.U. Arm	4	4	4	4	4			
L.U. Arm	4	4	4	4	4			
R.L. Arm	3	3	3	3	3			
L.L. Arm	3	3	3	3	3			
R. Hand	$2\frac{1}{2}$	$2\frac{1}{2}$	$2\frac{1}{2}$	$2\frac{1}{2}$	$2\frac{1}{2}$			
L. Hand	$2\frac{1}{2}$	$2\frac{1}{2}$	$2\frac{1}{2}$	$2\frac{1}{2}$	$2\frac{1}{2}$			
R. Thigh	$5\frac{1}{2}$	$6\frac{1}{2}$	$8\frac{1}{2}$	$8\frac{1}{2}$	$9\frac{1}{2}$			
L. Thigh	$5\frac{1}{2}$	$6\frac{1}{2}$	$8\frac{1}{2}$	$8\frac{1}{2}$	$9\frac{1}{2}$			
R. Leg	5	5	$5\frac{1}{2}$	6	7			
L. Leg	5	5	$5\frac{1}{2}$	6	7			
R. Foot	$3\frac{1}{2}$	$3\frac{1}{2}$	$3\frac{1}{2}$	$3\frac{1}{2}$	$3\frac{1}{2}$			
L. Foot	$3\frac{1}{2}$	$3\frac{1}{2}$	$3\frac{1}{2}$	$3\frac{1}{2}$	$3\frac{1}{2}$			
					Total			

Weight _____

Height _____

Inhalation Injuries

Inhalation injuries accounted for more than half of the 4,500-plus burn-related deaths in the United States in 1998. Inhalation injuries are classified as carbon monoxide poisoning, heat inhalation injuries, or smoke (toxic) inhalation injuries. Most frequently, inhalation injuries occur when a patient is injured in a confined space or is trapped; however, even victims of fires in open spaces may have inhalation injuries. Flash explosions (no fire) practically never cause inhalation injuries.

Carbon monoxide poisoning and asphyxiation are by far the most common causes of early death associated with burn injury. Carbon monoxide is a by-product of combustion and is one of the numerous chemicals in common smoke. It is present in high concentrations in auto exhaust fumes and fumes from some types of home space heaters. Since it is colorless, odorless, and tasteless, its presence is virtually impossible to detect. Carbon monoxide binds to hemoglobin (257 times stronger than oxygen), resulting in the hemoglobin being unable to transport oxygen. Patients quickly become hypoxic even in the presence of low concentrations of carbon monoxide, and an alteration in their level of consciousness is the predominant sign of this hypoxia (see Table 14-4). A cherry-red skin color or cyanosis is rarely present as a result of carbon monoxide poisoning and, therefore, cannot be used in the assessment of patients for carbon monoxide poisoning. Pulse

TABLE 14-3	Injuries That Benefit from Care at a Burn Center.

1. Second- and third-degree burns, 10% body surface area if age <10 or >50
2. Second- and third-degree burns, 20% body surface area, any age
3. Burns of face, hands, feet, genitalia, perineum, and skin overlying major joints
4. Third-degree burns, ≥ 5% total body surface area
5. Specialized burn types
   a. Electrical, including lightning
   b. Chemical
   c. Inhalation injury
   d. Circumferential chest or extremity injury
6. Presence of significant preexisting medical disorders
7. Presence of significant other injuries

Source: American Burn Association.

oximetry will remain normal to high in the presence of carbon monoxide and cannot be used to assess these patients. Death usually occurs because of either cerebral or myocardial ischemia or myocardial infarction due to progressive cardiac hypoxia. Treat patients suspected of having carbon monoxide poisoning with high-flow oxygen by mask. If such a patient loses consciousness, begin ventilation using 100% oxygen. If a patient is simply removed from the source of the carbon monoxide and allowed to breathe fresh air, it takes up to 7 hours to reduce the carbon monoxide–hemoglobin complex to a safe level. Having the patient breathe 100% oxygen decreases this time to about 90 to 120 minutes, and use of hyperbaric oxygen (100% oxygen at 2.5 atmospheres) will decrease this time to about 30 minutes (see Figure 14-7). All suspected cases of carbon monoxide poisoning or toxic inhalation should be transported to an appropriate hospital. The decision to transport the patient to a hyperbaric chamber should be made by Medical Direction.

TABLE 14-4	Symptoms Associated with Increasing Levels of Carboxyhemoglobin Binding.

Carboxyhemoglobin Level (%)	Symptoms
20	Headache common, throbbing in nature; shortness of breath on exertion
30	Headache present; altered central nervous system function with disturbed judgment; irritability, dizziness; decreased vision
40–50	Marked central nervous system alteration with confusion, collapse; also fainting with exertion
60–70	Convulsions; unconsciousness; apnea with prolonged exposure
80	Rapidly fatal

Heat inhalation injuries are confined to the upper airway, since breathing in flame and hot gases does not result in heat transport down to the lung tissue itself. The water vapor in the air in the tracheal–bronchial tree effectively absorbs this heat. Steam inhalation is the exception to this rule, as steam is superheated water vapor. A second exception to this rule is if the patient has inhaled a flammable gas which then ignites and causes thermal injury to the level of the alveoli (example: a painter in a closed space where the paint fumes are ignited by a spark). As a result of the heat injury, tissue swelling occurs just as it does with surface burns. The vocal cords themselves do not swell because they are dense fibrous bands of connective tissue. However, the loose mucosa in the supraglottic area (the hypopharynx) is where the swelling occurs, and can easily progress to complete airway obstruction and death (see Figure 14-8). There is usually some time between the injury and the development of airway edema, so loss of airway due to direct thermal injury is rare in the initial prehospital phase. Be aware that once the swelling begins, the airway can obstruct rapidly.

During secondary transport to a burn center, the risk of airway swelling can become significant and can cause airway obstruction as volume-resuscitation IV fluids are being administered. For this reason, if there is any potential for airway burns, the patient should be sedated and intubated before a transfer. Figure 14-9 lists signs that should alert you to the danger of your patient having upper airway burns. Swollen lips indicate the presence of thermal injury at the airway entrance, and hoarseness (indicating altered airflow through the larynx area) is a warning of early airway swelling. Stridor (high-pitched inspiratory breathing and/or a seal-bark cough) indicates severe airway swelling with pending airway obstruction and *represents an immediate emergency*. The only appropriate treatment is airway stabilization, and immediate transport.

Smoke inhalation injuries (see Figure 14-10) are the result of inhaled toxic chemicals that cause structural damage to lung cells. Smoke may contain hundreds of toxic chemicals that damage the delicate alveolar cells. Smoke from plastic and synthetic products is the most damaging. Tissue destruction in the bronchi and alveoli may take hours to days. However, as these toxic products in the smoke are very irritating, they may precipitate bronchospasm or coronary artery spasm in susceptible individuals.

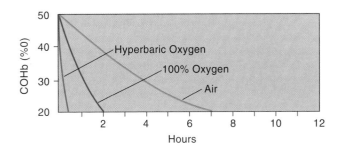

Figure 14-7 Decay curve for disappearance of carboxyhemoglobin from 50% lethal level to 20% acceptable level in air, 1 atm. O_2 (100% oxygen) and 2.5 atm. O_2 (hyperbaric oxygen—100% at 2.5 atmospheres).

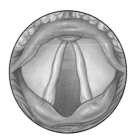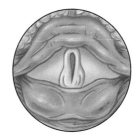

Figure 14-8 Heat inhalation can cause complete airway obstruction by swelling of the hypopharynx. Left side—normal anatomy; right side—swelling proximal to cords.

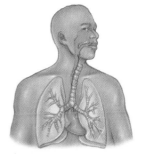

- Burns of the face
- Singed eyebrows or nasal hair
- Burns in the mouth
- Carbonaceous (sooty) sputum
- History of being confined in a closed space while being burned
- Exposure to steam

Figure 14-9 Danger signs of upper airway burns.

Chemical Burns

There are thousands of different types of chemicals that can cause burn injuries. Chemicals may not only injure the skin, but also may be absorbed into the body and cause internal organ failure (especially liver and kidney damage). Volatile forms of chemicals

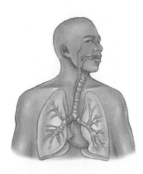

- Victims exposed to smoke in an enclosed place

- Victims who were unconscious while exposed to smoke or fire

- Victims with a cough after being exposed to smoke or fire

- Victims short of breath after being exposed to smoke or fire

- Victims with chest pain after being exposed to smoke or fire

Figure 14-10 Patients in whom you should suspect smoke inhalation.

may be inhaled and cause lung tissue damage with subsequent severe life-threatening respiratory failure. The effects of the chemical agents on the other organ systems, such as the lung or liver, may not be immediately apparent after exposure. Chemical injuries are frequently deceiving in that initial skin changes may be minimal even when a severe injury is present. This may lead to secondary contamination of rescuers. Minimal burns on the patient may not be obvious. As a result you can get these chemicals on your own skin unless appropriate precautions are taken. Factors that lead to tissue damage include chemical concentration, amount, manner and duration of skin contact, and the mechanism of action of the chemical agent. The pathologic process causing the tissue damage continues until the chemical is either consumed in the damage process, detoxified by the body, or is physically removed. Attempts at inactivation with specific neutralizing chemicals are dangerous because the process of neutralization may generate other chemical reactions (heat) that may worsen the injury. Therefore, you should aim treatment at chemical removal by following these four steps:

PROCEDURE

1. Wear appropriate protective gloves, eyewear, and respiratory protection if needed.

2. Remove all the patient's clothing. Place in plastic bags to limit further contact.

3. Flush chemicals off the body by irrigating copiously with any source of available water or other irrigant. If dry chemicals are on the skin, they should first be thoroughly brushed off before performing copious irrigation. "The solution to pollution is dilution."

4. Remove any retained agent adhering to the skin by any appropriate physical means such as wiping or gentle scraping. Follow this by further irrigation (see Figures 14-11 and 14-12).

Ideally, all contaminated patients should be decontaminated prior to transport, so as to limit skin damage *and* prevent contamination of the ambulance or hospital. Critical interventions including airway management can be initiated prior to and during the

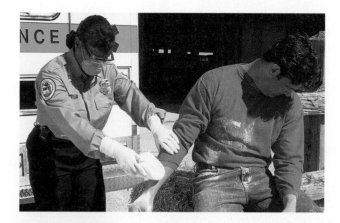
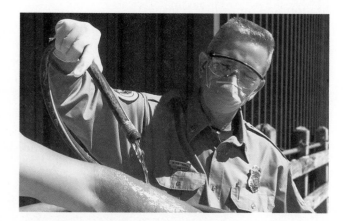

Figure 14-11 For a chemical burn, (A) brush away dry powders, and then (B) flood the area with water.
(Photos courtesy of Michael Heron)

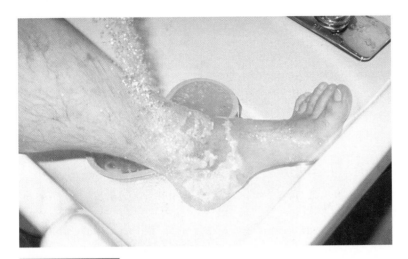

Figure 14-12 Acid burn of the ankle being irrigated.
(Courtesy of Roy Alson, M.D.)

decontamination process. If the patient has not been fully decontaminated prior to transport, notify the receiving hospital as soon as possible, so that they can be prepared to manage the patient.

Irrigation of caustic chemicals in the eye is exceptionally important because irreversible damage will occur in a very short period of time (less than the transport time to get to the hospital). Irrigation of injured eyes may be difficult because of the pain associated with eye opening. However, you must begin irrigation to prevent severe and permanent damage to the corneas (see Figure 14-13). Check for contact lenses or foreign bodies and, if present, remove them early during irrigation. A nasal cannula hooked to an IV bag and placed over the bridge of the nose makes an excellent bilateral eye wash system during transport.

PEARLS

Remember that dealing with hazardous materials requires proper training and equipment. You must use appropriate personal protective equipment.

Electrical Burns

In cases of electrical burns, damage is caused by electricity entering the body and traveling through the tissues. Injury results from the effects of the electricity on the function of the body organs and from the heat generated by the passage of the current. Extremities are at risk for more significant tissue damage, versus the torso, because their small size results in higher local current density (see Figure 14-14). The factors that determine severity of electrical injury include the following:

1. The type and amount of current (alternating versus direct and the voltage)
2. Path of the current through the body
3. Duration of contact with the current source

The most serious and immediate injury that results from electrical contact is cardiac arrhythmia. Any patient who receives an electric current injury, regardless of how stable he looks, should have a careful immediate evaluation of his cardiac status and continuous monitoring of cardiac activity. The most common life-threatening arrhythmias are premature ventricular contractions, ventricular tachycardia, and ventricular fibrillation. Aggressive Advanced Life Support management of these arrhythmias should be undertaken, since these patients usually have normal healthy hearts and the chances for resuscitation are excellent. For a patient in ventricular fibrillation with only basic life support available, start cardiopulmonary resuscitation (CPR) and transport immediately to a hospital facility. Most of these victims do not have preexisting cardiovascular disease, and their

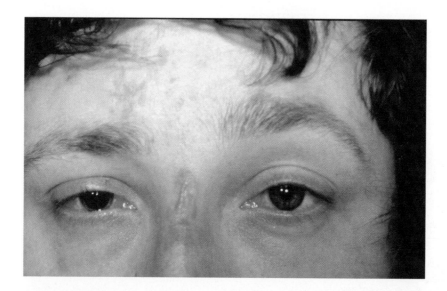

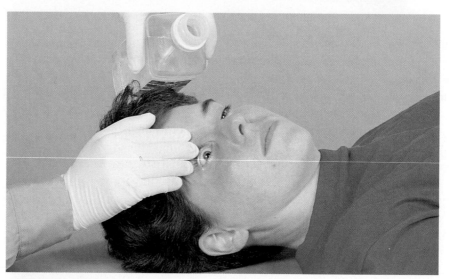

Figure 14-13 (A) Chemical burns to the eyes; (B) emergency care of chemical burns to the eye.

heart muscle tissue is usually not damaged as a result of the electricity. Even under circumstances of prolonged CPR, resuscitation is often possible. Once those efforts at managing cardiac status are complete, provide field care as previously described for thermal burns.

Electrical injuries cause skin burns at the entrance and exit sites because of high temperatures generated by the electric arc (2,500 degrees centigrade) at the skin surface. Additional surface flame burns may result if the patient's clothing is ignited. Fractures and/or dislocations may be present due to the violent muscle contractions that electrical injuries cause. Often victims are involved in construction and may sustain fractures or other injuries due to falls after an electric shock. Internal injuries usually involve muscle damage, nerve damage, and possible intravascular blood coagulation due to electrical current passage. *Internal chest or abdominal organ damage due to electrical current is exceedingly rare.*

At the scene of an electrical injury, your first priority is scene safety. Determine if the patient is still in contact with the electrical current. If so, you must remove the patient from contact without becoming a victim yourself (see Figure 14-15). Handling high-voltage electrical wires is extremely hazardous. Special training and special equipment are

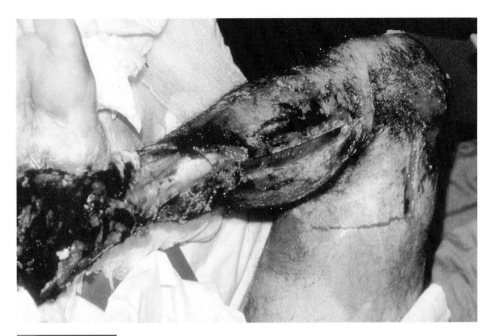

Figure 14-14 Electrical burn of the lower leg and foot. *(Courtesy of Roy Alson, M.D.)*

needed to deal with downed wires; *never attempt to move wires with makeshift equipment.* Tree limbs, pieces of wood, and even manila rope may conduct high-voltage electricity. Even firefighter's gloves and boots do not offer adequate protection in this situation. If possible, leave the handling of downed wires to power company personnel or develop a special training program with your local power company to learn how to use the special equipment designed to handle high-voltage lines.

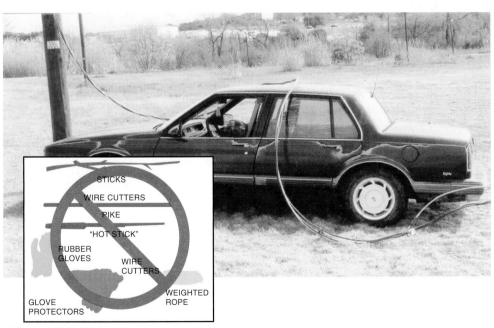

Figure 14-15 Removal of high-voltage electrical wires. Do not try to remove wires with safety equipment (or sticks) unless specially trained. Turn off the electricity at the source or call the power company to remove the wires. *(Courtesy of Leon Charpentier, EMT-P)*

In the field setting, it is impossible to tell the total extent of the damage in electrical burns; all electrical burn patients should be transported for hospital evaluation. Due to the potential for arrhythmia development you should monitor the heart, if you have this capability.

Lightning Injury

Lightning kills more persons in North America each year than any other weather-related phenomenon. Injuries from lightning are very different from other electrical injuries in that lightning produces extremely high voltages (>10,000,000 volts) and currents (>2,000 amps), but has a very short duration (<100 msec) of contact.

Lightning produces a "flashover" phenomenon, in which the current flows around the outside of the victim's body. Consequently, the internal damage from current flow seen with generated electricity is not seen in a lightning strike. Most of the effects from a lightning strike are the result of the massive DC (direct current) shock that is received. Classic lightning strike burns produce a fern-like or splatter pattern across the skin (see Figure 14-16). The victim does not need to be struck directly to sustain an injury. Lightning may strike an adjacent object or nearby ground and still produce an injury to a victim. Often the victim's skin is wet, from either sweat or rain. This water, when heated by the lightning current, is quickly vaporized, producing superficial and partial-thickness burns, and may literally explode the clothing off the victim. As these burns are superficial, aggressive fluid resuscitation is not required.

The most serious effect of a lightning strike is cardiorespiratory arrest, with the massive current acting like a defibrillator to briefly stop the heart. Cardiac activity often spontaneously resumes within minutes. However, the respiratory drive centers of the brain are also depressed by the current discharge, and these areas take longer to recover and resume the normal respiratory drive. Consequently, the victim remains in respiratory arrest, which is followed by a hypoxic cardiac arrest.

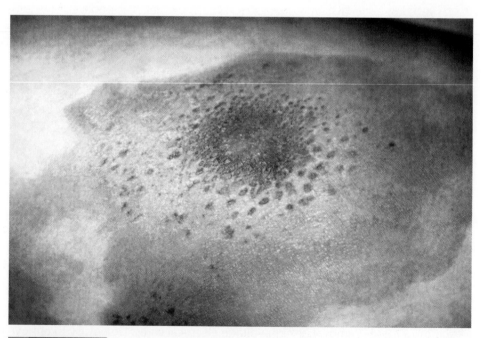

Figure 14-16 Flashover pattern of burns on the skin of a victim of a lightning strike.

The essential component of the management of the lightning strike victim is restoration of cardiorespiratory function, while protecting the cervical spine. Follow standard guidelines for CPR. Since lightning strikes can occur at sporting events and other outdoor gatherings, strikes often become multiple-casualty events. It must be stressed that in a multiple-casualty lightning strike, the conventional triage approach of a pulseless or non-breathing patient equaling a dead patient should not be followed. If a patient is awake or breathing after a lightning strike, she will most likely survive without further intervention. Resuscitative efforts should concentrate on those victims who are in respiratory or cardiac arrest, since prompt CPR represents the only chance that these victims have for survival.

Long-term problems have been seen in lightning strike patients, such as the development of cataracts, or neurological and/or psychological difficulties. Perforation of the eardrum is quite common, and rarely long bone or scapular fractures, as seen in the victims of generated high-voltage electrical injuries, may be seen. These fractures are managed as described in Chapter 12.

There are over 200 reported deaths in North America each year due to lightning strike. This represents only 30% of lightning strike victims; thus it is possible that you will have to care for such a victim. These events often involve multiple victims, with varying degrees of severity. Prompt CPR greatly improves the chances of survival. When confronted with a naked (or partially unclothed) unconscious or confused patient, with perforated eardrums and a fern-like or splatter burn pattern on his body, think: lightning strike!

Secondary Transport

Major burns often do not occur in locations where immediate transport to a burn center is possible. As a result, transport from a primary hospital to a burn center is commonly necessary. After the initial stabilization, prompt transfer to a burn center can improve patient outcome. During this transport, it is important for the ambulance crew to continue resuscitation initiated at the referring facility.

Prior to secondary transport, the transferring physician should have completed the following:

1. Stabilization of respiratory and hemodynamic function. This may include intubation and IV access for fluid administration.

2. Assessment and management of associated injuries

3. Review of appropriate lab data (specifically, blood gas analysis)

4. A nasogastric tube is usually inserted in patients having burns covering more than 20% of the body surface area.

5. Placement of a Foley (urinary) catheter allows measurement of urine output, which can assist in determining the adequacy of ongoing fluid resuscitation.

6. Assessment of peripheral circulation and appropriate wound management

7. Proper arrangements with the receiving hospital and physician

You should specifically discuss the transport with either the referring or the receiving physician to determine what special functions may need monitoring and to determine the appropriate range for fluid administration, since burns often require extremely large hourly IV rates for appropriate cardiovascular support. Initial resuscitative fluid needs in a burn patient are calculated using the Parkland Formula:

$$4 \text{ cc/kg of Ringers lactate or normal saline} \times \% \text{ burn area}$$
$$\times \text{ body weight (kg)} = \text{fluid needs in first 24 hours.}$$

Half of this fluid is given in the first eight (8) hours and the remainder over the next 16 hours.

PEARLS

1. Maintain appropriate safety when removing patients from the source of a burn injury.
2. Treat burn patients as trauma patients—BTLS Primary Survey, critical interventions, and transport decision, Detailed Exam, and Ongoing Exam.
3. Properly cool the surface thermal injury if early after burn event—don't cause hypothermia.
4. Any type of burn can have some degree of inhalation injury.
5. Early deaths from burns are not due to burn injury but to airway compromise. Perform frequent Ongoing Exams of the airway and be prepared to secure the airway.
6. Chemical injuries, in general, require prolonged and copious irrigation.
7. Immediately check cardiac status of victims of electrical injury.
8. Plan all secondary transports to burn centers and effectively continue resuscitation during such transports.
9. Do not begin a secondary transport of a patient with a possible airway burn without the patient being intubated before transport.

It is important for you to maintain careful records indicating patient condition and treatment during transport. You should also make an in-depth report to the receiving facility.

PEDIATRIC BURNS

Children represent nearly one-half of all patients who seek treatment for burns. Because of their thinner skin, they are at greater risk for severe injury following a burn. Postburn problems, such as hypothermia, are more likely to occur in children because of their larger surface area to body mass ratio. Because of differences in anatomy, the rule of nines must be modified, as in small children the head represents a larger portion of the body surface (see Figure 14-5). The Lund and Browder chart is better for estimating burn size in children (see Table 14-2). The palmar surface (1%) rule applies to children as well as adults.

Sadly, burns in children may be the result of intentional abuse and, in fact, 10% of abuse cases in the United States involve burns. You should be alert for signs of abuse. These include burns that match shapes of objects such as curling irons, irons, or cigarette burns. Also suspicious for abuse are multiple stories of how the injury occurred or stories of the burn being caused by activities by the child that are inconsistent with the child's development. Burns to the genitalia, perineum, or in a stocking or glove distribution (see Figure 14-17) should also raise suspicion. If there is a suspicion of abuse, this must be reported to child protective services or law enforcement.

Fire and EMS personnel can help reduce burns in children through community education. Programs to teach parents about limiting the temperature on household water heaters to 120 degrees Fahrenheit and programs to teach children about fire safety can make a significant impact on the incidence of pediatric burns in your community. You should also be aware that the elderly may also be victims of abuse by burns (see Chapter 16).

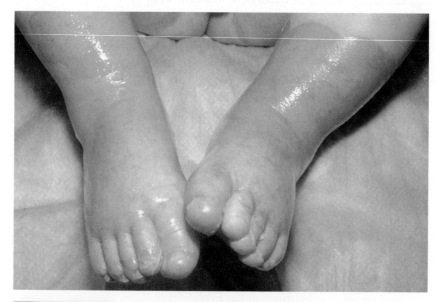

Figure 14-17 Scald burns on a child. This is a typical pattern of child abuse burns. *(Courtesy of Roy Alson, M.D.)*

CASE STUDY

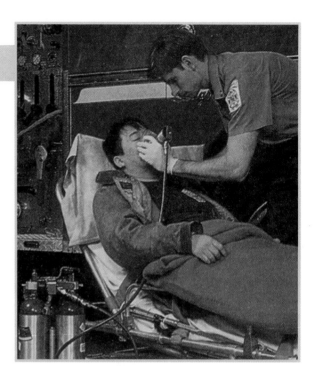

Dan, Joyce, and Buddy of the Emergency Transport System have been called to the scene of a warehouse fire. They are told that the watchman has just been rescued from an upstairs bathroom. During travel to the scene they decide that Buddy will be team leader and they prepare to care for a patient with burns and/or inhalation injuries.

They arrive in the industrial district to find a large warehouse engulfed in flames. The victim has been removed from the area of the fire to a local staging area. As they approach their general impression is bad, as the patient appears to be having difficulty breathing. He is alert but can only speak in one- and two-word sentences because of dyspnea. His voice is hoarse and there is audible wheezing. Initial assessment reveals that his airway is open but he is having wheezing and rapid, stridorous respiration. There are obvious burns of the face. He has a strong but rapid pulse at the wrist. Dan applies an oxygen mask attached to a demand valve (flow-restricted oxygen powered ventilation device—FROPVD) while Buddy continues the BTLS Rapid Trauma Survey. There is erythema and some blistering of the face. The nose hairs are singed. There is soot in the mouth and nose. There is no deformity of the neck and the neck veins are flat. The chest has no apparent injuries but there are inspiratory and expiratory wheezes bilaterally. Heart sounds are rapid and faint. The abdomen is soft and the patient denies pain with palpation. The pelvis is stable and nontender. There is some erythema of the hands but no blistering. There is normal PMS of the extremities.

Buddy gets the team to immediately move the patient to the ambulance and they begin transport. Vital signs are: BP 160/100, pulse 140, respiration 40 per minute. His pulse oximeter saturation is 100%, but Buddy realizes that the pulse oximeter is worthless in carbon monoxide inhalation victims so he attaches no significance to the reading. The patent states he is 45 years old and has a history of asthma. He denies any allergies and his medication is an Albuterol inhaler that he uses as needed. He was upstairs making his rounds when he heard a loud explosion. When he opened the door to the stairs they were engulfed in flames. He went to the back of the building, where he was eventually rescued by the fire department. He complains of burning of his face and hands and also has chest pain and severe dyspnea. He had just finished eating his evening meal when the explosion occurred. Because of the wheezing and stridor, Dan assists the patient in using his Albuteral inhalor. Afterwards he is improved but still has stridor and some wheezing.

Given the injuries found by the crew, Medical Direction instructs them to transport the patient to the regional burn center in the next county. The burn team meets them at the emergency department of the burn center. Because of the rapid treatment the patient eventually makes a complete recovery.

CASE STUDY WRAP-UP

A blast of flame can cause upper airway burns leading to loss of the airway from swelling. The patient with facial burns and burns in the mouth or nose and who has stridor is in danger of immediate loss of the airway. Not only does smoke inhalation cause hypoxia and poisoning by multiple toxic gases, it can precipitate bronchospasm in susceptible individuals. The hypoxia can precipitate a myocardial infarction in individuals who already have borderline coronary arteries. The toxic gases can precipitate coronary spasm leading to myocardial infarction or arrhythmias. Giving 100% oxygen is the best prehospital treatment of carbon monoxide poisoning. The pulse oximeter is unable to tell the difference between oxyhemoglobin and carboxyhemoglobin, so will give false results and is not to be trusted in this case.

SUMMARY

Burn injuries are potentially deadly for both you and your patient. You must never forget the rules of scene safety. Half of all burn deaths are from inhalation injuries; do not forget the airway. Give 100% oxygen if there is any chance of inhalation injury. Cool the burn to halt the burning process, but do not cause hypothermia. You must begin irrigating chemical burns in the field, or the burn damage will continue during transport. This is one of the few instances in trauma care when extra time spent in the field may be beneficial to the patient. Electrical burns are commonly associated with cardiac arrest, but rapid evaluation and management are usually lifesaving. High-voltage electricity is extremely dangerous; get trained personnel to turn it off. Do not begin secondary transfer of a burn patient until the patient has been properly stabilized and the airway protected.

BIBLIOGRAPHY

1. Alson, R. "Thermal Burns." *Emedicine: On-line Emergency Medicine Text.* Boston: Boston Medical Publishers, 1998.

2. Committee on Trauma, American College of Surgeons. "Injuries Due to Burns and Cold." *Advanced Trauma Life Support.* Chicago: The College, 1997.

3. Criss, E., and others. "Not Just Blowing Smoke." *Emergency Medical Services* (March 1998), pp. 27–39.

4. Wald, D. A. "Burn Management: Systematic Patient Evaluation, Fluid Resuscitation, and Wound Management." *Emergency Medicine Reports*, Vol. 19 (1998), pp. 45–52.

Trauma in Children

Ann Marie Dietrich, M.D., F.A.C.E.P., F.A.A.P.
Jon Groner, M.D.

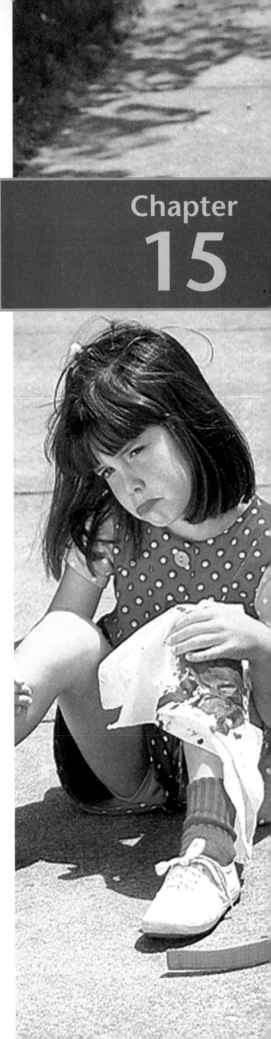

Objectives

Upon completion of this chapter, you should be able to:

1. Describe effective techniques for gaining the confidence of children and their parents.

2. Predict pediatric injuries based on common mechanisms of injury.

3. Describe the Primary Survey and Detailed Exam in the pediatric patient.

4. Demonstrate understanding of the need for immediate transport in potentially life-threatening circumstances, regardless of lack of immediate parental consent.

5. Differentiate equipment needs of pediatric patients from those of adults.

6. Describe the various ways to immobilize a child and how this differs from an adult.

7. Discuss the need for involvement of EMS personnel in prevention programs for parents and children.

   Note: Because of increasing demand for further training in management of the injured child, BTLS has developed a one-day course (Pediatric BTLS) that covers this subject in greater detail. You may get more information about this course by calling BTLS International at: 1-800-495-2875.

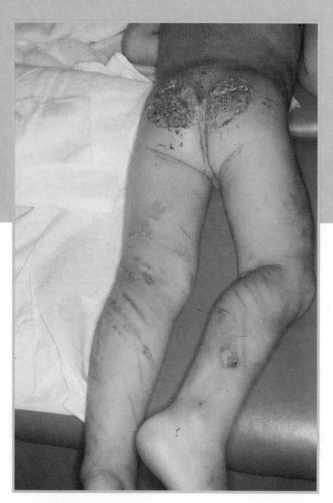

CASE STUDY

Joyce, Dan, and Buddy have received a call to a home for an injured child. They are told that the child had a wreck on his bicycle and is unconscious. As they respond to the scene they decide that Joyce will be team leader. What sort of injuries should they expect from this mechanism? How does evaluating and treating a child differ from an adult? Keep these questions in mind as you read the chapter. The case study will continue at the end of the chapter.

COMMUNICATING WITH THE CHILD AND FAMILY

An injured child is still part of a family unit. Family-centered care is critical for the child, and the one constant factor in their life is their family. Remember that the caregiver of a child will not always be a parent, but for simplicity we will use the generic term "parents" when referring to the guardian of a child. Following an injury, parents should be involved as much as possible in the care their child receives. The parents should be directed and supported in efforts to provide love and concern to their child. Parents who receive careful instructions and guidance are the best assets in the field. Explain to the parents what you are doing and why you are doing it, and use their trust relationship with the child to enhance your history, physical examination, and care of the patient. Inclusion and respect of the family will improve the performance of all aspects of stabilization of an injured child.

The best way to get the parents' confidence is to demonstrate your competence and compassion in managing the child. Parents are more likely to be cooperative if they see that you are confident, organized, and are using equipment that is designed for children. Show the parents you know how important they are by involving them in the care of their child. Whenever possible, keep parents in physical and verbal contact with the child. They can perform simple tasks such as holding a pressure dressing or holding the child's hand. Parents can explain to the child what is going on or sing their favorite songs.

Show your concern for the child—but don't freeze. One technique is to pretend that the parent is one of your examiners. You can then talk your way through the examination using language that is understandable to both the child and family. You will also be able to better assess mental status. A child who can be consoled or distracted by a person or a toy has a normal mental status (most sensitive indicator of adequate perfusion). On the other hand, a child who cannot be consoled or distracted may have a head injury, be in shock, be experiencing hypoxia, or be in severe pain. Changes in distractibility and consolability are important observations about the level of consciousness of a child. Record and report them just as you would report changes in level of consciousness of an adult. Since they are familiar with a child's baseline mental status, the parents are your best resource for detecting subtle changes in the child's level of consciousness. They will notice when the child is "not acting right" before you will.

A child less than nine months old likes to hear "cooing" sounds, the tinkle and sight of keys, and often feels more comfortable when swaddled. For the child under two, the flashlight is a good distraction. Use appropriate language for the development of the child. Children less than one year of age know many "ah" sounds, like "mama" and "papa." Try to use those. Older children, especially two-year-olds, are typically negative and often difficult to distract or comfort. Expect all questions to be answered by "no." Therefore, tell the child and the parents what you are going to do and do it. For example, "We are going to hold your head still. Mom, this is important in case he has hurt his neck." Speak simply, slowly, and clearly. Be gentle and firm. The toddler and young child can benefit from a toy or doll being with them. Ask the parent to get one favorite belonging, if easily available, for the ride to the hospital. It will make the trip to and through the hospital easier. If time allows and the patient is stable, you can make an airplane out of two tongue blades or a doll out of a rubber glove (if child is over 3 years old and won't choke on the rubber).

Don't get caught in the trap of asking the child if he wants to take a trip in the ambulance or to be placed in a cervical collar. The child will answer "no" most of the time. Tell the child what you are doing with a smile on your face. Show it does not hurt, perhaps by doing it to a parent or yourself. Size is intimidating. When approaching a child, try to make yourself small by getting on the child's level. In the care of the child, it is appropriate that paramedics spend much field time on their knees. Frightened children, especially around the ages of two to four, may try to defend themselves by biting, spitting, or hitting. They are acting out of fear. Stay calm, recognize that the behavior is normal, reassure the child, and use firm, not painful, physical control of the patient as needed. Parents and children do not understand packaging, which makes them more likely to resist it. Explain why packaging is necessary. Most parents will understand if you explain that even though the chances are low that there is anything seriously wrong with the spine, the stakes are high if there is. Make a game of packaging with the child. If the parent refuses to let you package the child, write it down on your run report and get the parent to sign it.

Many states have consent laws that exist to protect children. Although consent is necessary for children who are stable, and desirable in children who are injured, any critically injured child should NOT have care delayed while attempting to obtain consent. Paramedics have to make a decision on whether it will take too long to find a parent to obtain consent. In a situation in which a child needs emergency care (e.g., a child in a bicycle–auto collision and no parent present), you must treat that child appropriately. Transport before you receive permission, document why you are transporting without permission, and notify Medical Direction of this action. If the parents or legal guardians do not want you to transport or treat, try to persuade them. If you cannot, document your actions on the written report and try to get them to sign it. If the child has a critical injury and the parents refuse transport, notify law enforcement and the appropriate social authorities *immediately* and try to continue your care of the child until they arrive. If you suspect abuse, notify authorities at the appropriate time.

Whenever possible, allow parents to accompany their child in the vehicle. It is very frightening for a child and a family to be separated, especially if the injuries are severe. Give the parents specific instructions and position them to provide comfort and support to their child without interfering with the care that must be given.

Before you leave the scene with the child, be sure to ask the parent about other children. Sometimes they are so concerned about one that they forget other small children who may be in a high-risk situation, such as alone in the house.

EQUIPMENT

Table 15-1 contains a list of suggested pediatric equipment for the prehospital provider. You would not want to approach a 170-pound man having a heart attack with a pediatric backboard, nor would you approach a child with adult equipment. Pediatric equipment should be kept in a separate trauma box. Equipment for each size child could be kept in different trauma boxes, so that everything for that size child would be at your fingertips. However, lack of storage space makes multiple boxes impractical for most rescue vehicles and ambulances. In addition, it is impractical to make multiple trips back to the vehicle if the dispatch information was inaccurate. There are length-based tapes (Broselow or Standard Pediatric Aid to Resuscitation Card system [SPARC]) that, when used to measure the length of a child, gives you the estimated weight of the child, precalculated doses of fluid and medications, and estimated sizes of common equipment needed. You could have equipment and supplies sorted into boxes or bags coded to the color panels on the length-based tape (compact color-coded bags are commercially available).

Using a length-based drug dose chart or tape (i.e., the Broselow tape or SPARC system) has become an essential component for determining the appropriate equipment for a child (see Figure 15-1a and b). These devices allow you to focus on the patient instead of remembering the correct equipment size. These tape systems estimate weight better than emergency medicine professionals.

TABLE 15-1	Prehospital Pediatric Equipment and Supplies.
BLS Equipment and Supplies	
Essential	**Desirable**
Oropharyngeal airways: infant, child, and adult sizes (sizes 00–5) with tongue blades for insertion	Infant car seat
Self-inflating resuscitation bag, child and adult sizes	Glasgow Coma Score reference
Masks for bag-valve mask device: infant, child, and adult sizes	Small stuffed toy
Nonrebreathing mask: pediatric and adult sizes	Finger-stick blood glucose device
Stethoscope	Pulse Oximeter
Pediatric femur traction splint	
Pediatric backboard with head immobilizer	
Pediatric cervical collars (rigid)	
Blood pressure cuff, infant and child	
Portable suction unit with a regulator	
Suction catheter: tonsil-tip and 6F–14F	
Extremity splints: pediatric size	
Bulb syringe	
Obstetric pack	
Thermal blanket	
Length-based tape or chart (Broselow or Sparc)	

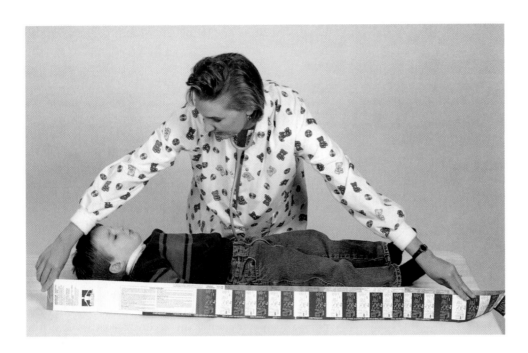

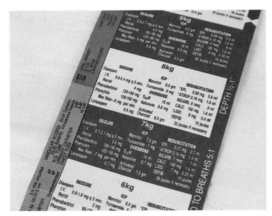

Figure 15-1a Use of Broselow tape.

PATIENT ASSESSMENT (see Figure 15-2)

Common Mechanisms of Injury in Children

Children are most commonly injured from falls, MVCs, auto–pedestrian accidents, burns, airway obstruction from a foreign body, and child abuse. Children who fall usually land on their heads because the head is the largest and heaviest part of a small child's body. You should anticipate head injury when a child falls. Auto collisions, especially if lap belt restraints are improperly used, may injure the liver, spleen, or intestines. Any situation in which the injury pattern and mechanism differ may be child abuse. Suspect abuse if the history doesn't match the injury, if there is a delay in seeking health care, or if the story keeps changing.

Airway with Cervical Spine Stabilization and Initial Level of Consciousness

This aspect of assessment is easier in the child than in the adult. It is true that the child's tongue is large, the tissue is soft, and the airway is easy to obstruct, but other characteristics make it easier to manage the child's airway. For example, neonates are obligatory nose

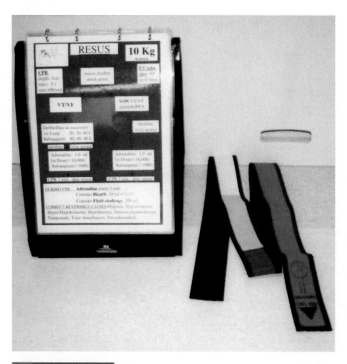

Figure 15-1b Standard Pediatric Aid to Resuscitation Card System has color-coded tape and booklet of precalculated doses of fluids, medications, and equipment. *(Photo Courtesy of Kyee Han, M.D.)*

breathers, so just opening the mouth or clearing the nose with a bulb syringe can be lifesaving. To use the bulb syringe, collapse the bulb end of the syringe, put the point end in the nose of the child, and release the bulb. Remove the syringe from the nose; squeeze the bulb to empty the mucus, blood, or vomit, and repeat. The bulb syringe can be used to remove secretions from the posterior pharynx of infants as well.

Be sure to stabilize the neck in a neutral position with your hands. Do not take time to apply a cervical collar until you have finished the BTLS Primary Survey. Recognize the signs of airway obstruction in children: apnea, stridor, or "gurgling" respiration. So that the neck does not have to be moved, the jaw thrust should be the first airway maneuver in the unconscious child who has sustained trauma. In small children, the occiput is so big that it will flex the neck and may occlude the airway when the child is lying flat. It is often necessary to place a pad underneath the torso to keep the neck in a neutral position (see Figure 15-3 and Chapter 9). Hyperextension of the neck also may cause airway occlusion. For the unconscious child with no gag reflex, an oral airway is very helpful to get the tongue out of the way and keep the airway open (see Chapter 5). If a tooth is loose, be sure to remove it from the mouth so that the child does not choke on it. The oral airway can stimulate a gag reflex, which is very sensitive in the conscious child, thus limiting the use of this airway to unconscious children with no gag reflex. Nasopharyngeal airways are too small to work predictably in children; do not use them. Give ventilation instructions as soon as you complete your evaluation of breathing.

Check the neck for signs of injury (bruises, marks, and lacerations), carotid pulse, and distended neck veins, and feel for a deviated trachea. What appears to be minor blunt trauma to the neck can be life threatening. A deviated trachea is difficult to detect in a small child, but has the same significance as in adults. Make a mental note of the child's initial level of consciousness as you begin your survey. Although a sleeping preschool child can look unconscious, remember that most children will not sleep through the arrival of emergency vehicles. Ask the parents to awaken the child to get an initial assessment of their airway and level of consciousness. Following a traumatic event, a decreased level of consciousness may suggest hypoxia, shock, head trauma, or seizure.

Assessment of Breathing

Assess the child for breathing difficulty. Count the child's respiratory rate. Most children breathe fast when they are having trouble and then, when they can no longer compensate, they have periods of apnea or a very slow respiratory rate. Note whether the child is "working" to breathe, demonstrated by retractions, flaring, or grunting. Look at the chest rise, listen for air going in and out, and feel the air coming out of the nose. If there is no movement, you must breathe for the child. If ventilation is inadequate, you must assist the child. When performing mouth-to-mouth ventilation for a small child, you may cover both the child's nose and mouth with your mouth. If the face mask does not fit well when performing bag-valve mask ventilation, try turning the mask upside down for a better seal. Pay attention to your hand placement (see Figure 15-4). Your large hands can easily

Patient Assessment Using Priority Plan

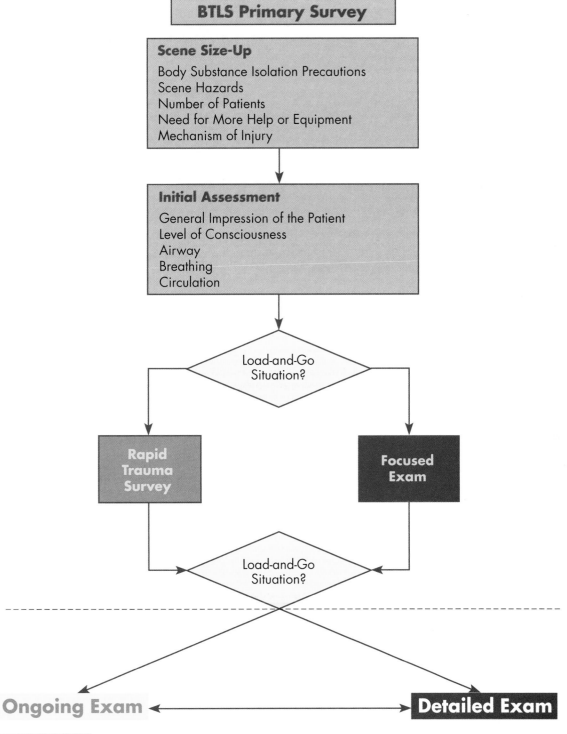

BTLS Primary Survey

Scene Size-Up

Body Substance Isolation Precautions
Scene Hazards
Number of Patients
Need for More Help or Equipment
Mechanism of Injury

Initial Assessment

General Impression of the Patient
Level of Consciousness
Airway
Breathing
Circulation

Load-and-Go
Situation?

Rapid Trauma Survey

Focused Exam

Load-and-Go
Situation?

Ongoing Exam   **Detailed Exam**

Figure 15-2 Steps in the assessment and management of the trauma patient. This is the same for both children and adults.

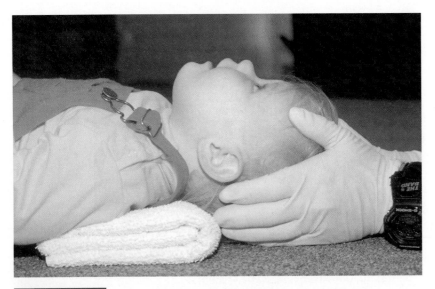

Figure 15-3 Most children require padding under their back and shoulders to keep the C-spine in a neutral position.
(Courtesy of Bob Page, NREMT-P)

obstruct the airway or injure the child's eyes. Give the breaths slowly at low pressure, less than 20 cm H_2O, to keep from inflating the stomach or causing a pneumothorax. The rates are 30 per minute for a child less than a year of age, 20 per minute for greater than one year of age, and 15 per minute for an adolescent. Most important, watch for chest rise when you ventilate. If the chest is rising, air is getting into the lungs. Check air entry on both sides of the chest with your stethoscope. *Gentle* cricoid pressure (Sellick maneuver; see Chapter 4) is useful and recommended in a child. Some self-inflatable bag-valve masks have a pop-off valve at about 40 cm H_2O pressure. The pressure generated by these devices is more than adequate most of the time. However, lungs are sometimes stiff from a near-drowning, bronchospasm, or aspiration, and more pressure is needed. Be familiar with your equipment. Make sure that your bag-valve mask does not have a pop-off valve.

As you package a child, you will often have to improvise. Tape and straps can restrict the child's chest movement, so assess ventilation frequently en route. Any child with a significant injury should receive supplemental oxygen (as close to 100% oxygen as possible), even if there seems to be no difficulty breathing. Injury, fear, and crying all increase oxygen demands on tissues. Children with any type of injury are likely to vomit; be prepared. Remember to give ventilation instructions to your teammate before moving to assessment of circulation.

Assessment of Circulation

Early shock is more difficult to diagnose in a child than an adult. *Persistent tachycardia is the most reliable indicator of shock in a child.* As pulses may be difficult to find and judge in a child, practice feeling them on most of your pediatric runs and on your children. In a child, the brachial pulse is usually easy to feel, whereas the carotid is not. Feeling a dorsalis pedis pulse causes less anxiety and may be easier to find than a femoral pulse. A weak rapid pulse with a rate over 130 is usually a sign of shock in all children except neonates (see Table 15-2). Prolonged capillary refill and cool extremities may manifest decreased tissue perfusion. Capillary refill may be used along with other meth-

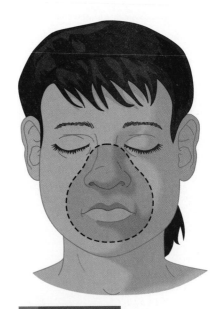

Figure 15-4a

The mask should fit on the nose and the cleft above the chin.

ods to assess the circulation, but do not depend on it alone to diagnose shock. Although currently controversial, capillary refill should still be included as part of the Initial Assessment for shock in a child. To test capillary refill, compress the nailbed, the entire foot, or the skin over the sternum for two seconds and release to see how quickly the blood returns. Skin color should return to the precompressed state within two seconds. If it does not, the child has vasoconstriction, which can be a sign of shock.

Individual variances may make some of the signs of shock normal for a particular child. Tachycardia may occur because of fear or fever. Mottling may be normal in an infant less than six months of age, but it also may be a sign of poor circulation, so note it. Extremities may be cold because of nervousness, cold weather, or poor perfusion. Capillary refill may be prolonged in a child who is cold. In general, a child should be carefully evaluated and assumed to have signs of shock if there is persistent tachycardia or signs of poor peripheral perfusion (prolonged capillary refill or cool extremities).

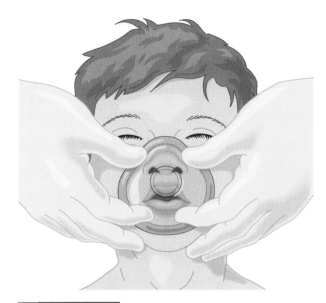

Figure 15-4b Two-handed face mask seal.

The child's level of consciousness is also a useful indicator of circulatory status, yet note that circulation can be poor even though the child appears awake. As mentioned earlier, if the child is able to focus on their parent, or is consolable by the parent or a member of the EMS team, there is enough circulation to allow the child's brain to be working.

Low blood pressure is a sign of late shock, but measuring blood pressure in a frightened child can be time-consuming, especially for the inexperienced. To make it easier and more reliable to obtain blood pressure in an emergency, practice taking it at every opportunity. The rule of thumb for cuff size is to use the largest one that will fit snugly on the patient's upper arm. If there is too much noise, you can perform a blood pressure by palpation. Find the radial pulse, pump up the blood pressure cuff until you no longer feel the pulse, and allow air to leak slowly while observing the dial on the blood pressure cuff. Record the pressure at which you first feel the pulse and label it "p," for palpation. This will be a systolic blood pressure only and will be slightly lower than a blood pressure that can be auscultated. A systolic blood pressure less than 80 in children, and less than 70 in young infants, is a sign of shock.

Shock may be secondary to occult bleeding in the abdomen, chest, or in a femur fracture. Also, although we teach that patients don't go into shock from intracranial blood loss, this can happen in the young infant. Thus, if you see an infant in shock with no obvious source of bleeding, consider intracranial blood loss.

The antishock garment (MAST or PASG) is no longer recommended for treatment of shock except in special circumstances (see Chapter 7). Remember, older children wearing tight-fitting pants are already wearing a form of antishock garment. Cutting these off, like deflating a traditional antishock garment, may produce a drop in blood pressure. Thus, in children with signs of shock, it is wise to delay cutting off tight pants until after you arrive at the hospital.

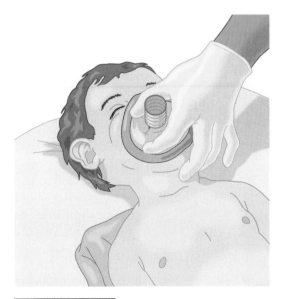

Figure 15-4c One-handed face mask seal.

TABLE 15-2	Ranges for Vital Signs.			
Age	Weight (kg)	Respirations	Pulse	Systolic Blood Pressure (mmHg)
Newborn	3–4	30–50	120–160	>60
6 mo.–1 yr.	8–10	30–40	120–140	70–80
2–4 yr.	12–16	20–30	100–110	80–95
5–8 yr.	18–26	14–20	90–100	90–100
8–12 yr.	26–50	12–20	80–100	100–110
> 12 yr.	>50	12–16	80–100	100–120

Control of Bleeding

Obvious bleeding sources must be controlled to maintain circulation. Remember, the child's blood volume is about 80 to 90 cc per kilogram, so a 10-kg child has less than 1 L of blood. Three or four lacerations can cause a 200-cc blood loss, which is about 20% of the child's total volume. Therefore, pay closer attention to blood loss in a child than you do in an adult. Use pressure firm enough to control arterial bleeding if necessary. If you ask the parent or a bystander to help hold pressure, monitor them to be sure they are applying enough pressure to stop the bleeding. Use a bandage tight enough to control venous bleeding, not one that will just soak up the blood so that you do not see it. Elevating an injured extremity also can help to control bleeding.

Decision: Is There a Critical Trauma Situation Present?

If you have found a critical trauma situation, the child needs rapid transport. Log-roll the child onto a pediatric backboard and go. Remember to use a pad under the torso to align the neck in a neutral position. Appropriately sized rigid cervical collars are useful, especially in children over one year of age, and can help remind the patient and the providers not to move the head. Do not depend on the cervical collar alone; restrict motion of the head with tape and a head motion-restriction device. Children are portable and they can (and should) be transported rapidly. *There are very few procedures that should be done in the field.* Minutes count, especially in children. On-scene times of less than 5 minutes are desirable. Administer 100% oxygen to all critical pediatric patients. Not all emergency departments have the equipment or personnel to handle pediatric emergencies. Transfer arrangements for more severe problems should be worked out in advance so that when the injury occurs, confusion will be minimized and time will be saved. See Table 15-3 for a partial list of mechanisms of injury that are criteria for transport to an emergency department approved for pediatrics or a pediatric trauma center. These, plus pediatric burns, near-drowning, and head injuries with loss of consciousness should go to facilities qualified to handle major pediatric trauma.

If, after completing the Primary Assessment, you find no critical trauma situation, place the child on a backboard and do a methodical Detailed Exam.

Detailed Exam

As in adults, record accurate vital signs, take a SAMPLE history, and perform a complete head-to-toes exam, including a more detailed neurological exam. During your neurological exam make a notation of whether the child is consolable or distractible. Finish bandaging and splinting, and transport the child while continuously monitoring. Notify

TABLE 15-3	Suggested Criteria for Transfer to an Emergency Department Approved for Pediatrics or a Pediatric Trauma Center.

Criteria
Obstructed airway
Need for an airway intervention
Respiratory distress
Shock
Altered mental status
Dilated pupil
Glasgow Coma Score < 13
Pediatric Trauma Score < 8
Mechanism of injury (less reliable indicators) associated with severe injuries:
1. Fall from a height of 15 feet or more
2. An accident with fatalities
3. Ejected from an automobile in a MVC
4. In a MVC, the engine entered the passenger compartment
5. Hit by a car as a pedestrian or bicyclist
6. Fractures in more than one extremity
7. Significant injury to more than one organ system

Medical Direction. Calculate the Glasgow Coma Score (GCS) and Pediatric Trauma Score during transport (Tables 15-4 and 15-5).

INJURIES
Head Injury

Head injuries are the most common cause of death in pediatric patients. The head is the primary focus of injury in the child because the child's head is proportionately larger than the adult's. The force of impact does some damage to the brain, but much of the brain damage from head injuries comes after impact, from preventable causes. To avoid this, you must do three things:

1. *Give oxygen.* Head injury increases brain cell metabolic rate and decreases blood flow in at least part of the brain.

2. *Keep blood pressure up.* Blood must get to the brain to carry oxygen, so systolic pressure must be at least 80 mmHg in the preschool child and 90 mmHg in older children. It is therefore critical to recognize early signs of shock (tachycardia and poor perfusion).

3. *Be prepared to prevent aspiration.* Head-injury patients frequently vomit. The Sellick maneuver should be used during bag-valve mask ventilation. Suction should be readily assessable for any child with a head injury.

Changing level of consciousness is the best indicator of head trauma. A child entering the emergency department with a GCS of 10 that has come down from 13 will be approached very differently from the child who has a GCS of 10 that has come up from 7. Assessments using vague words like "semiconscious" are not helpful. Instead, note specific

TABLE 15-4		Glasgow Coma Score.		
		> 1 year	**< 1 year**	
Eyes Opening	4	Spontaneously	Spontaneously	
	3	To verbal command	To shout	
	2	To pain	To pain	
	1	No response	No response	
		> 1 year	**< 1 year**	
Best Motor Response	6	Obeys		
	5	Localizes pain	Localizes pain	
	4	Flexion-withdrawal	Flexion-normal	
	3	Flexion-abnormal (decorticate rigidity)	Flexion-abnormal (decorticate rigidity)	
	2	Extension (decerebrate rigidity)	Extension (decerebrate rigidity)	
	1	No response	No response	
		> 5 years	**2–5 years**	**0–23 Months**
Best Verbal Response	5	Oriented and converses	Appropriate words and phrases	Smiles, coos, cries appropriately
	4	Disoriented and converses	Inappropriate words	Cries
	3	Inappropriate words	Cries and/or screams	Inappropriate crying and/or screaming
	2	Incomprehensible sounds	Grunts	Grunts
	1	No response	No response	No response

points such as whether the child is distractible, consolable, reaches for the parent, or reacts to pain or voice. Assessment of pupils is as important in the child as in the adult. Note also whether the eyes are moving both left and right or whether they remain in one position. Do not move the head to determine this!

Children with head injury often fare much better than adults with the same degree of injury. Children with head trauma and low GCS may do well if they receive aggressive medical management that focuses on maintenance of oxygenation, ventilation, and perfusion of the brain. Pediatric patients, similar to adults, should not be hyperventilated unless they have evidence of the cerebral herniation syndrome (see Chapter 8). Children with certain types of head injuries, such as epidural hematoma, may need immediate surgical intervention to give the brain the maximum chance of complete healing. Transport children with serious head injuries to a trauma center equipped to provide definitive care.

TABLE 15-5	Pediatric Trauma Score.		
Score	+2	+1	−1
Weight	>44 lb (>20 kg)	22–44 lb (10–20 kg)	<22 lb (<10 kg)
Airway	Normal	Oral or nasal airway	Intubated tracheostomy invasive airway
Blood pressure	Pulse at wrist >90 mmHg	Carotid or femoral pulse palpable 50–90 mmHg	No palpable pulse <50 mmHg
Level of consciousness	Completely awake	Obtunded or any loss of consciousness	Comatose
Open wound	None	Minor	Major or penetrating
Fractures	None	Closed fracture	Open or multiple fractures

Chest Injury

Children generally give visible signs of respiratory distress, such as tachypnea, grunting, nasal flaring, and retractions. Be aware that children's normal respiratory rates are higher than adults' (Table 15-2). A child breathing faster than 40, or an infant faster than 60, usually has respiratory distress and would benefit from supplemental oxygen. A few grunts are not significant, but persistent grunting indicates a need for ventilatory assistance. A child in respiratory distress often breathes with his nose like a rabbit, which is called *flaring*. Retractions relate to caving in of the suprasternal, intercostal, or subcostal areas with inspiration. Retractions suggest the child is straining to breathe. If any of these signs are persistent, they should alert you to something wrong with the respiratory system (pneumo/hemothorax, foreign body, pulmonary contusion).

Children with blunt chest injury are at risk for pneumothorax. Because the chest is small, a difference in breath sounds from side to side may be more subtle than in the adult. You may not be able to tell a difference, even by listening carefully. It is also difficult to diagnose tension pneumothorax in young children, who usually have short, fat necks that mask both neck vein distension and tracheal deviation. If a tension pneumothorax develops, the heart and trachea should eventually shift away from the side of the pneumothorax. To help detect a shift of a child's heart, place an "X" over the point of maximum impulse (PMI) of the heart. Repeatedly check the location of the PMI.

Children in the preadolescent age group have highly elastic chest walls. Rib fractures, flail chest, pericardial tamponade, and aortic rupture are, therefore, seldom seen in this group. However, pulmonary contusion is common. If a child does have rib fractures or a flail chest, he has sustained a significant force to his chest and should be assumed to have internal injuries.

Abdominal Injury

The second leading cause of traumatic death in most pediatric centers is internal bleeding secondary to rupture of the liver and/or spleen. In children, the liver and spleen both protrude below the ribs, exposing the organs to blunt trauma. This poor protection and the relatively large size of the liver and spleen in children allow these organs to be easily torn.

PEARLS

1. Children require special equipment. Without this equipment, you cannot provide the pediatric patient with adequate care. See essential equipment in Table 15-1.
2. Because of strong compensatory mechanisms, children can look surprisingly good in early shock. When they deteriorate, they often "crash." If the mechanism of injury or the assessment suggests the possibility of hemorrhagic shock, load and go.
3. You are the only one to see the scene of the injury. Be alert to signs of child abuse.

Abdominal injuries are difficult to diagnose in the field. A child may have a severe abdominal injury with minimal signs of trauma. Any child with seat belt marks or bruises to the abdomen should be assumed to have internal injuries. If a child has blunt injury to the chest or abdomen, be prepared to treat for shock. The capsule of a child's liver and spleen are thicker than an adult's; therefore, bleeding is often contained within the organ. If a child with blunt trauma is in shock with no obvious source of bleeding, your decision should be to load-and-go. Any child who has been crying or suffered an abdominal injury will develop gastric distention and a tendency to vomit; be prepared.

Spinal Injury

Although children have short necks, big heads, and loose ligaments, cervical spine injuries are uncommon before adolescence. Cervical spine injuries do occur, however, and you should perform SMR on all children with a potential spinal injury. A cervical collar is not necessary if the head is properly restricted in a padded device. Again, try to make a game of packaging the child. You can promise you will give him a ride in the ambulance as a reward after you get him all wrapped up and ready. Use a parent or other familiar person, if possible. Be sure your packaging does not restrict chest movement. As mentioned before, children up to about eight years of age will need a pad under the torso to keep the neck in a neutral position.

CHILD RESTRAINT SEATS

A child in a wreck while properly restrained is much less likely to have a serious injury than an unrestrained passenger. If the child is in a car seat, he can usually be transported without being removed from the device. Assess the child as you would other trauma patients. If no injury is found and the seat is undamaged, place padding around the child's head, and tape the head directly to the car seat (see Figure 15-5). This method of transportation should only be used after a complete assessment that has revealed NO injury to the child. If the child has evidence of any serious injuries, he should be removed from the car seat and packaged. Some new-model cars have built-in infant restraint seats. These seats cannot be removed, so the child who is restrained in one of these will have to be extricated and placed on a pediatric SMR device.

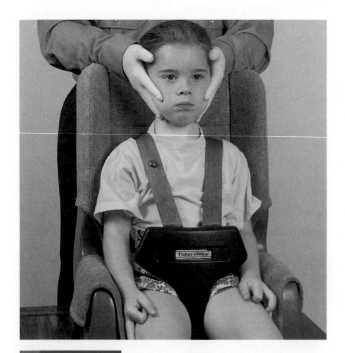

Figure 15-5a One paramedic stabilizes the car seat in an upright position and applies and maintains manual in-line stabilization throughout the SMR process.

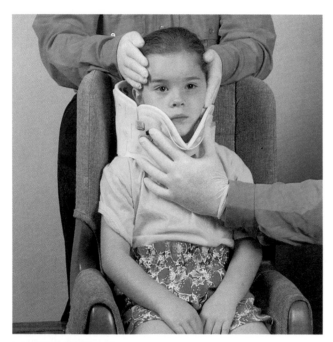

Figure 15-5b A second paramedic applies an appropriately sized cervical collar. If one is not available, improvise using a rolled hand towel.

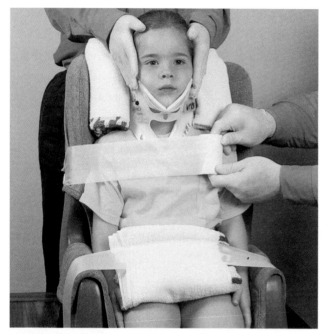

Figure 15-5c The second paramedic places a small blanket or towel on the child's lap, then uses straps or wide tape to secure the chest and pelvic areas to the seat.

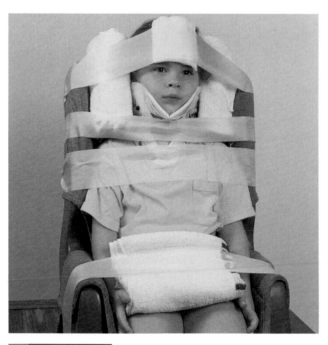

Figure 15-5d

The second paramedic places towel rolls on both sides of the child's head to fill voids between the head and seat. The medic tapes the head into place, taping across the forehead and the collar, but avoiding taping over the chin, which would put pressure on the neck. The patient and seat can be carried to the ambulance and strapped to the stretcher, with the stretcher head raised.

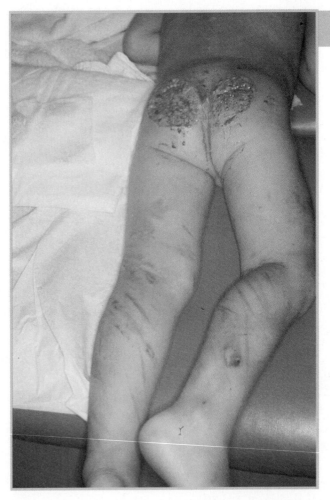

(Photo Courtesy of Scott and White Hospital and Clinic)

CASE STUDY

In the afternoon Joyce, Dan, and Buddy receive a call to a home for an injured child. They are told that the child had a wreck on his bicycle and is unconscious. As they respond to the scene they decide that Joyce will be team leader.

They arrive at an apartment. There is no bicycle seen and the child is inside the apartment. A man who identifies himself as the stepfather says, "Donnie was riding his bike too fast and he wrecked right in front of the apartment. He skinned himself up pretty bad and must have hit his head. He didn't have nothing on but some shorts and was not wearing no helmet. I picked him up and brought him inside and called ya'll." They see an eight-year-old male lying on the couch. The general impression is not good, as the child is neither awake nor moving. He is not clothed and there are obvious old full-thickness burns of his buttocks and multiple bruises of varying ages on his body. They are not injuries that would have come from a bicycle wreck.

Donnie does not respond to Joyce as she speaks to him. She immediately checks the airway and finds it open but respiration is slow and shallow. Donnie has a slow but strong pulse at the wrist. Dan immediately places a clean sheet on the backboard and they carefully log-roll Donnie onto the backboard. Buddy stabilizes the neck with his knees and begins ventilation with a bag-valve mask as Joyce performs the Rapid Trauma Assessment. The child has an obvious hematoma of the right temporal area, with bruising of the face. As he begins ventilation, Buddy notes that the right pupil is slightly larger than the left. The neck has no obvious deformities; the neck veins are flat and trachea is in the midline. The chest has multiple bruises and abrasions and there is crepitation of the ribs on the left side. Donnie moans in pain when his ribs are palpated and localizes with his hands. Buddy notes that he opens his eyes to pain. Breath sounds are present and equal. The heart can be heard and the rate is about 60 beats per minute. Donnie does not respond when Joyce palpates his abdomen. She notes that the abdomen is not distended but has several bruises in a loop pattern such as an electrical cord would make. The pelvis feels stable. Examination of the extremities reveals normal PMS, but there are multiple bruises in linear and loop patterns and some small burns that look like they might have been made with a cigarette. Buddy reports that Donnie has a gag reflex, so he will not insert an oral airway. He keeps suction immediately available.

Joyce decides to transport immediately both because it is a load-and-go situation and she knows she must leave now before her building rage causes her to attack the beast that was responsible for these injuries. As they are going out the front door they meet a woman with a bruise on her cheek. She appears to be coming home from work. She sees the child and cries, "My God! Lester, what have you done to Donnie now?" He glares at her and she begins crying. Neither asks to ride in the ambulance, but she asks where they are taking him and says she will be there soon. Dan drives. Joyce takes vital signs: BP 110/70, respiration 8 per minute when Buddy is not ventilating, and pulse 60 per minute. She calculates the GCS as 9 (eyes, 2; motor, 5; and verbal 2). She also attaches the cardiac monitor (sinus bradycardia) and pulse oximeter (95% on 100% oxygen). She performs the Detailed Exam that reveals no new information except that the eyes both react to light.

Joyce notifies Medical Direction that they have an unconscious eight-year-old child with multiple injuries including blunt head trauma, burns, bruises, and broken ribs. When they arrive she immediately notifies the doctor and nurse of what they saw and heard at the scene. The police and social services were notified; the mother and live-in boyfriend were both arrested. The boyfriend was convicted of child abuse and sent to jail but the mother, because she was also an abuse victim, was placed on probation with loss of child custody. The child required surgery for his epidural hematoma and skin grafting for his burns but eventually recovered and went to live with his grandparents. Joyce suffered nightmares, and the whole team went though critical incident stress debriefing.

CASE STUDY WRAP-UP

Some humans (if they can be called such) can inflict unspeakable torture on children. The common thread among EMS providers is care for others. When confronted with child abuse, our initial reaction can be rage. We must be alert to the signs of child neglect or abuse but never let our emotions prevent us from focusing on treatment of the child (always transport the child to the hospital if you have suspicions of abuse). The investigation is better left to those trained to do so. Most countries have laws requiring the reporting of suspected child abuse and providing legal protection for those who do so. It is extremely important that you report suspicions, as you may be the last chance that child has for survival. There is nothing as tragic as an abused child being saved by good medical care and then returned to be abused again. If you report your suspicions to the emergency physician or nurse and they ignore them, you must make your report directly to the appropriate organization. When making a report, always include local law enforcement. Most social service organizations do an excellent job, but many carry heavy workloads and some do not include local law enforcement in their investigation. Child abuse is not just poor social skills; it is the basest and cruelest of crimes.

SUMMARY

To provide good trauma care for children, you must have the proper equipment, know how to interact with frightened parents, know the normal vital signs for various ages (or have them posted in your trauma box), and be familiar with the injuries that are more common in children. Fortunately, the assessment sequence is the same for children as for adults. If you perform your assessment well, you will obtain the information needed to make the right decisions in management. Focusing on assessment and management of the child's airway (with cervical spine control), breathing, and circulation will result in the best possible outcome.

While assessment and management of the injured child are life-saving skills, all of us involved in the care of the seriously injured child should be concerned also about prevention (see Appendix H). Car seats, bicycle helmets, seat belts, all-terrain vehicle injuries, water safety, scald burn injuries, firearm safety, and fire drills are within our area of concern. We should donate our time to teaching safety (see Figure 15-6), and we should speak out for laws (infant seat restraints, seat belts, drunk driving) that save lives.

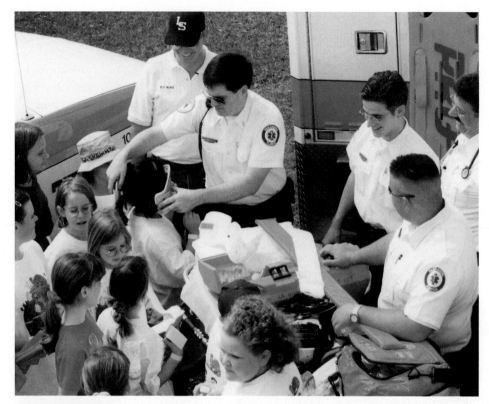

Figure 15-6 It is important to organize or participate in programs that educate children about injury prevention and health care. *(Photo © Craig Jackson/In the Dark Photography)*

BIBLIOGRAPHY

1. Dietrich, A., S. Shaner, and J. Campbell. *Pediatric Basic Trauma Life Support.* Oakbrook Terrace, IL: Basic Trauma Life Support International, 1998.

2. Gausche M., Lewis R. J., et al. "Effect of Out-of-Hospital Pediatric Endotracheal Intubation on Survival and Neurological Outcome: A Controlled Clinical Trial." *JAMA* 2000; 283(6):783.

Trauma in the Elderly

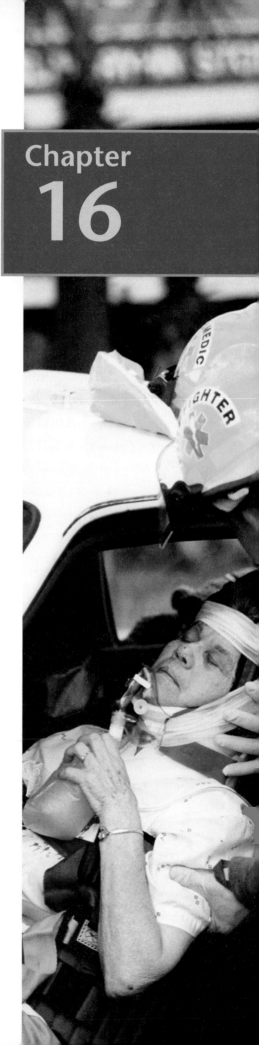

Leah J. Heimbach, R.N., NREMT-P, J.D.

Jere F. Baldwin, M.D., F.A.C.E.P., F.A.A.F.P.

Objectives

Upon completion of this chapter, you should be able to:

1. Describe the changes that occur with aging, and explain how these changes can affect your assessment of the geriatric trauma patient.

2. Describe the assessment of the geriatric trauma patient.

3. Describe the management of the geriatric trauma patient.

(Photo courtesy of Eddie M. Sperling/Eddie Sperling Photography)

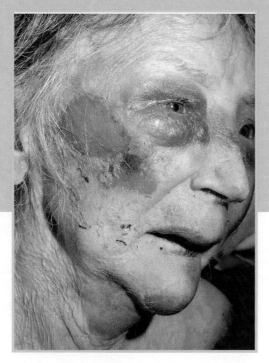

CASE STUDY

Dan, Joyce, and Buddy are dispatched to the home of an elderly woman whose neighbor called 911 and said she was hurt. The dispatcher asked the neighbor to remain with the patient until they arrived. As they respond, they decide that Dan will be team leader and they discuss common home injuries in the elderly. What should you be expecting if you answered this call? How does evaluation of the elderly differ from younger adult patients? Keep these questions in mind as you read the chapter. The case study will continue at the end of the chapter.

By the twenty-first century, it is estimated that citizens over the age of 65 will comprise one-fifth of the U.S. population. The geriatric population already comprises a significant number of the patients being transported by ambulance. In the United States, over 30% of all patients transported by ambulance are over the age of 65.

"Elderly" is often understood as being 65 years or older because retirement benefits are usually initiated at this point in life. However, chronological age is not the most reliable definition of "elderly." It is more appropriate to consider the biologic processes that change with time, for example, the fewer number of neurons, the decreased functioning of the kidneys, and the decreased elasticity of the skin and tissues.

As a group, geriatric patients tend to respond to injury less favorably than the younger adult population. Geriatric patients who are injured are more likely to experience fatal outcomes, even if the injury is of a relatively low severity. According to the U.S. National Safety Council, falls, thermal injury, and MVCs have been identified as common causes of traumatic death in the geriatric population.

Falls account for the majority of injuries in the geriatric population, the most common pathology being fractures of the hip, femur, and wrist, and head injuries. MVCs account for approximately 25% of geriatric deaths, although the elderly drive fewer miles. The geriatric population has a higher incidence of collision than other age groups, second only to that group under the age of 25. Eight percent of deaths are attributable to thermal injuries. These injuries include inhalation, contact with the heat source resulting in scalding and flame burns, and electrical injury.

Little has been written on the response of the geriatric patient to trauma. By gaining an understanding of the normal physiologic changes involved in the aging process, you will be better prepared to provide optimum care to the geriatric trauma victim.

This chapter addresses these processes, highlights illnesses to which the geriatric patient is susceptible, and shows how these processes and illnesses make it difficult to predict the physiological response to trauma in the geriatric patient.

PATHOPHYSIOLOGY OF AGING

Aging is a gradual process whereby changes in bodily functions may occur. These changes are in part responsible for the greater risk of injury in the geriatric population.

Airway: Changes in airway structures of the geriatric patient may include tooth decay, gum disease, and use of a dental prosthesis. Caps, bridges, dentures, and fillings all present potential airway obstructions in the geriatric trauma patient.

Respiratory System: Changes in the respiratory system begin to appear in the early adult years and increase markedly after the age of 60. Circulation to the pulmonary system decreases 30%, reducing the amount of carbon dioxide and oxygen exchanged at the alveolar level. There is a decrease in chest wall movement and in the flexibility of the muscles of the chest wall. These changes cause a decreased inhalation time, resulting in rapid breathing. There is a decreased vital capacity (or decrease in the amount of air exchanged per breath) because of an increased residual volume (volume of air in the lungs after deep exhalation). Overall breathing capacity and maximal work rate may also decrease. If there is a history of cigarette smoking, or a history of working in an area with pollutants, these changes in breathing are even more significant.

Cardiovascular System: Circulation is reduced due to changes in the heart and the blood vessels. Cardiac output and stroke volume may decrease, and the conduction system may degenerate. The ability of the valves of the heart to operate efficiently may decline. These changes may predispose the patient to congestive heart failure and pulmonary edema. Arteriosclerosis occurs with increasing frequency in the course of the aging process, resulting in an increased peripheral vascular resistance (and perhaps systolic hypertension). There may be a normally higher blood pressure in the elderly. Thus a significant change may occur in a patient when the normal blood pressure of 160 drops to 120 as a result of trauma. There may be a decreased blood flow to the periphery, making the capillary refill an inaccurate indicator of shock.

Neurological and Sensory Function: Several changes occur in the brain with age. The brain shrinks, and the outermost meningeal layer, the dura mater, remains tightly adherent to the skull. This creates a space or an increased distance between the brain and the skull. Instead of protecting the brain during impact, this space allows an increased incidence of subdural hematoma following trauma. There is also a hardening, narrowing, and loss of elasticity of some arteries in the brain. A deceleration injury may cause blood vessel rupture and potential bleeding inside the skull. There is decreased blood flow to the brain. The patient may experience a slowing of sensory responses such as pain perception and decreases in hearing, eyesight, or in other sensory perceptions. Many older patients may have a higher pain tolerance from living with conditions such as arthritis, or from being on analgesic medications chronically. This can result in their failure to identify areas in which they have been injured. Other signs of decreased cerebral circulation due to the aging process may include confusion, irritability, forgetfulness, altered sleep patterns, and mental dysfunctions such as loss of memory and regressive behavior. There may be a decrease in the ability, or even an absence of the ability, to compensate for shock.

Thermoregulation: Mechanisms to maintain normal body temperature may not function properly. The geriatric patient may not be able to respond to an infection with a fever, or the patient may not be able to maintain a normal temperature in the face of injury. The geriatric patient with a broken hip who has been lying on the floor in a room where the temperature is 64 degrees Fahrenheit can experience hypothermia.

Renal System: A decrease in the number of functioning nephrons in the kidneys of the geriatric patient can result in a decrease in filtration and a reduced ability to excrete urine and drugs.

Musculoskeletal System: The geriatric patient may exhibit signs of changes in posture. There may be a decrease in total height due to the narrowing of the vertebral discs. There may be slight flexion of the knees and hips. There may be decreased muscle strength. This may result in a kyphotic deformity of the spine, resulting in the "s" curvature of the spine often seen in the stooped elderly. The geriatric patient may also have advanced osteoporosis—a thinning of the bone resulting in a decrease in bone density. This renders the bone more susceptible to fractures. Finally, there may be a weakening in the strength of the muscle and bone from the decrease in physical activity; this will also render the geriatric patient more susceptible to fractures with only a slight fall.

Gastrointestinal System: Saliva production, esophageal motility, and gastric secretion may decrease. This may result in decreased ability to absorb nutrients. Constipation and fecal impactions are common. The liver may be enlarged because of disease processes or may be failing due to disease or malnutrition. This may result in a decreased ability to metabolize medications.

Immune System: As the aging process continues, the geriatric patient may be less able to fight off infection. The patient in a poor nutritional state will thus be more susceptible to infection from open wounds, IV access sites, and lung and kidney infections. The geriatric trauma patient who is not otherwise severely injured may die from sepsis from an impaired immune system.

Other Changes: The total body water and total number of body cells may be decreased, and there is an increase in the proportion of the body weight as fat. There may be a loss in the capacity of the systems to adjust to illness or injury.

Medications: Many geriatric patients take several medications that can interfere with their ability to compensate after sustaining trauma. Anticoagulants may increase bleeding time. Antihypertensives and peripheral vasodilators can interfere with the body's ability to vasoconstrict blood vessels in response to hypovolemia. Beta-blockers can inhibit the heart's ability to increase the rate of contraction even in hypovolemia shock.

A number of the aging processes contribute to the increased risk of injury to the geriatric patient. The changes that may increase susceptibility to injury include the following:

1. Slower reflexes
2. Failing eyesight
3. Hearing loss
4. Arthritis
5. Fragile skin and blood vessels
6. Fragile bones

Causative factors related to the aging process have been linked with specific injuries such as tripping over furniture and falling down stairs. Further investigation reveals that these falls are often related as much to a decrease in the function of special senses, such as loss in peripheral vision, as they are to syncope, postural instability, transient impairment of cerebrovascular perfusion, alcohol ingestion, or medication usage. Alterations in perception and delayed response to stressors may also contribute to injury in the geriatric patient. When treating the geriatric trauma patient, remember that the priorities are the same as for all trauma patients. However, you must give consideration to three important issues:

1. General organ systems may not function as effectively as those in the younger adult, especially the cardiovascular, pulmonary, and renal systems.

2. The geriatric patient also may have a chronic illness that may complicate the effectiveness of trauma care.

3. Bones may fracture more easily with less force.

ASSESSMENT AND MANAGEMENT OF THE ELDERLY TRAUMA PATIENT

Geriatric patient assessment, as any assessment, must take into account priorities, interventions, and life-threatening conditions. However, *you must be acutely aware that geriatric patients can die from less severe injuries than younger patients.* In addition, it is often difficult to separate the effects of the aging process or of a chronic illness from the consequences of the injury. The chief complaint may seem trivial because the patient may not report truly important symptoms. You must search for important signs or symptoms. In the geriatric patient, it is not uncommon for the patient to suffer from more than one illness or injury at the same time. Remember that the elderly patient may not have the same response to pain, hypoxia, or hypovolemia as a young person. Don't underestimate the severity of the patient's condition.

You may have difficulty communicating with the patient. This could result from the patient's diminished senses, hearing or sight impairment, or depression. The geriatric patient nonetheless should not be approached in a condescending manner. Do not allow others to take over the reporting of events from the patient who is able and willing to communicate reliable information. Unfortunately, the patient may minimize or even deny symptoms out of fear of becoming dependent, bedridden, institutionalized, or even of losing a sense of self-sufficiency. It is important that you explain any actions, including removing any clothing, before initiating the physical assessment.

There are other considerations in assessing the geriatric trauma patient. Peripheral pulses may be difficult to evaluate. Older patients often wear many layers of clothing, which can impede physical assessment. You must also distinguish between signs and symptoms of a chronic disease and an acute problem, for instance:

1. The geriatric patient may have nonpathologic rales.
2. The loss of skin elasticity and the presence of mouth breathing may not necessarily represent dehydration.
3. Dependent edema may be secondary to venous insufficiency with varicose veins or inactivity rather than congestive heart failure.

Pay attention to deviation from expected ranges in vital signs and other physical assessment findings in the geriatric patient. An injury that is isolated and noncomplicated in the young adult may be debilitating in the older adult. This may be due to the patient's overall condition, lowered defenses, or inability to keep the effects of an injury localized.

When obtaining the past medical history, it is important to note what medications the patient may be taking. Medications may not only account for an abnormal pulse, but may also mask normal circulatory responses that would indicate deterioration in the circulatory system. The result can be a rapid decompensation without warning. Knowledge of the medications that the patient is taking can alert you to the fact that the patient's condition may be more unstable than that presented by current signs and symptoms. Antihypertensives, anticoagulants, beta-blockers, and hypoglycemic agents may profoundly influence the response of the geriatric patient to traumatic injury.

Primary Survey

Scene Size-Up: Survey the scene to decide if it is safe, to determine the number of patients, and to obtain the mechanism of injury. After the Primary Survey, it may be helpful to obtain further information and to verify the patient's history from reliable family members or neighbors. This is best done in an area where the patient is unable to overhear the conversation; otherwise it may suggest that the geriatric patient is less than a competent adult. Observe the surrounding area for indications that the patient is able to provide his own care, for signs of alcohol abuse or ingestion of multiple medications, and for signs of violence, abuse, or neglect. Abuse and/or neglect of the elderly are common. When your assessment of the patient and surroundings is suspicious for abuse or neglect, do not fail to notify the proper authorities. *Be sure to gather the patient's medications and bring them to the hospital.*

Evaluate Airway, Cervical Spine Control, and Initial Level of Consciousness: As with any trauma patient, you must evaluate and provide an adequate airway and maintain motion restriction of the cervical spine while assessing the initial level of consciousness. The initial level of consciousness has more significance with elderly patients than with younger patients. Subsequent health care providers may attribute a decreased level of consciousness to a pre-existing condition rather than to the trauma. This is more likely to occur if you have not clearly indicated that the patient was clear, lucid, and cooperative at the scene.

If patients respond appropriately to the initial verbal statements, they have an open airway and are conscious. If they do not respond, gently open the airway with a modified jaw thrust while maintaining the neck in a neutral position. This position may be difficult to determine with certainty because of arthritis and kyphosis of the spine. It is important to recognize this and not to forcibly place the occiput flat on the backboard or ground. You should add padding to the backboard to maintain the patient's usual spinal position.

The airway is likely to be partially obstructed. Clear the airway, being alert to possible teeth fragments due to decay and gum disease and dental devices such as caps, bridges, dentures, and fillings. Look, listen, and feel for movement of air. Ensure that the rate and volume of air exchange is adequate. The geriatric patient with unresolved airway difficulty or a decreased level of consciousness should be transported immediately. In such a case, frequently monitor the respiratory effort and level of consciousness (remember to check a blood glucose).

Breathing and Circulation: Place your face over the patient's mouth to look at the chest rise, to listen to the quality of the breath sounds from the mouth, and to feel the patient's breath against your ear. If the breathing is so fast that there is inadequate air exchange (more than 24 breaths per minute), or if it is too slow (fewer than 10 breaths per minute), or if the volume of air being exchanged is inadequate, provide assisted ventilation with 100% supplemental oxygen. Check the rate and quality of the pulse at the wrist (check at the neck if there is no pulse at the wrist). Evaluate skin color and condition. Scan the patient for bleeding, and control any bleeding with pressure.

RAPID TRAUMA SURVEY OR FOCUSED EXAM

The choice between the Rapid Trauma Survey and the Focused Exam depends on the mechanism of injury and/or the results of the Initial Assessment. If there is a dangerous generalized mechanism of injury (auto crash, fall from a height, etc.) or if the patient is unconscious, you should perform the BTLS Rapid Trauma Survey. If there is a dangerous focused mechanism of injury suggesting an isolated injury (bullet wound of thigh, stab wound to the chest, etc.), you may perform the Focused Exam limited to the area of injury. If there is no significant mechanism of injury (dropped rock on toe) and the Initial Assessment was normal (alert with no history of loss of consciousness, breathing normally, radial pulse less than 120, not complaining of dyspnea or chest, abdominal, or pelvic pain), you may move directly to the Focused Exam based on the patient's chief complaint.

Rapid Trauma Survey

Examine the Head, Neck, Chest, Abdomen, Pelvis, and Extremities: Briefly assess the head and neck for injuries and to see if the neck veins are flat or distended and the trachea is in the midline. You may apply a rigid extrication collar at this time. Now look, feel, and listen to the chest. Look for both asymmetrical and paradoxical movement. Note if the ribs rise with respiration or if there is only diaphragmatic breathing. Look for signs of blunt trauma or open wounds. Feel for tenderness, instability, or crepitation (TIC). Now listen to see if breath sounds are present and equal bilaterally. Make appropriate interventions for chest injuries. Remember that chest injuries are more likely to cause serious problems in older people with poor pulmonary reserve. Be especially alert to problems in patients with chronic lung disease. They usually have borderline hypoxia even when not injured. Briefly notice the heart sounds so you will have a baseline for changes such as development of muffled heart sounds. Rapidly expose and look at the abdomen (distention, contusions, penetrating wounds), and gently palpate the abdomen for tenderness, guarding, and rigidity. Check the pelvis and extremities for wounds, deformity, and TIC. Note whether the patient can move his fingers and toes before transferring to a backboard.

Critical Transport Decisions: There are a few procedures that may be initiated onscene, but do not delay transport. Examples of critical interventions that may be initiated at the scene are the following:

1. Provide airway management.
2. Assist ventilation.
3. Begin CPR.
4. Control major bleeding.
5. Seal sucking chest wounds.
6. Stabilize flail chest.
7. Stabilize impaled objects.

Consider whether the time delay in initiating these procedures outweighs the risks of delaying transportation. As mentioned elsewhere, the chance of survival decreases with a corresponding increase in the length of scene time. The same indications for immediate transport apply for the elderly as for younger patients (see Chapter 2), but remember that you may not have as dramatic a response to injury in the elderly, so you should have a low threshold for early transport. If one of the critical conditions is present, immediately transfer the patient to a long backboard with appropriate padding, apply oxygen, load the patient into the ambulance, and transport rapidly to the nearest appropriate emergency facility.

Packaging and Transport: Package or prepare the elderly patient for transport as quickly and gently as possible. Take extra care when performing SMR on the geriatric trauma patient. This includes padding void areas that may be exaggerated due to the aging process. The elderly patient with kyphosis will require padding under the shoulders and head to maintain the neck in its usual alignment (see Figure 16-1). Do not force the neck into a neutral position if it is painful to do so, or if the neck is obviously fused in a forward position. Remember to

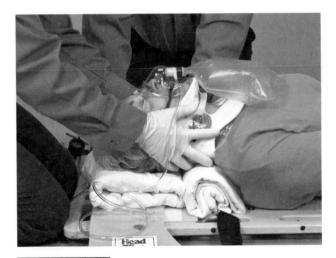

Figure 16-1 Elderly patients with kyphosis require padding under the shoulders and head to maintain the spine in its usual alignment.

treat and transport the geriatric trauma patient, as you do all trauma patients, gently and quickly.

Detailed Exam and Ongoing Exams: Perform a Detailed Exam on-scene if the patient is stable. If there is any question as to the patient's condition, you should transport and perform the Detailed Exam en route. Perform frequent Ongoing Exams. Frequently assess the patient's pulmonary status, including lung sounds and cardiac rhythm. All elderly patients should have cardiac monitoring and pulse oximetry, if available.

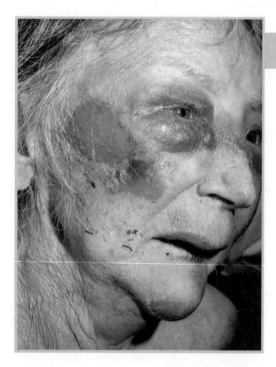

CASE STUDY

Dan, Joyce, and Buddy are dispatched to the home of an elderly woman whose neighbor called 911 and said she was hurt. The dispatcher asked the neighbor to remain with the patient until they arrived. As they respond, they decide that Dan will be team leader and they discuss common home injuries in the elderly. When they arrive, the neighbor meets them at the door and takes them to the patient's room. She is a 96-year-old woman (Mrs. Mary Higginbotham) who has bruises all over and appears to have been bed-bound for some time. She is awake but confused and unable to answer any of the questions. The room and bed linen are filthy. The sheets smell of urine and there are dried feces on the patient's legs. The neighbor states that the woman is usually alert and ambulatory and able to care for herself.

Because of Mary's failing eyesight, her grandson came to live with her about six months ago. The neighbor states that her grandson does not work but lives off her retirement (Mary is a retired college professor). "He drinks," she said. Mary's husband died 10 years ago and she has suffered from depression, but seemed to be doing better until her grandson came to live with her. She began having frequent bruises soon after he arrived, but she always explained them by saying "I fall a lot." The neighbor (and long-time friend) said that Mrs. Higginbotham has a history of type II diabetes and mild hypertension, and takes medication for both. She said that Dexter (the grandson) had discouraged her visiting and lately would not let her talk to Mary on the phone. In response to this she had begun waiting until he went out and then coming over to visit and check on Mary. The neighbor (Mrs. Bixby) said that she had been away for a week and was anxious to see Mary. When she saw Dexter leave this morning she came over, and was appalled to see that Mary could not get out of bed and didn't even recognize her.

Dan began his exam while Buddy and Joyce looked for medicine bottles. Mrs. Bixby was not sure about allergies, but said that she did not know of any. Dan is still not sure if this is a medical or trauma call but decides to do a trauma survey. The airway is open and the respiratory rate is a little fast and shallow. The mucous membranes look dry. The breath sounds are present and equal and the peripheral pulse is weak and rapid. There is a large bruise and abrasion of the right cheek and periorbital area. The pupils are equal and reactive to light but there are obvious cataracts in both eyes. The pharynx is edentulous but Dan can't find the dentures. The neck is nontender but there is marked dorsal kyphosis. There is equal expansion of the chest and no rales or wheezing is noted. The heart rate is fast but he hears no murmurs. The abdomen is thin and scaphoid with no obvious tenderness or masses. The pelvis is stable but she is tender over the left hip and the left leg is shortened. Peripheral pulses are present in both legs. There is very poor skin turgor. She follows commands and moves all extremities but complains of pain when the left leg is moved. By the time Dan is finished, Joyce has taken the vital signs and tells him that the blood pressure is 170/110, pulse 110, and respiration is 26 per minute. Pulse oximeter reading is 96% on room air. Buddy has found a half-empty bottle of Diabeta® (oral diabetes medication) open by the bedside table and a full, unopened bottle of Tenormin® (beta-blocker antihypertensive medication) in the kitchen on the counter. Both bottles were filled a week ago.

They carefully move Mrs. Higginbotham to a vacuum backboard and mold it to her to support her neck and hip. They then move her to the ambulance, where Dan applies nasal oxygen at 3 L/min. Buddy drives and Joyce does a fingerstick glucose. The glucose is 55. Dan gives her a tube of glucose paste and soon Mrs. Higginbotham is alert and oriented. She complains of pain in her left hip. When asked how she hurt it she lowers her eyes and says "I fall a lot." She does not remember about her medicine but says that sometimes Dexter gives it to her and sometimes she takes it on her own. She has been unable to walk for five days. "Dexter has to be out a lot so I haven't been able to keep the place cleaned up. He is really a good boy but he is forgetful and he has to be gone on business a lot." (Mrs. Bixby had told them that his "business" is drinking at the local pub.) Mrs. Higginbotham denies allergies and cannot remember when she last ate. The Detailed Exam revealed no new findings. At the hospital Mrs. Higginbotham is found to be dehydrated and malnourished with a fracture of her left hip and multiple bruises and abrasions. Dan reports their suspicion of abuse and neglect. An investigation later confirmed those suspicions. Mrs. Higginbotham survived her hip repair and upon recovery moved into an assisted living facility.

PEARLS

1. When performing SMR on an elderly patient, take into consideration the fact that they might remain on a hard backboard for extended periods of time. You should use some extra padding, such as a folded blanket, for the entire body. The vacuum backboard is far superior to a hard backboard for use in the elderly patient.

2. Extra padding may also be required under the head and shoulders in order to maintain the cervical spine in its normal alignment.

3. Organ systems in the elderly patient may not function as effectively as in the younger patient.

4. Chronic illnesses such as CHF, COPD, etc., should be taken into account as you make judgments about interventions needed to care for the elderly trauma patient.

5. Bones in the elderly patient may fracture more easily. Fractures of major bones such as hips or femurs can be life-threatening even with proper care.

6. Elderly patients with altered mental status should always be checked for hypoglycemia, shock, and head trauma, rather than assuming they are senile.

CASE STUDY WRAP-UP

Dealing with the very elderly can be very challenging, especially if you are not already familiar with the patient (many are transported so regularly that you are on a first-name basis.). If the patient has an altered mental status it is always helpful if there are family members or friends who can give you pertinent history. In this case, the neighbor said that the patient was usually alert and ambulatory. She voiced accusations against the grandson that may or may not have been true but the Scene Size-up suggested that the patient was at best being neglected, and at worst being physically abused. It became obvious that she had taken too much of her diabetes medication (hypoglycemic, with half of her tablets gone a week after the bottle was filled) and none of her blood pressure medication (Tenormin® is a beta-blocker that causes decrease in heart rate and blood pressure; she was hypertensive and tachycardic). The team was misled by the evidence of trauma and mistakenly assumed that the altered level of consciousness was caused by age and head trauma. They correctly picked up the hypoglycemia when they checked the blood glucose. No matter what the age, if the patient is not abusing alcohol or drugs, the most common cause of altered mental status is hypoglycemia. Just as with children, you have a moral obligation to report suspicion of elderly abuse. *You may be their last hope.*

SUMMARY

You will be called upon to treat and transport an increasing number of geriatric trauma patients. Although the mechanisms of injury may be different from those of younger adults, the prioritized evaluation and treatment is the same. As a general rule, elderly patients have more serious injuries and more complications than younger patients. The physiologic processes of aging and frequent concurrent illnesses make evaluation and treatment more difficult. You must be aware of these differences to provide optimal care to the patient.

BIBLIOGRAPHY

1. Diku, M., and K. Newton. "Geriatric Trauma." *Emergency Medicine Clinics of North America,* Vol. 16, No. 1 (Feb. 1998).

2. Fleisher, F., L. White, M. McMullen, and others. "The Geriatric Obstacle Course: A Training Session Designed to Help Prehospital Personnel Recognize Geriatric Stereotypes and Misconceptions." *Journal of Emergency Medicine,* Vol. 14, No. 4 (1996), pp. 439–444.

3. Gubler, K. D., R. Davis, T. Koepsell, and others. "Long-Term Survival of Elderly Trauma Patients." *Archives of Surgery,* Vol. 132 (September 1997).

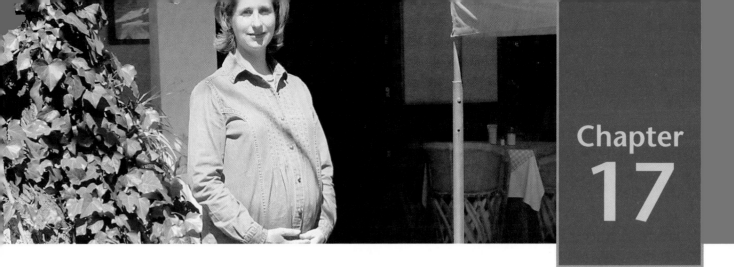

Trauma in Pregnancy

Walter J. Bradley, M.D., M.B.A., F.A.C.E.P.

Objectives

Upon completion of this chapter, you should be able to:

1. Understand the dual goals in managing the pregnant trauma patient.
2. Describe the physiological changes associated with pregnancy.
3. Understand the pregnant trauma patient's response to hypovolemia.
4. Describe the types of injuries most commonly associated with the pregnant trauma patient.
5. Describe the initial assessment and management of the pregnant trauma patient.
6. Discuss trauma prevention in pregnancy.

(Photo courtesy of Eduardo Romero Hicks, M.D. and Patricia Hicks, M.D.)

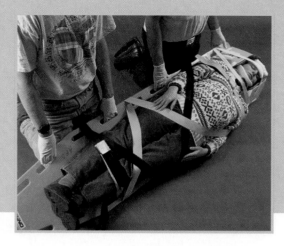

CASE STUDY

Joyce, Dan, and Buddy are dispatched to a single auto accident. During the response they decide that Buddy will be team leader. Upon arrival they find that the scene is safe. A local rescue squad has arrived and extricated the driver onto a long backboard. She is the only person involved. Her auto has run off the road and into a power pole. There are no downed wires. Since she is already packaged, they move her into the ambulance and begin the exam. The patient, Ms. Prunella Schmackengruber, states she was talking on her cell phone and took her eyes off of the road. She was not restrained ("I heard that seat belts might kill the baby") and the car was not equipped with airbags. She says that she is 25 years old and is six months pregnant. She denies any loss of consciousness. She complains of head, back, and lower abdominal pain. What is different about caring for this patient? What sort of injuries should Buddy suspect? Keep these questions in mind as you read the chapter. The case study will continue at the end of the chapter.

When the crossroads of pregnancy and trauma meet, this presents unique challenges. The vulnerability of the pregnant trauma patient and potential injuries to the unborn child serve as reminders of the dual roles of providing care to both mother and fetus. In addition, the pregnant patient is often at risk for a higher incidence of accidental trauma. The increase in fainting spells, hyperventilation, and excess fatigue that are commonly associated with early pregnancy, as well as the physiological changes that affect balance and coordination, add to risks. It is estimated that accidental injury may complicate 6 to 7% of all pregnancies. Minor injuries rarely present problems for you; the following discussion will concentrate on the more severe traumatic injuries to the pregnant patient.

EPIDEMIOLOGY

Trauma is a leading cause of morbidity and mortality in pregnancy. Approximately 6 to 7% of all pregnant women experience some degree of trauma. Significant trauma occurs in approximately one in 12 patients who are injured. Pregnant women with injuries requiring ICU admission occurs in three to four pregnancies per 100 deliveries. Motor vehicle collisions account for 65–70% of trauma in pregnant patients. Falls, abuse and domestic violence, penetrating injuries, and burns follow this.

PHYSIOLOGICAL CHANGES IN PREGNANCY

Dramatic physiological changes occur during pregnancy. The changes that are unique to the pregnant state affect and sometimes alter the physiologic response by both the mother and fetus.

The fetus is formed during the first three months of pregnancy. After the third month of gestation, the fully formed fetus and uterus grow rapidly, reaching the umbilicus by the fifth month and the epigastrium by the seventh month (see Figure 17-1 and Table 17-1). The fetus is considered viable at 24 weeks.

There are physiological changes that occur with respect to blood volume (increase), cardiac output (increase), and blood pressure (decrease) during pregnancy (see Figure 17-2a and b). The respiratory status also has significant changes due to an enlarging uterus that will elevate the diaphragm and decrease the overall volume of the thoracic cavity. This leads to a relative alkalosis and predisposes the patient to hyperventilation. There is, in addition, an increase in both red blood cells and plasma. With the increase of plasma greater than red blood cells, the patient will appear to be anemic (physiologic anemia of pregnancy). However, many pregnant patients have poor nutritional intake during pregnancy and develop an absolute anemia. Gastric motility is also decreased; thus, always assume the stomach of a pregnant patient is full. Always guard against vomiting and aspiration. Table 17-2 illustrates the changes during pregnancy.

RESPONSES TO HYPOVOLEMIA

Acute blood loss results in a decrease in circulating blood volume. The cardiac output decreases as the venous return falls. This hypovolemia causes the arterial blood pressure to fall, resulting in an inhibition of vagal tone and the release of catecholamines. The effect of this response is to produce vasoconstriction and tachycardia. This vasoconstriction profoundly affects the uterus. Uterine vasoconstriction leads to reduction

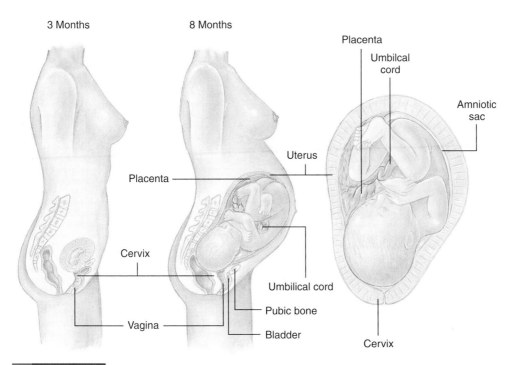

Figure 17-1 Anatomy of pregnancy: Uterus at 3 months and at 8 months gestation.

TABLE 17-1	Assessment of a Pregnancy.		
	First Trimester (1–12 weeks)	Second Trimester (13–24 weeks)	Third Trimester (25–40 weeks)
Viability	Fetus not viable	Potential viability	Fetus viable
Vaginal bleeding	Potential for miscarriage	Potential miscarriage	Potential preterm birth
Fetal heart tones	Not obtainable	120–170 beats per minute	120–160
Fundal height symphysis pubis to fundus	Difficult to measure	Half-way to umbilicus equals 16 weeks To the umbilicus equals 20 weeks	1 cm equals 1 week until 37 weeks, then uterus size decreases with dates

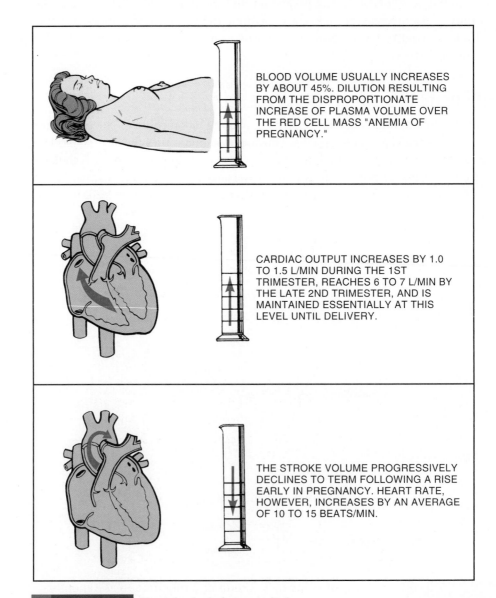

BLOOD VOLUME USUALLY INCREASES BY ABOUT 45%. DILUTION RESULTING FROM THE DISPROPORTIONATE INCREASE OF PLASMA VOLUME OVER THE RED CELL MASS "ANEMIA OF PREGNANCY."

CARDIAC OUTPUT INCREASES BY 1.0 TO 1.5 L/MIN DURING THE 1ST TRIMESTER, REACHES 6 TO 7 L/MIN BY THE LATE 2ND TRIMESTER, AND IS MAINTAINED ESSENTIALLY AT THIS LEVEL UNTIL DELIVERY.

THE STROKE VOLUME PROGRESSIVELY DECLINES TO TERM FOLLOWING A RISE EARLY IN PREGNANCY. HEART RATE, HOWEVER, INCREASES BY AN AVERAGE OF 10 TO 15 BEATS/MIN.

Figure 17-2a Physiological changes during pregnancy.

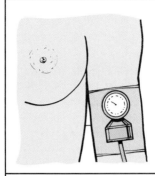

THE MEAN LEVEL OF BLOOD PRESSURE IS CHARACTERISTICALLY 10 TO 15 MMHG LOWER DURING PREGNANCY, THE DECLINE USUALLY APPARENT BY THE END OF THE 1ST TRIMESTER. WIDENED PULSE PRESSURE RESULTS FROM A PROPORTIONATELY GREATER REDUCTION IN THE DIASTOLIC COMPONENT.

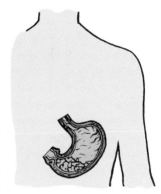

PERISTALSIS IS SLOWED; THUS, THE STOMACH MAY STILL CONTAIN FOOD HOURS AFTER A MEAL. BE ALERT TO THE DANGER OF VOMITING AND ASPIRATION.

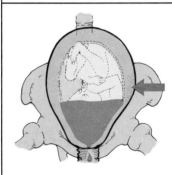

INJURY TO THE UTERUS OR PELVIS MAY CAUSE MASSIVE HEMORRHAGE.

Figure 17-2b Physiological changes during pregnancy *(continued)*.

TABLE 17-2	**Physiological Changes During Pregnancy.**	
Parameter Monitored	**Normal Female**	**Change**
Blood volume	4000 ml	Increased 40–50%
Heart rate	70	Increased 10–15%
Blood pressure	110/70	Decreased 5–15 mmHg
Cardiac output	4–5 L/minute	Increased 20–30%
Hematocrit/hemoglobin	13/40	Decreased
PCO_2	38	Decreased
Gastric motility	Normal	Decreased

in uterine blood flow by 20 to 30%. The pregnant patient may lose up to 1,500cc of blood before any detectable change is noted in the blood pressure of the mother. The fetus reacts to this hypoperfusion by a drop in the arterial blood pressure and a decrease in heart rate. The fetus now begins to suffer from reduced oxygen concentration in the maternal circulation. Therefore, it is important to give 100% oxygen to the mother in order to provide sufficient oxygen to the fetus, who suffers from both oxygen starvation and inadequate blood supply. A shock state in the mother is associated with an 80% fetal mortality rate.

INITIAL ASSESSMENT AND MANAGEMENT

The major goal in managing the pregnant trauma patient is the evaluation and stabilization of the mother. The BTLS Rapid Trauma Survey is the same for the pregnant patient as for other patients (see Chapter 2). All prehospital interventions are directed toward optimizing both fetal and maternal outcome. If the patient is pregnant there are two patients being treated. *Optimal care for the fetus is appropriate treatment of the mother.* Oxygen administration (100% by non-rebreather mask) should be prompt. Monitoring of this patient should be immediate and constant because the anatomic and physiologic changes of pregnancy make the trauma assessment more difficult. Acute hypotension in the pregnant patient due to decreased venous return requires special mention. This "supine hypotension syndrome" usually occurs when the patient is in a supine position with a 20-week (uterus up to umbilicus) or larger uterus (see Figure 17-3). This can lead to maternal hypotension, syncope, and fetal bradycardia. Therefore, the transport of all pregnant trauma patients, if no contraindication exists, should be by one of the following methods to alleviate vena cava compression:

1. Tilt or rotate the backboard 15–30° to the left.
2. Elevate the right hip four to six in. with a towel and manually displace the uterus to the left.

You must be very careful when strapping a term pregnant patient onto a long backboard and then tilting it 15–30° to the left. Many patients (and backboards) will roll right

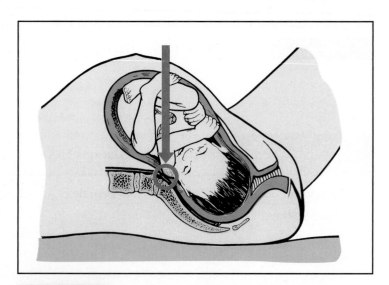

Figure 17-3 Venous return to the maternal heart may be decreased up to 30% because of vena cava compression by the fetus. Transport the patient on her left side or tilt the backboard to the left.

over onto the ambulance floor if the backboard is not secured to the stretcher. The vacuum backboard (see Figure 17-4) is more comfortable and makes it easier to maintain SMR of the pregnant patient than the hard backboard.

Table 17-3 illustrates evaluation of uterine size and its effect on management of the pregnant patient.

TYPES OF TRAUMA
Motor Vehicle Collisions

The most common cause of fetal death in trauma is maternal death. Motor vehicle collisions account for most of 65–75% of pregnancy-related trauma. Fetal distress, fetal death, placental abruption, uterine rupture (see Figure 17-5), and preterm labor are often seen in pregnant patients who have been in MVCs. A review of the literature indicates that fewer than 1% of pregnant patients will sustain injury when there is minor damage to the vehicle. Head injury is the most common cause of death in pregnant patients involved in MVCs. This is closely followed by uncontrolled hemorrhage. Pregnant victims of MVCs have associated injuries, such as pelvic fractures, that often result in concealed hemorrhage within the retroperitoneal space. The retroperitoneal area, because of its low-pressure venous system, can accommodate the loss of four or more liters of blood into that area with few clinical signs. *Seat belt use with both a shoulder restraint and lap belt can significantly decrease patient mortality and has not shown any increase in uterine injuries.*

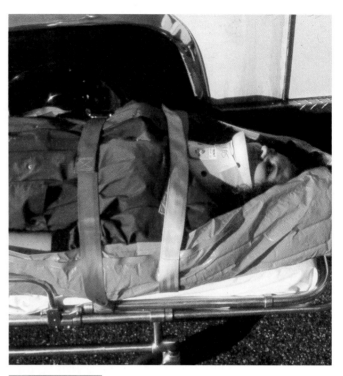

Figure 17-4 The pregnant patient is better stabilized and more comfortable in a vacuum backboard than a hard backboard.

Penetrating Injuries

Gunshot sounds and stabbings are the most common injuries encountered. If the path of entry is below the fundus, the uterus will often offer protection to the mother, absorbing the force of the bullet or knife. Upper abdominal wounds will often injure the bowel due

TABLE 17-3	BTLS Primary Survey (ABC) Brief Evaluation of Uterine Size.
Uterine Size < 20 Weeks	**Uterine Size > 20 Weeks**
Uterus Not to Umbilicus	Uterus to Umbilicus or Higher
↓	↓
Pregnancy Management Unchanged	Lateral Displacement of Uterus
↓	↓
Maternal Stabilization	Brief Confirmation of Fetal Heart Activity (if possible)
	↓
	Maternal Stabilization
	Secondary Fetal Stabilization

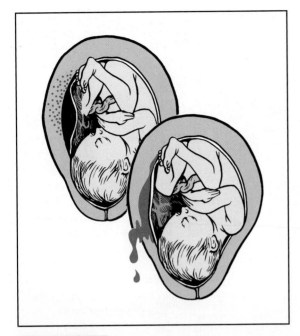

Figure 17-5 Blunt trauma to the uterus. Blunt trauma may cause separation of the placenta or rupture of the uterus. Massive bleeding may occur, but there may not be visible vaginal bleeding early.

PEARLS

1. Do not mistake normal vital signs in pregnant patients as signs of shock. The pregnant patient has a normal resting pulse that is 10 to 15 beats faster than usual and the blood pressure is 10 to 15 mmHg lower than usual. However, it is also important to realize that a blood loss of 30 to 35% can occur in these patients before there is a significant change in blood pressure. Therefore, be especially alert to all signs of shock, and monitor the vital signs with frequent Ongoing Exams.

2. Trauma to the abdominal compartment can cause occult bleeding in either the intrauterine or retroperitoneal area. Keep in mind

(continued)

to its compression in a smaller than normal space by the uterus.

Studies have shown that gunshot wounds to the pregnant abdomen carry a high mortality rate for the fetus (40–70%). They are lower for the mother (4–10%) because the large uterus usually protects vital organs. Stab wounds follow much the same pattern of outcome, with fetal mortality rates of about 40%. Definitive care will depend on several factors, involving degree of shock, associated organ injury, and time of gestation.

Domestic Violence

A large percentage of pregnant women experience domestic violence that appears to worsen as pregnancy progresses. Through the second and third trimesters, it is estimated that one in 10 pregnant women experiences abuse during pregnancy. Physical abuse is more likely to be manifest with proximal and midline injuries than the distal injuries of accidental trauma. The face and neck are most common. Domestic abuse has also been associated with low birth weight. The pregnant patient who is under great stress produces hormones (high circulating adrenalin levels, etc.) that are not good for her pregnancy. The "old wives' tale" that pregnant patients should be shielded from frightening or disturbing situations is probably true. Spouses and boyfriends are the perpetrators of the violence in 70–85% of cases.

Falls

The incidence of falls increases with the progression of pregnancy. This is in part due to an alteration in the patient's center of gravity. The incidence of significant injury is proportionate to the force of impact and the specific body part that sustains the impact. Pelvic injuries may result in placental separation and fetal fractures. Emergency department evaluation and monitoring is recommended.

Burns

Of the 2.2 million patients that suffer burn injuries in the United States annually, less than 4% are pregnant. The overall mortality and morbidity resulting from thermal injuries to the pregnant patient is not markedly different from the nonpregnant patient. However, it is important to remember that the fluid requirement for the pregnant patient is greater than that of the nonpregnant female. Fetal mortality increases when the maternal surface burn exceeds 20%.

TRAUMA PREVENTION IN PREGNANCY

Upon reviewing major causes of trauma in pregnancy, it is clear that specific recommendations such as seat belt use in motor vehicles, reporting and counseling for domestic violence, as well as education of the multiple physiologic, anatomical, and emotional changes associated with pregnancy, will all serve to reduce trauma in pregnancy. Some patients get very little if any prenatal care, and even less prenatal education. If the situation is not critical, you should not hesitate to educate your pregnant patients when you are called to see them.

CASE STUDY

Joyce, Dan, and Buddy are dispatched to a single auto accident. During the response they decide that Buddy will be team leader. Upon arrival they find that the scene is safe. A local rescue squad has arrived and extricated the driver onto a long backboard. She is the only person involved. Her auto has run off the road and into a power pole. There are no downed wires. Buddy notes that the windshield is starred and the steering wheel is bent. Since she is already packaged, they move her into the ambulance and begin the exam. Dan is told to transport to the hospital as soon as Buddy finishes the BTLS Primary Survey. The patient, Ms. Prunella Schmackengruber, states she was talking on her cell phone and took her eyes off of the road. She was not restrained ("I heard that seat belts might kill the baby") and the car was not equipped with airbags. She says that she is 25 years old and is six months pregnant. She denies any loss of consciousness. She complains of head, back, and lower abdominal pain.

Buddy asks Joyce to tilt the backboard about 20° to the left and strap it down well so it does not flip over onto the floor of the ambulance. Prunella obviously has an open airway and seems to be breathing normally. She has bruising and a laceration of the forehead where she struck the windshield. The cervical collar is opened to examine the neck. There is tenderness and spasm but no deformity noted. Neck veins are flat and the trachea is in the midline. The cervical collar is replaced. The chest has no obvious deformities but is tender over the sternum. Breath sounds are present and equal, heart sounds are easily heard, and she has a strong rapid peripheral pulse. The uterus is felt halfway between the umbilicus and the xyphoid, and it is hard and very tender. Buddy can't hear fetal heart tones with his stethoscope and does not have a Doppler. The pelvis is stable and nontender. She has good PMS of the extremities. Joyce reports that the vital signs are: BP 100/60, pulse 120, respiration 24, and the pulse oximeter reading is 95% on ambient air. Joyce applies a non-rebreather oxygen mask. Prunella says she feels as if she has wet herself but when Joyce checks there is a large bloodstain on her pants. Joyce notifies Medical Direction and asks her to have the emergency department send for a sonogram machine to assess the fetus on arrival. She also asks for the trauma team and the obstetrician on-call to be present on arrival. She then applies the cardiac monitor (sinus tachycardia) while Buddy does the Detailed Exam.

The patient denies any medical problems or allergies and is taking only prenatal vitamins. She has not eaten today because she was a little nauseated. The Detail Exam reveals that the neurological exam is normal but that the abdomen is more tender, with obvious constant spasm of the uterus. The BP has dropped to 90/50 and the Pulse is up to 130. When they arrive at the emergency department a sonogram reveals that the fetus is still alive but the abdomen is full of fluid. Prunella is taken to surgery where a ruptured uterus is found; 2,000 cc of blood is suctioned from the abdomen. Prunella has to have a hysterectomy to stop the bleeding. The baby requires a month in the neonatal ICU, but lives. Prunella is so appreciative of the care given by Buddy's team that she names the baby "Buddy Jodan Schmackengruber."

PEARLS (continued)

that gradual stretching of the abdominal wall during pregnancy, along with hormonal changes within the body, make the peritoneal surface less sensitive to irritable stimuli. Therefore, bleeding can occur intraperitoneally, and the signs of rebound, guarding, and rigidity may not be present.

3. You are treating two patients; however, the mortality of the fetus is related to the treatment provided to the mother. The goal of prehospital intervention is to maximize the chances of maternal survival, which will provide the fetus with the best chance for survival.

4. Hypoxemia of the fetus may go unnoticed in the injured pregnant patient. Treatment should include high-flow oxygen.

5. Transport must include appropriate spinal motion restriction, extremity splints, and prevention of vena cava compression.

6. If the mother dies, continue CPR and notify the hospital to be prepared for immediate cesarean section. Have them bring a sonogram machine to the emergency department for immediate evaluation of the fetus.

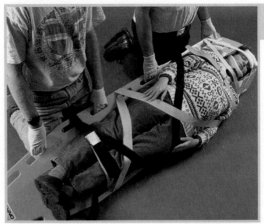

CASE STUDY WRAP-UP

Because of the rapid treatment and transport of this patient she survived what would have been a fatal injury. She was transported with the backboard tilted to the left to prevent compression of the inferior vena cava by the gravid uterus. Her shock was treated by oxygen, load and go and by rapid evaluation and surgery at the hospital. If she had worn her seat belt, she would probably have had only minor injuries.

SUMMARY

Management of the pregnant trauma patient requires knowledge of the physiological changes that occur during pregnancy. Pregnant patients require rapid evaluation and also rapid interventions for stabilization. They require special techniques in packaging and transport to prevent the vena cava compression syndrome. Because of the difficulty in early diagnosis, you should have a low threshold for load-and-go if there is any danger of the development of hemorrhagic shock. Pregnant patients with serious injuries should be directly transported to a facility (trauma center) capable of managing these complex patients. Optional fetal care is dependent on care of the mother.

BIBLIOGRAPHY

1. Agnoli, F .L., M. E. Deutchman. "Trauma in Pregnancy." *J Fam Prac* 37:588–592, 1993.

2. Bickell, W. H., J. F. Wall, P. E. Pepe, et al. "Immediate versus Delayed Fluid Resuscitation for Hypotensive Patients with Penetrating Torso Injuries." *N Engl J Med* 331:1105–1109, 1994.

3. Bock, J., J. Courtney, M. Pearlman, et al. "Trauma in Pregnancy." *Ann Emerg Med* 17:829–834, 1988.

4. Bowman, M., W. Giles, S. Deane. "Trauma during Pregnancy: A Review of Management." Aust/NZ: *J Obstet Gynaecol* 29:389, 1989.

5. Dahmus, M. A., B. M. Sibai. "Blunt Abdominal Trauma: Are There Any Predictive Factors for Abruptio Placenta or Maternal-Fetal Distress?" *Am J Obstet Gynecol* 169:1054–1059, 1993.

6. Esposito, T. J. "Trauma During Pregnancy." *Emerg Med Clin North Am* 12:167–199, 1994.

7. Fildes J., L. Reed, N. Jones et al. "Trauma: The Leading Cause of Maternal Death." *J Trauma* 32:643, 1992.

8. George E. R., T. Vandekwaak, D. J. Scholten. "Factors Influencing Pregnancy Outcome after Trauma." *Am Surgeon* 58:594, 1992.

9. Helton, A. S., J. McFarlane, E. T. Anderson. "Battered and Pregnant: A Prevalence Study." *Am J Public Health* 77:1337, 1987.

10. Hill, D. A., J. J. Lense. "Abdominal Trauma in the Pregnant Patient." *Am Fam Physician* 53:1269–1274, 1996.

11. Kuhlmann, R. S., D. P. Cruikshank. "Maternal Trauma During Pregnancy." *Clin Obstet Gynecol* 37:274–293, 1994.

12. Lavery, J. P., M. Staten-McCormick. "Management of Moderate to Severe Trauma in Pregnancy." *Obstet Gynecol Clin North Am* 22:69–90, 1995.

13. Lavin, J. P., S. S. Polsky. "Abdominal Trauma during Pregnancy." *Clin Perinatol* 1:423, 1983.

14. Neufield, J. D. G. "Trauma in Pregnancy: What If . . . ?" *Emerg Med Clin North Am.* 11:207, 1993.

15. Pearlman, M.D., E. Tintinalli. "Evaluation and Treatment of the Gravida and Fetus Following Trauma During Pregnancy." *Obst Gynecol Clin North Am* 18:371, 1991.

16. Pimentel, L. "Mother and Child: Trauma in Pregnancy." *Emerg Med Clin North Am* 9:549, 1991.

17. Pons, P. T. "Prehospital Considerations in the Pregnant Patient." *Emerg Med Clin North Am* 12:1–7, 1994.

18. Poole, G. V., J. N. Martin, K. G. Perry, et al. "Trauma in Pregnancy: The Role of Interpersonal Violence." *Am J Obstst Gynecol* 174:1873–1878.

19. Rose, P. G., P. L. Strohm, F. P. Zuspan. "Fetomaternal Hemorrhage Following Trauma." *Am J Obstst Gynecol* 153:844, 1985.

20. Rothenberger, D., F. W. Quattlebaum, J. F. Perry et al. "Blunt Maternal Trauma: A Review of 103 Cases." *J Trauma* 18:173, 1978.

21. Scorpio, R. J., T. J. Esposito, L. G. Smith, et al. "Blunt Trauma During Pregnancy: Factors Affecting Fetal Outcome." *J Trauma* 32:213, 1992.

22. Sherman, H. F., L. M. Scott, A. S. Rosemurgy. "Changes Affecting the Initial Evaluation and Care of the Pregnant Trauma Victim." *J Emerg Med* 8;575–582, 1990.

23. Timberlake, G. A., N. E. McSwain. "Trauma in Pregnancy: A 10-Year Perspective." *Am Surg* 55:151, 1989.

24. Vaizey, C. J., Jackson M. J., Cross F. W. "Trauma in Pregnancy." *Br J Surg* 81:1406–1415, 1994.

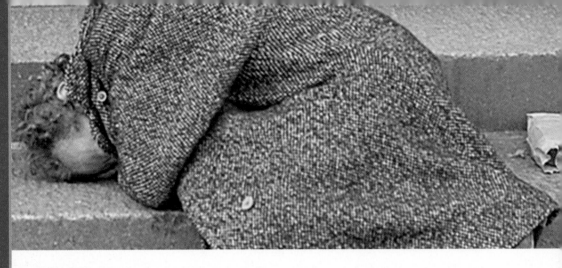

Chapter 18

Patients Under the Influence of Alcohol or Drugs

Jonathan G. Newman, M.D., F.A.C.E.P., NREMT-P

Objectives

Upon completion of this chapter, you should be able to:

1. List signs and symptoms of patients under the influence of alcohol and/or drugs.

2. Describe the five strategies you would use to best ensure cooperation during assessment and management of a patient under the influence of alcohol and/or drugs.

3. Describe situations in which you would restrain patients and tell how to handle an uncooperative patient.

4. List the special considerations for assessment and management of patients in whom substance abuse is suspected.

CASE STUDY

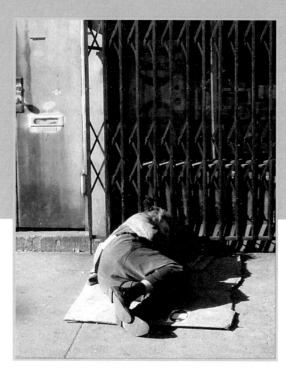

J oyce, Buddy, and Dan have been dispatched to a run-down section of town after the police called to report a man being stabbed. They have been to this area many times before to pick up patients after altercations over alcohol or drugs. They are told that the patient is covered in blood but is not cooperative. What injuries would you expect in this situation? What strategies would you use to get this patient to cooperate with treatment? Keep these questions in mind as you read the chapter. The case study will continue at the end of the chapter.

The relationship between alcohol and trauma is well documented. For instance, it is reported that car crashes involving alcohol result in injuries to about 500,000 people a year. The involvement of drugs in trauma has not been as well examined. However, substance abuse, which includes individuals who have abused alcohol, drugs, or both, has been associated with a number of traumatic events. The trauma caused by substance abuse often results from accidents, car crashes, suicides, homicides, and other violent crimes. Therefore, it would not be surprising to find that a number of trauma patients are under the influence of alcohol or some other substance. This group of trauma patients often presents with unique challenges that can require some special patient management techniques along with good BTLS care.

A high index of suspicion, combined with the results of the physical exam, the history obtained from the patient or bystanders, and evidence at the scene, can clue you into whether your patient is under the influence of alcohol or drugs. Table 18-1 includes some commonly abused drugs, along with signs and symptoms of their use.

ASSESSMENT AND MANAGEMENT

While your Primary Survey and Detailed Exam should follow the BTLS guidelines that have been described in this book (see Chapter 2), there are some particular aspects to be aware of when conducting the exam.

When you suspect the patient has abused substances, pay particular attention to mental status, pupils, speech, and respiration, and note any needle marks you may discover. An altered mental status can be seen in every form of substance abuse. However, remember that an altered level of consciousness is due to a head injury, shock, or hypoglycemia until proven otherwise. Pupils are often constricted in patients who have abused opiates. Dilated pupils are common in patients exposed to amphetamines, cocaine, hallucinogens, and marijuana. Patients who use barbiturates will have pupils that are constricted early on; however, if high doses have been consumed, the pupils can eventually become fixed and dilated. Speech can be slurred when patients use alcohol or sedatives, and patients

TABLE 18-1	Commonly Abused Drugs with Their Associated Signs and Symptoms.

Drug Category	Common Names	Signs and Symptoms of Use or Abuse
Alcohol	Beer, whiskey, wine	Altered mental function, confusion, polyuria, slurred speech, coma, hypertension, hyperthermia, tachycardia
Amphetamines	Bennies, ice, speed, uppers, dexies	Excitement, hyperactivity, dilated pupils, hypertension, tachycardia, tremors, seizures, fever, paranoia, psychosis
Cocaine	Coke, crack, blow, rock	Same as amphetamines plus chest pain; lethal dysrhythmia
Hallucinogens	Acid, LSD, PCP	Hallucinations, dizziness, dilated pupils, nausea, rambling speech, psychosis, anxiety, panic
Marijuana	Grass, hash, pot, tea, weed	Euphoria, sleepiness, dilated pupils, dry mouth, increased appetite
Opiates	Heroin, horse, big H, Darvon, codeine, stuff, morphine, smack	Altered mental status, constricted pupils, bradycardia, hypotension, respiratory depression, hypothermia
Sedatives	Thorazine; barbiturates; benzodiazepines, e.g., Librium, Valium, Xanax, Ativan	Altered mental status, dilated pupils, bradycardia, hypotension, respiratory depression, hypothermia

who are under the influence of hallucinogens may seem to ramble when they talk. Respiration can be significantly depressed with opiates and sedatives.

The history supplied by the patient or bystanders can also help to establish whether substance abuse is involved. Try to find out what was used, when it was taken, and how much was taken. However, be aware that patients often deny that they have used or abused any substance. If possible, inspect the patient's surroundings for clues that drugs or alcohol may have been used. Note any alcoholic beverage bottles, pill containers, injection equipment, smoking paraphernalia, or unusual odors.

Trauma patients under the influence of alcohol or drugs can challenge the provider not only by their traumatic injuries but by their attitudes. *The way in which you interact with patients who have abused substances can determine if the patient will be cooperative or uncooperative.* How you speak to these patients can be as important as what you are doing for them. Your interaction style, if offensive, can make patients uncooperative and lose you both precious minutes of the golden hour. If your interactive style is positive and nonjudgmental, the patient is more likely to be cooperative and to allow all the appropriate medical interventions, thus decreasing on-scene time. As noted before, all the substances that are abused can cause an altered mental state. When interacting with patients you must be prepared to deal with euphoria, psychosis, paranoia, or confusion and disorientation. Some strategies to help you gain your patient's cooperation follow:

1. Identify yourself to patients and orient them to their surroundings. Tell them your name and your title, for example, "EMT, Paramedic." Ask them their name and how they would like to be addressed. Avoid using generic names like "Bub" or "Honey." With this patient population it may be necessary to orient them to place, date, and what is going on. These patients may need to be reoriented frequently.

2. Treat the patient in a respectful manner and avoid being judgmental. Often a lack of respect can be heard in the tone of your voice or how you say things, not just in what you say. Never forget that you are there to save lives; this includes all patients. You are not a police officer (don't gather or destroy evidence), and you are not there to pass judgment on the patient's worth to society.

3. Acknowledge the patient's concerns and feelings. The patient who is scared or confused may be more comfortable with what is taking place if you recognize and address these feelings. Be gentle but firm. Explain all treatment interventions before they are performed. Be honest. Backboards and extrication collars are uncomfortable.

4. Let your patients know what will be required of them. For instance, they may be confused and not realize that they need to hold still while you are trying to stabilize them on a backboard.

5. Ask closed-ended questions when getting your history from the patient. These are questions that can be answered with a yes or no. These patients may only be able to concentrate for short periods of time, and they may ramble when asked open-ended questions that require a full answer. Consider getting as much of the history as you can from relatives, friends, or bystanders. This may help improve the reliability of what you discover. Get as much relevant history as you can, *but do not delay transport.*

THE UNCOOPERATIVE PATIENT

A small percentage of your patients may be uncooperative. You must be firm with these patients. Set limits to their behavior, and let them know when their behavior is inappropriate. Consider physical restraint only if you are not able to secure enough cooperation to provide adequate care for your patient. Often a show of force may be enough to convince an uncooperative patient to allow medical care to be provided. First, check with your local jurisdiction to determine what protocol you must use when restraining patients against their will. Most municipalities allow police officers to place people in custody if they are a threat to themselves or others. Severely injured trauma patients who refuse or will not cooperate with care can be considered a threat to themselves. Once the decision has been made to restrain the patient, it must be carried out with care. Securely strapping a patient to a backboard with use of a cervical collar and head motion-restriction device will serve to restrain most patients. Caution must be taken not to worsen any current injuries or to inflict any new ones. *There is often no good solution to this predicament.* Restrained patients may struggle so hard that spinal motion restriction is rendered ineffective. The Reeves sleeve is one of the few pieces of equipment that is very effective in providing both restraint and motion restriction (see Figure 18-1). Crews should plan and practice procedures for restraining patients. The trauma scene is not the place to learn new skills. Reassess restrained patients often. A review of the literature notes at least two cases of drug-impaired patients dying by asphyxiation during prehospital restraint.

The standard BTLS approach to patient care will work well, even with patients under the influence of alcohol or drugs. Ensure that the scene is safe, determine the number of injured, and discover the mechanism of injury. Use universal precautions. This patient population includes people who are at high risk for infection with hepatitis B, hepatitis C,

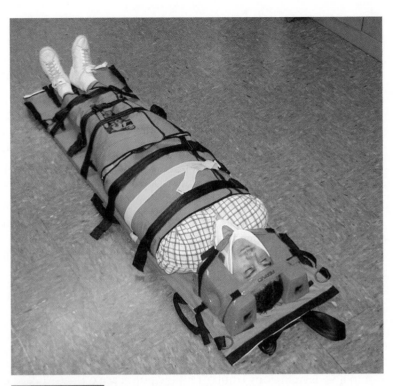

Figure 18-1 Reeves sleeve.

and HIV. Follow the Primary Survey and Detailed Exam as recorded in Chapter 2. Remember to note any mental status changes that might be associated with substance abuse. When performing the Detailed Exam, be sure to include the specific areas that can provide clues to substance abuse. As with all trauma patients, treatment includes the consideration of oxygen, cardiac monitoring (if available), and O_2 saturation monitoring. Table 18-2 lists some drug categories and associated specific treatments or areas to pay close attention to when substance abuse is suspected.

TABLE 18-2	Drug Categories and Specific Treatments to Consider or Areas to Assess Closely.
Drug Category	**Specific Treatments and Areas to Assess**
Alcohol	Watch for hypothermia.
Amphetamines	Monitor for seizures and dysrhythmias.
Cocaine	Monitor for seizures and dysrhythmias.
Hallucinogens	Provide reassurance.
Marijuana	Provide reassurance.
Opiates	Watch for hypothermia, hypotension, and respiratory depression.
Sedatives	Watch for hypothermia, hypotension, and respiratory depression.

CASE STUDY

Joyce, Buddy, and Dan have been dispatched to a run-down section of town after the police called to report a man being stabbed. They have been to this area many times before to pick up patients after altercations over alcohol or drugs. They are told that the patient is covered in blood but is not cooperative. As they respond, they decide to have Joyce act as team leader since she is good at interacting with uncooperative patients. They carefully don personal protective equipment since the police described a lot of blood, and hepatitis and HIV were known to be present among the regulars they treated in this area.

When they arrive they see that the police have the scene under control and are putting a cursing, struggling, handcuffed man into a patrol car. There is a very unkempt man lying on a pallet on the sidewalk. He is actively bleeding from lacerations of the chest and abdomen. There is an impressive amount of blood on the front of his shirt and trousers. There are several empty wine bottles strewn about. Joyce introduces herself and asks him what happened? "We were drinking together and he hogged all of his wine down and then reached for my bottle. I told him to get his own G—d—wine and the SOB cut me!" Joyce asks him his name (Cuthbert Mulford), and assures him that he is not in any trouble and the police are only there to arrest the SOB who cut him. She explains that the paramedics are there to help him and take care of his wounds. She asks for permission to examine him and he grudgingly agrees. Since there was no mechanism for spinal injury, they do not apply spinal motion restriction precautions.

He obviously has an open airway and seems to be in no respiratory difficulty (the odor of stale wine on his breath makes Joyce dyspneic), so she proceeds with the Rapid Trauma Survey. There are no apparent injuries of the head or face. His neck is nontender, the neck veins flat, and the trachea in the midline. There is equal expansion of the chest, with breath sounds present and equal. There are two 8–10 cm lacerations across his left anterior chest but they do not appear to go into the chest cavity. Heart sounds are heard and the rate is rapid, with a weak peripheral pulse. There is a deep laceration across the left upper quadrant of the abdomen with protruding intestines. Cuthbert looks at it as Joyce lifts his shirt and says "He gutted me, didn't he?" Joyce has Buddy apply a saline moistened dressing and then an occlusive dressing. She continues her assessment. She finds no other injuries and so she explains to Cuthbert that they will have to take him to the hospital to fix his intestines. He seems markedly more sober after looking at his intestines and readily agrees. They carefully move him to the stretcher and transport immediately. During transport Joyce bandages his lacerations while Buddy takes vital signs: BP 110/70, pulse 110, respiration 24, and oxygen saturation 96%. Cuthbert states his only medical history is seizures (alcohol withdrawal?) for which he takes no prescription medications, has no allergies, and hasn't eaten in the last 24 hours. "I get my nourishment from cigarettes and a bottle of Sly Fox!" The Detailed Exam reveals no new findings. Cuthbert's recovery is complicated by delirium tremens and a wound infection, but he lives to ride with Joyce on many more occasions.

PEARLS

1. It is extremely difficult to differentiate between patients under the influence and those experiencing a medical and/or trauma emergency. You may have to alter your usual management techniques. Many patients will initially refuse treatment. You may have to consult local protocol, medical direction, and appropriate law enforcement personnel for assistance.

2. The standard BTLS approach to patient care will work well, even with patients under the influence. Your attitude can help determine if your patient approach will be accepted or not. Be positive and nonjudgmental.

3. Check finger-stick glucose on every patient with altered mental status.

4. In this population, hypothermia, hypotension, and respiratory depression are common and must be treated aggressively.

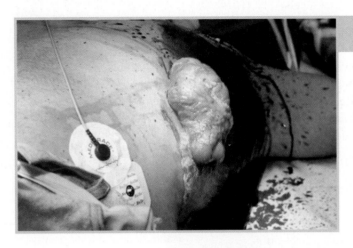

(Photo courtesy of Roy Alson, M.D.)

CASE STUDY WRAP-UP

Because people who abuse alcohol and drugs frequently are the victims of trauma (and often the cause of trauma to people who don't abuse alcohol and drugs) you will have to treat them on almost a daily basis. A patient, caring attitude will save you much grief, but we all know that some people who are intoxicated are sociopathic and no matter what you do they will not cooperate. Many confrontations will not go as well as the case study above. The Reeves Sleeve is invaluable for the patient that must be restrained for his own safety. It does not require placing the patient prone and it allows you to manage the airway and give medication and IV fluids. It can be carried rolled up in storage until you need it; slide a backboard into it, and you have a total body restraint system. Whether the patient is sober enough to refuse treatment may be the hardest decision to make. Sometimes you, the police, and Medical Direction have to make the best decision based on the situation. As mentioned above, sometimes there is no good answer.

SUMMARY

Knowing the signs and symptoms of alcohol and drug abuse will allow you to recognize the patient who may be impaired from their use. Assessing the patient for signs and symptoms outlined in this section can help you confirm your suspicions. Determining that your patient has abused some substance will allow you to pay attention to specific areas for critical changes as well as provide lifesaving interventions that may be indicated for individual substances. The five interaction strategies for improving patient cooperation are very important when dealing with the patient under the influence of alcohol or drugs, but these strategies should also be used with all patients. Remember that the patient's safety is a primary concern. If you must restrain a patient for his or her safety, do so in a preplanned manner that is most sensitive to your patient's needs.

BIBLIOGRAPHY

1. Bledsoe, B., R. Porter, and B. Shade. *Paramedic Emergency Care,* pp. 795–800. Upper Saddle River, NJ: Prentice Hall, 1991.
2. Caroline, N. *Emergency Care in the Streets,* 4th ed., pp. 628–637. Boston: Little, Brown, 1991.

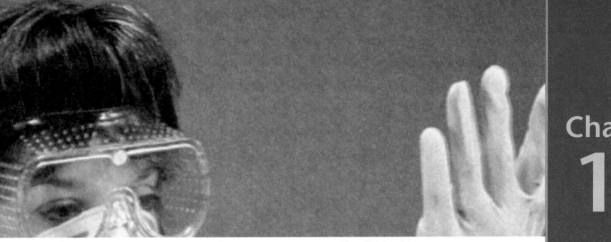

Chapter 19

Blood and Body Substance Precautions in the Prehospital Setting

Howard Werman, M.D., F.A.C.E.P.

Richard N. Nelson, M.D., F.A.C.E.P.

Katherine West, BSN, MSEd, CIC

Objectives

Upon completion of this chapter, you should be able to:

1. State the three most common bloodborne viral illnesses that EMS providers are likely to be exposed to in the provision of patient care.

2. Discuss the signs and symptoms of tuberculosis and describe protective measures to take to reduce possible exposure to TB.

3. Describe precautions EMS providers can take to prevent exposure to blood and other potentially infectious materials (CSF, synovial fluid, amniotic fluid, pericardial fluid, pleural fluid, or any fluid with gross visible blood).

4. Identify appropriate use of personal protective equipment.

5. Describe procedures for EMS providers to follow if they are accidentally exposed.

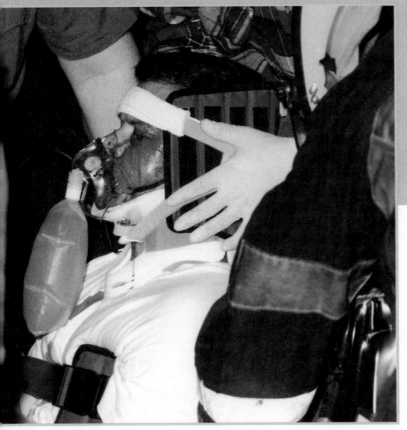

CASE STUDY

Joyce, Buddy, and Dan have been dispatched to a local gay bar where a man has been injured in a fight. As they respond, they decide that Buddy will be team leader and they don personal protective equipment, since they expect the patient to be bloody. When they arrive they find that the police are already there and have the scene under control. Sitting in a chair is a young male who has been beaten and "stomped" by a motorcycle gang after he made a pass at the leader's boyfriend. As they approach, Buddy's initial impression is not good; the patient is bloody and is struggling to breathe. He is confused and combative. Joyce stabilizes his neck with her hands and asks Dan to apply a non-rebreather oxygen mask. The airway is open but there is poor movement of air. There is a rapid, weak peripheral pulse and there is an obvious large flail chest on the left side. Buddy instructs Dan to get the Reeves sleeve and to also get the KED short backboard device to use to splint the flail chest. He begins the Rapid Trauma Survey. The face has bruises and abrasions all over and there is dried blood in the nose, but the active bleeding has stopped. He appears to have facial fractures but the airway is not compromised. The neck is bruised and tender but with no obvious deformities. Neck veins are flat and the trachea is midline. The breath sounds are decreased on the left side but heart sounds are normal. The abdomen is tender to palpation but not distended, and there are no masses felt. The pelvis is stable and nontender. The extremities are bruised but there is good PMS. The patient (Poochie) has good sensation and movement in his fingers and toes.

Buddy applies the Kendrick Extrication Device in order to stabilize the flail chest. The team then moves the patient onto theReeves sleeve and transports immediately. Joyce drives. Vital signs taken en route are: BP 90/50, pulse 140, respiration 36, and pulse oximeter reading 95% on 100% oxygen. The cardiac monitor shows sinus tachycardia. As Buddy is checking a laceration on his lip, Poochie bites him. There is blood on his teeth. What should Buddy do now? What tests will need to be done? What sort of information should be recorded? What is the worst that can happen? Keep these questions in mind. The case study will continue at the end of the chapter.

EMS personnel have always faced risks when carrying out their jobs. These risks have mostly involved highway hazards, fires, downed electrical wires, toxic substances, and scene security problems. However, you must also assume you are also at risk of acquiring certain diseases from the patients you are treating. Fortunately, there are many precautions that may be taken to markedly reduce these risks. Additionally, if personal protective equipment could not be used or failed, treatment offered can be taken to reduce the risk of acquiring these diseases following an exposure event.

The spectrum of diseases to which you are potentially exposed is beyond the scope of this book. However, the three most common types of viral infections are appropriate to discuss in conjunction with trauma management, since their modes of spread are primarily by contaminated blood and other potentially infectious material (blood/opim): hepatitis B (HBV), hepatitis C (HCV), and HIV infection. *Body fluids that do NOT pose a risk for HBV, HCV, and HIV are: tears, sweat, saliva, urine, stool, vomitus, nasal secretions, and sputum.*

HEPATITIS B

The term *viral hepatitis* is used to describe a group of viral infections involving the liver. At least five types of viruses have been described: hepatitis A, B, C, D, and E. Hepatitis A and E are spread primarily through contact with contaminated fecal material and are not bloodborne. Hepatitis D is transmitted through blood and body fluid exposure to patients already infected with hepatitis B. Because of their frequent contact with blood and needles, health care workers are considered at intermediate risk of becoming infected with the hepatitis B virus (HBV). Fortunately, hepatitis B is the one form of hepatitis for which there is an effective vaccine.

HBV is a major cause of acute and chronic hepatitis, cirrhosis, and liver cancer. An estimated 3,000 persons in the United States are infected each year. In 1995, OSHA reported that about 800 health care workers acquired the disease through occupational exposure. Because of the universal vaccination program, these numbers are markedly reduced from in the past. Following acute infection, 5 to 10% of these patients continue to be chronic carriers of the virus. These carriers are potentially infectious. HBV is spread by contact with contaminated blood/opim, sexual transmission and direct contact with a contaminated item and non-intact skin. Infection usually occurs from contaminated needle sticks or through sexual contact. It is estimated that there is a 6–30% chance that health care workers who are exposed to a needlestick by HBV-contaminated blood will develop hepatitis B infection if they have not received their vaccine or have not reported the exposure. Infection can also occur by contacting infectious bloody secretions with open skin lesions or mucosal surfaces. Routine testing of donor blood for HBV makes transmission from blood transfusion very rare.

Although HBV infection is uncommon in the general population, members of certain groups are considered much more likely to harbor the virus. High-risk groups are immigrants from areas where HBV is prevalent (Asia, Pacific Islands), incarcerated individuals, institutionalized patients, intravenous drug users, male homosexuals, hemophiliacs, household contacts of HBV patients, and hemodialysis patients.

In the United States, the Occupational Safety and Health Administration (OSHA) mandated in 1991 that all departments are required to offer HBV vaccine to any health care worker who is at risk of occupational exposure to blood /opim. This happens within 10 days of being hired. This vaccine offers lifelong protection. Vaccines available today are recombinant—they contain no human components. The vaccine is safe and produces immunity in over 90% of persons vaccinated. The second form of protection is hepatitis B immunoglobulin (HBIG). This preparation contains antibodies to HBV and provides temporary, passive protection against HBV. HBIG is only 70% effective and only for six months. HBIG is used only when there has been a significant exposure to HBV in an unimmunized person. It is given in conjunction with hepatitis B vaccine.

HEPATITIS C

The hepatitis C virus (HCV) was identified in 1988–1989. This virus is thought to be responsible for the majority of what had been identified as non-A, non-B hepatitis infections. The incubation period is six to seven weeks. Antibodies to the HCV have been used to identify patients with previous HCV infection. Those exposed to HCV are test positive five to six weeks after exposure.

Prior to 1992, HCV was the leading cause of hepatitis resulting from blood transfusions. In addition to being spread by blood transfusion, the virus also appears to be spread by sharing of intravenous needles, sexual contact, tattooing, and body piercing, much like HBV. Health care workers can acquire infection though hollow-bore needlesticks with contaminated needles. The likelihood of becoming infected with HCV after a single needlestick is estimated at 1.8%.

HCV infection tends to be less severe than HBV during the initial infection. However, there appears to be a greater likelihood of becoming a chronic carrier of HCV following infection, placing the health care worker at an increasing risk of exposure. Liver failure and cirrhosis occur in 10 to 20% of chronic HCV carriers.

There is currently no vaccine available to protect against HCV infection. Evidence suggests that there is no protective effect provided by administering immune globulin following exposure to HCV. However, post-exposure testing can answer the question of whether or not one contracted the disease in four to six weeks following the exposure event. The new test is a test for the virus itself. This reduces the concern about having acquired the disease to four to six weeks instead of six months of follow-up. Treatment is available for persons who acquire the disease.

HUMAN IMMUNODEFICIENCY VIRUS INFECTION

HIV infection is caused by the human immunodeficiency virus (HIV). Patients with HIV infection develop a defect in their immune system. This predisposes the HIV-infected patient to a variety of unusual infections that are not generally seen in healthy patients of similar age. Patients infected with HIV can present with a wide spectrum of clinical manifestations. Many patients with HIV infection are asymptomatic carriers. Any *untreated* patient who carries HIV, whether he manifests symptoms of AIDS or is asymptomatic, can transmit the virus. HIV patients being treated with current drugs may be virus negative and they pose a minute risk. HIV appears to be transmitted in a manner similar to HBV. Although the virus has been cultured from a variety of body fluids, only blood has been implicated in the transmission of the virus in the workplace. Semen and vaginal secretions have been shown to transmit the virus during sexual activity, but this should be of no concern in the workplace. *There is no evidence to suggest that the HIV is transmitted by casual contact.* Transmission to health care workers has been documented only after accidental parenteral exposure (needlestick) or exposure of mucous membranes and open wounds to large amounts of *infected blood.* Measurable risk data for occupational exposure is 0.32% for needlestick injuries and 0.09% for mucous membrane exposure. There are no documented cases of transmission from infected blood on non-intact skin since 1985.

HIV appears to be different from the hepatitis B virus in two ways:

1. HIV does not survive outside the body. No special cleaning agents are required.

2. HIV is transmitted far less efficiently than HBV. An unimmunized person with a parenteral exposure to HBV has one chance in four of contracting the disease. The same person with a parenteral exposure to HIV would have three chances in 1,000 and if a mucous membrane exposure would be less than one chance in 1,000.

Several groups have been identified as having a high risk of HIV infection. These include male homosexuals or bisexuals, intravenous drug abusers, patients who have received blood transfusions or pooled-plasma products (e.g., hemophiliacs), and heterosexual contacts of HIV carriers. However, because of the difficulty in identifying HIV-infected patients, all contacts with blood/opim should be considered a potential HIV exposure. This concept (all patients are potentially infective) is why body substance isolation precautions are "universally" applied.

There is currently no available vaccine to protect against HIV infection. Anti-retroviral drug regimens, though not a cure, have been shown to prolong the life of HIV/AIDS patients. Some studies have suggested that anti-retroviral agents may reduce the risk of HIV transmission in health care workers immediately following a significant exposure to HIV-infected blood/opim. The decision to administer such agents should be based on the nature of the exposure, the likelihood that the patient is infected with HIV, and the duration of time following exposure (see Figure 19-1). In general, hollow needle exposures are more significant than solid instruments (such as a scalpel). Those studies that have shown a benefit in using these agents suggest that the drug effectiveness declines after a period of hours after exposure.

TUBERCULOSIS

From 1985 to 1993, the incidence of active tuberculosis increased significantly, to over 25,000 cases in the United States. This was the result of an increase in cases among persons infected with HIV and an increase in immigration of people from areas where tuberculosis infection is endemic (Asia, Latin America, the Caribbean, Africa). Because of better public health measures, tuberculosis has been declining in the last several years. Cases decreased by 36% from 1990–1997. Risk factors for tuberculosis include homeless patients, certain immigrant populations, patients at risk for HIV infection, and persons who live in congregate settings (correction facilities, nursing homes, homeless shelters).

Tuberculosis is caused by a bacterium, *Mycobacterium tuberculosis,* which is spread from an infected person to susceptible persons through the air, especially by coughing or sneezing. *This is* NOT *a highly communicable disease.* Contracting tuberculosis requires prolonged direct contact, as in a family living situation. Only persons with active infection of the lung or throat spread tuberculosis. It is estimated that up to 5% of health care workers will test positive for tuberculosis when working in high-prevalence environments. Clinical manifestations of the disease become apparent only when the patient's immune system fails to keep the bacteria in check. The bacteria then begins to infect the lungs and may spread to other portions of the body, particularly the kidneys, spine, or brain. (These cases are termed "extrapulmonary" and are not communicable to the care provider.) Another type of TB is called *atypical.* This form is common in HIV-infected individuals. Atypical TB is not communicable. Symptoms of tuberculosis are most prominent in the lungs and include a bad cough that lasts longer than two weeks, pain in the chest, or coughing up bloody sputum. Other symptoms of tuberculosis are weakness or fatigue, weight loss, loss of appetite, fever, chills, or night sweats. A person suspect for TB should present with persistent cough for two to three weeks plus two other signs/symptoms.

Treatment of tuberculosis includes antibiotic agents. *TB infection* means a positive skin test. This means no active disease. *TB disease* is the term for active disease. If there is a positive skin test but no symptoms of active TB, Isoniazid (INH) or Rifampin is used for a period of six to nine months to eradicate the infection. Three to four antibiotic agents are used when TB disease is confirmed. While some strains of TB are developing resistance to many of the agents used to treat the disease, multi-drug resistant TB is still treatable and is rare (140 cases in the United States in 2000).

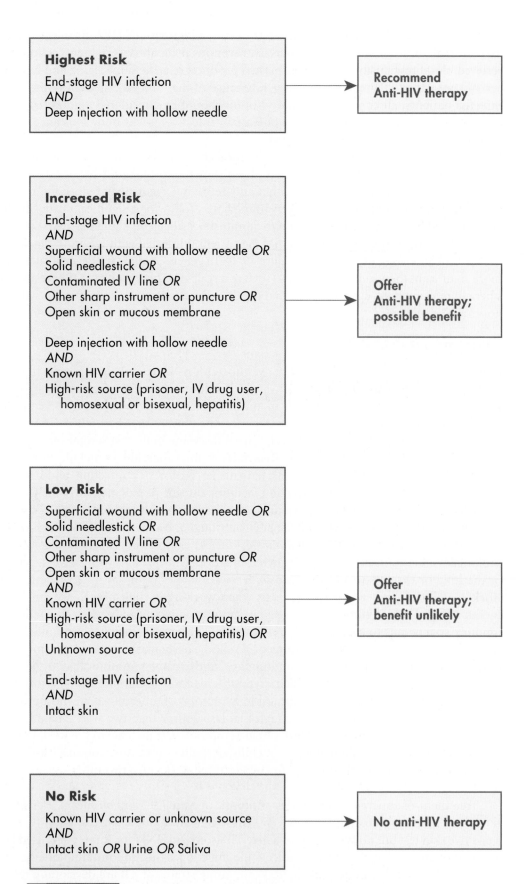

Figure 19-1 Risk assessment for anti-HIV therapy following blood and body fluid exposure.

Since 1995, the U.S. Center for Disease Control and Prevention has recommended placing a surgical mask on any patient suspected of having TB. Thus the care provider does not need to wear a mask of any kind. Health care workers should receive tuberculin skin testing prior to employment and periodically thereafter to ensure that tuberculosis has not been acquired.

PRECAUTIONS FOR PREVENTION OF HEPATITIS B, HEPATITIS C, AND HIV TRANSMISSION

BSI (Body Substance Isolation) refers to treating everyone (including you) as if they are infectious. Your goal is to prevent the spread of infection from you to the patient and from the patient to you. In today's environment, you must use precautions for each and every patient. Equipment used is task based (see Table 19-1).

🖐 PROCEDURE

✳ A. General Considerations

1. You should be knowledgeable about infection from hepatitis B, hepatitis C, and HIV. You should understand their etiologies, signs and symptoms, routes of transmission, and epidemiology (relationships of the various factors determining the frequency and distribution of a disease).

2. If you have open or weeping lesions, take special precautions to prevent exposure of these areas to blood or opim. If these lesions cannot be adequately protected, avoid invasive procedures, other direct patient care activities, or handling of equipment used for patient care.

3. Perform routine handwashing before and after all patient contact. Wash hands as soon as possible following exposure to blood or opim. Alcohol-based foam or gel is best for in-field use. *No artificial nails or extensions for patient care providers (CDC 2002).*

4. Become immunized against the hepatitis B virus.

5. Report any exposure event to your Designated Infection Control Officer.

✳ B. Personal Protection During Patient Exposures

1. Wear gloves if exposure to blood or opim is anticipated. This precaution should be taken when performing an invasive procedure or handling any item soiled with blood or body fluids. Almost all trauma patients are risks for exposure to blood or body fluids.

2. Disposable gowns, masks, and eye coverings are necessary only when extensive contact with blood or body fluids is anticipated. These precautions are advised when spraying, or airborne spread of blood or body fluids is likely (e.g., endotracheal intubation, blind insertion airway device insertion, vaginal deliveries, and major trauma).

3. When treating any patient with respiratory complaints, mask the patient with a surgical mask or non-rebreather oxygen mask.

4. Direct mouth-to-mouth ventilation of patients during CPR is to be discouraged. Use disposable mouthpieces when mouth-to-mouth ventilation is indicated. However, if not available or not working, mouth-to-mouth is to be performed. *Don't let the patient die because you weren't prepared.*

TABLE 19-1	Recommended Personal Protective Equipment for Worker Protection Against HIV and HBV Transmission in Prehospital Settings (from U.S. OSHA Guidelines).			
Task or Activity	Disposable Gloves	Gown	Mask	Protective Eyewear
Bleeding control with spurting blood	Yes	Yes	Yes	Yes
Bleeding control with minimal bleeding	Yes	No	No	No
Emergency childbirth	Yes	Yes	Yes	Yes
Blood drawing	Yes	No	No	No
Starting IV line	Yes	No	No	No
ET intubation or use of BIAD	Yes	No	No, unless splashing is likely	No, unless splashing is likely
Oral/nasal suctioning, manually cleaning airway	Yes	No	No, unless splashing is likely	No, unless splashing is likely
Handling and cleaning instruments with microbial contamination	Yes	No, unless soiling is likely	No	No
Measuring blood pressure	No	No	No	No
Measuring temperature	No	No	No	No
Giving an injection	No	No	No	No

✳ C. Handling of Items Exposed to Blood or Other Potentially Infectious Materials

1. Consider any sharp instrument potentially infective after patient use. Place disposable syringes, needles, scalpel blades, and other sharp objects directly in puncture-resistant containers. Needles should not be recapped, bent, or otherwise manipulated following use. It is strongly recommended that you use exposure-proof parenteral injection sets. In the United States, federal law has mandated that all sharps be needle safe since 2001.

2. Any disposable equipment such as masks, gowns, gloves, mouthpieces, and airways that have been contaminated by blood or opim should be collected in an impervious plastic bag. These plastic bags should then be disposed of according to state definitions of medical waste, in proper waste containers available in hospital emergency departments or other health care locations. Nondisposable gowns can be laundered

using simple laundry procedures. Your hospital should have linen bags or linen containers designated for contaminated gowns, etc.

3. Wash, with a low-sudsing detergent with a neutral pH, any surface spills on nondisposable equipment that does not usually come in contact with skin or mucous membranes. The equipment should then be wet down or soaked for 10 minutes in a 1:100 dilution of household bleach (or 70% isopropyl alcohol). In this concentration, bleach will not cause corrosion of metal objects (U.S. CDC guidelines for public safety 1989).

4. Wash, using a low-sudsing detergent with a neutral pH, nondisposable medical devices that will frequently contact skin or mucous membranes. Then soak them for 30–40 minutes or more in 2% alkaline glutaraldehyde (e.g., Cidex) or similar solution, rinse in sterile water and package until reuse.

❖ D. Procedure After Accidental Exposure to Blood or Opim

1. Thoroughly wash or irrigate the exposed area immediately following an exposure to blood or contaminated body fluids. In the United States you must contact your Designated Officer (mandated by federal law March, 1994). Every department must have a designated officer. The designated officer will deal with the incident and the medical facility from this point.

2. The designated officer (DO) will make the first determination regarding whether or not an exposure occurred. The DO will notify the receiving facility of the possible exposure at the time of the incident. The DO will ask the facility to cooperate in determining the serologic status of the source. In some areas, informed consent need not be obtained to determine serologic status of the source. Know your local laws.

3. Write a report of the incident as soon as possible. The minimum information that should be recorded on the report is included in Figure 19-2. The written ambulance report may be used to supplement, but not replace, the incident report. In the United States you will fill out a confidential exposure report form. *Only the exposed employee, the DO, and the treating physician are allowed to see the form.*

4. Blood tests (if any) to be done on the exposed employee depend on reports of testing of the source patient. If the results of rapid HIV testing are negative, no further testing of the employee is needed. If the source patient is positive for HIV, the exposed employee should undergo HIV serology determination at the time of the incident. *Repeat testing should be done at one month, three months, and six months.* If the source patient is HCV positive, the exposed employee can be tested for HCV in four to six weeks. If the source patient is HBV positive and the exposed care provider has not already been immunized, hepatitis B vaccine should be administered. The administration of HBIG or IG should be determined by the serologic testing of both the source (where possible) and the exposed health care provider, as well as by the assessment of the risk of the exposure.

PEARLS

1. All patients are potential carriers of infectious disease; that is why Universal Precautions are universal and Body Substance Isolation is the EMS standard for practice.

2. If your patient has a persistent cough or is a patient with possible TB disease, place a mask on the patient, not on yourself. You should wear a mask if the patient requires oxygen and can't wear a mask.

3. Be prepared! Have needed equipment with you so you are not required to do mouth-to-mouth breathing. However, you have an obligation to perform mouth-to-mouth resuscitation if your patient needs it and you forgot your equipment.

4. Be prepared! Stay up to date on all of your immunizations.

5. Immediately report to your Designated Officer (know who this is) any possible exposure to blood/opim.

REPORT OF EXPOSURE TO BLOOD OR BODY FLUID

NAME OF EMS PERSONNEL _____

NAME OF EMS SERVICE _____

ADDRESS OF EMS SERVICE _____

_____

PHONE NUMBER (HOME) _____ (WORK) _____

DATE OF EXPOSURE _____ TIME OF EXPOSURE _____

NAME OF PATIENT _____

HOSPITAL ID NUMBER _____

PATIENT ADDRESS _____

_____

PHONE NUMBER (WORK) _____ (HOME) _____

ROUTE OF EXPOSURE:

(   ) Parenteral exposure (needlestick or sharp instrument)

(   ) Mucous membrane

(   ) Open skin

(   ) Intact skin

(   ) Other _____

TYPE OF FLUID:

(   ) blood   (   ) emesis   (   ) saliva

(   ) stool   (   ) urine   (   ) other _____

SOURCE OF EXPOSURE:

HIV:	( ) Yes	( ) No	( ) Unknown	
Hepatitis B:	( ) No	( ) Acute	( ) Chronic Carrier	( ) Unknown
Hepatitis C:	( ) No	( ) Acute	( ) Chronic Carrier	( ) Unknown
Tuberculosis:	( ) No	( ) Yes		

Figure 19-2 Sample Report Form.

RISK FACTORS:

(   ) Homosexual   (   ) IV Drug Abuser

(   ) Hemophilia   (   ) Dialysis Patient

(   ) Sexual Contact of the Above

(   ) Other _____

HIV Test: (   ) Pos.   (   ) Neg.   (   ) Unknown

Date of Test: _____

HBsAg: (   ) Pos.   (   ) Neg.   (   ) Unknown

Date of Test: _____

PERSONNEL DATA:

HBV Vaccine: (   ) No   (   ) Yes   TB skin test: (   ) No   (   ) Yes

Date Completed: _____

Doses: _____

HIV Test: (   ) Pos.   (   ) Neg.   (   ) Unknown

Date of Test: _____

HBsAg: (   ) Pos.   (   ) Neg.   (   ) Unknown

Date of Test: _____

HBsAb: (   ) Pos.   (   ) Neg.   (   ) Unknown

Date of Test: _____

Description of Circumstances Surrounding the Exposure, Including Measures
Taken After Exposure: _____

_____

_____

_____

INSTITUTION NOTIFIED: _____

PHYSICIAN OR RESPONSIBLE PERSON: _____

DATE OF NOTIFICATION: _____ TIME OF NOTIFICATION: _____

NAME OF EXPOSED PERSONNEL _____ DATE _____

SIGNATURE _____

Figure 19-2 Sample Report Form. (continued)

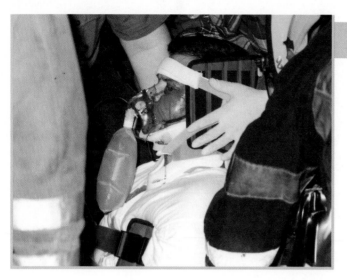

CASE STUDY

Joyce, Dan, and Buddy are transporting a homosexual male patient who has been beaten severely and has a flail chest. As Buddy is checking a lip laceration the patient bites him with bloody teeth. He immediately washes his hand thoroughly. He continues his care of the patient. The SAMPLE history reveals that Poochie was beaten by a gang of men but was never unconscious. He complains of pain "all over." He has a history of HIV infection but has never been told that he has AIDS. He also had "hepatitis," but does not know which kind. He takes several medications for his HIV but does not know their names and does not have them with him. He last ate an hour ago. He has no known allergies. Detailed exam reveals that the abdomen is becoming distended and more tender. The blood pressure has dropped to 70/40. Buddy reports all of this to Medical Direction, who instructs them to take him to the regional trauma center. The trauma team meets them at the emergency room and the patient is taken directly to surgery. He has a fractured liver and a hemothorax as well as the flail chest. He requires 10 units of blood and survives surgery but later dies of pneumonia. His blood is positive for HIV and for Hepatitis B. Buddy has already been immunized for Hepatitis B. Buddy is offered anti-HIV therapy but he declines. He is counseled by the medical director of Infectious Disease and is followed by him for a year. Buddy has HIV tests done immediately and at one, three, and six months afterwards. He remains seronegative.

CASE STUDY WRAP-UP

All health care workers should be immunized against Hepatitis B since the immunization is very effective and without it there is one chance in four of contracting Hepatitis B if exposed. In contrast, there is no immunization for HIV but there are only three chances in 1,000 of contracting the disease if exposed by a hollow-needle stick. This was a high-risk situation because of the blood on the patient and because the patient was in a group (homosexual males) who have a high risk for having Hepatitis B or C and for having HIV. In this case, the patient had HIV but not AIDS. This patient was a low risk for transmission because he was taking his anti-HIV medications and thus should not have had a viral load in his blood. Buddy's refusal of anti-HIV medication was based on his consideration of the toxicity of the antiviral drugs being offered and also the low risk of infection in this situation.

SUMMARY

Like most health care workers, you are at risk of exposure to many contagious diseases. Because of the presence of blood and contaminated secretions in many trauma victims, you must take extra precautions to avoid exposure to the viruses that cause hepatitis B, hepatitis C, and HIV and to the bacteria that cause tuberculosis. Knowledge of the modes of exposure, as well as adherence to barrier precautions, will reduce your risk of contracting any of these infections. In the United States, the recent standards released by OSHA make adherence to these precautions mandatory for health care workers at risk for exposure to contaminated blood and opim.

BIBLIOGRAPHY

1. CPL 2-2.69, Compliance Directive for Occupational Exposure to Bloodborne Pathogens. U.S. Department of Labor, November 27, 2001.

2. NIOSH *Alert*, Latex Allergy, June 1997.

3. Hand Hygiene Guidelines, U.S. Centers for Disease Control and Prevention, October 25, 2002.

4. Update, U.S. Public Health Service Guidelines for the Management of Occupational Exposures to HBV, HCV and HIV and Recommendations for Postexposure Prophylaxis, *MMWR*, June 29, 2001/50(RR11)1–42. Centers for Disease Control and Prevention, Atlanta, GA.

Appendix A
Optional Skills

Donna Hastings, EMT-P

OPTIONAL SKILL 1: Antishock Garment
Objectives
Upon completion of this skill station, you should be able to:
1. Recite the indications and contraindications for the use of the antishock garment.
2. Apply and inflate the antishock garment.
3. Deflate and remove the antishock garment.

Note: Antishock garments are also known as military antishock trousers (MAST) or pneumatic antishock garments (PASG).

INDICATIONS AND CONTRAINDICATIONS

Indications for Use of the Antishock Trousers in Trauma Patients
1. Shock secondary to hemorrhage that can be controlled.
2. Neurogenic shock without evidence of other internal injuries.
3. Isolated fractures of legs without evidence of other internal injuries (blow up to only air-splint pressures).
4. Systolic blood pressure less than 50 mm Hg (controversial).

Contraindications for Use of Antishock Trousers
1. *Absolute:*
   a. Pulmonary edema.
   b. Bleeding that cannot be controlled, such as penetrating chest or abdominal trauma.
2. *Conditional:* Pregnancy—May use leg compartments.

The National Association of EMS Physicians has developed a position paper on the use of antishock trousers in both medical and trauma situations. The reference for this position paper is recorded in the bibliography of Chapter 8.

TECHNIQUES

Application (see Figure A-1)
1. Evaluate the patient through at least the Primary Survey. Apply a blood pressure cuff to the patient's arm.
2. Have your partner unfold the trousers and lay them flat on a long backboard and place the backboard beside the patient.
3. Maintain mobility of the spine by log-rolling the patient (check the back quickly as you do this) onto the backboard. The top of the antishock garment should be just below the lowest rib.
4. Wrap the trousers around the left leg and fasten the Velcro® strips.
5. Wrap the trousers around the right leg and fasten the Velcro® strips.
6. Wrap the abdominal compartment around the abdomen and fasten the Velcro® strips. Be sure the top of the garment is below the bottom ribs.
7. Attach the tubes from the foot pump to the connections on the trousers.

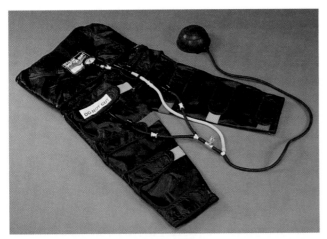

Adult garment and inflation pedal.

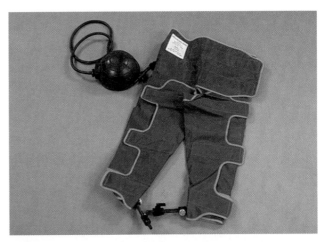

Pediatric garment.

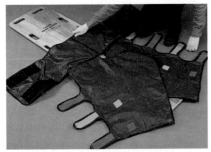

1. Unfold the garment and lay it flat. It should be smoothed of wrinkles.

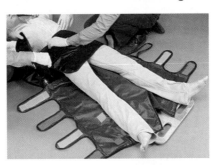

2. Log-roll the patient onto the garment, or slip it under him. The upper edge of the garment must be just below the rib cage.

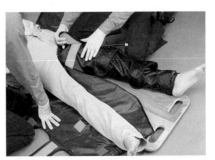

3. Check for a distal pulse and enclose the left leg, securing the Velcro® straps.

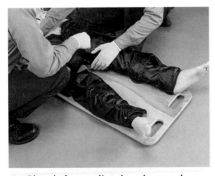

4. Check for a distal pulse and enclose the right leg, securing the Velcro® straps.

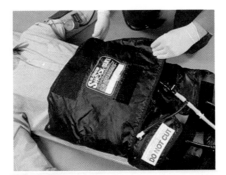

5. Enclose the abdomen and pelvis, securing the Velcro® straps.

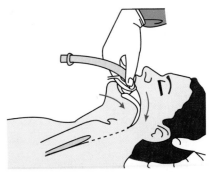

6. Check the tubes leading to the compartments and the pump.

Note: Patient's clothing remains on for demonstration purposes. In actual use, clothing should be removed.

Figure A-1 Application of an antishock garment.

Procedure for Inflation of Trousers

1. Recheck and record the vital signs.
2. Inflate the leg compartments while monitoring the blood pressure. If the blood pressure is not in the range 90 to 100 mmHg, inflate the abdominal compartment.
3. When the patient's blood pressure reaches 90 to 100 mmHg, turn the stopcocks to hold the pressure.

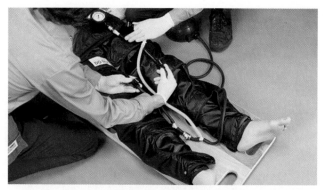

7. Open the stopcocks to the legs and close the abdominal compartment stopcock.

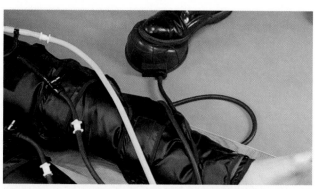

8. Use the foot pedal to inflate the lower compartments simultaneously. Inflate until air exhausts through the relief valves, the Velcro® makes a crackling noise, or the patient's systolic blood pressure is stable at 90–100 mmHg.

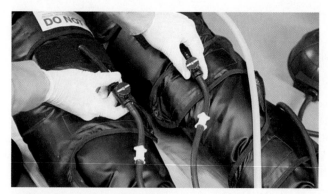

9. Close the stopcocks.

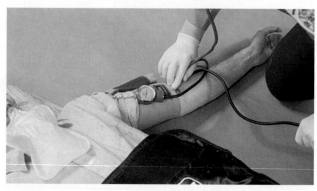

10. Check the patient's blood pressure.

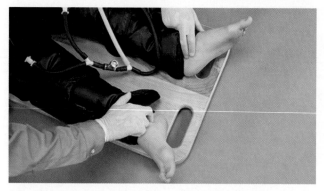

11. Check both lower extremities for a distal pulse.

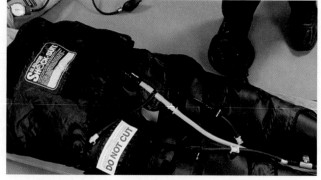

12. If blood pressure is below 90 mmHg, open the abdominal stopcock and inflate abdominal compartment. Close stopcock.

Figure A-1   Application of an antishock garment *(continued)*.

4. Remember, it is not the pressure in the trousers you are monitoring, but the patient's blood pressure.
5. Continue monitoring the patient's blood pressure, adding pressure to the trousers as needed.

Deflation of Trousers

Before deflation occurs, two large-bore IVs must be inserted and sufficient volume of fluids and/or blood given to replace the volume lost from hemorrhage. The antishock garment is usually deflated only at the hospital. The only reason to deflate it in the field is if it causes difficulty with breathing (pulmonary edema).

1. Record the patient's vital signs.
2. From Medical Direction, obtain permission to deflate the trousers.
3. Slowly deflate the abdominal compartment while monitoring the patient's blood pressure.
4. If the blood pressure drops 5 mmHg or more, you must stop deflation and infuse more fluid or blood until the vital signs stabilize again (this usually requires at least 200 cc).
5. Proceed from the abdominal compartment to the right leg and then left leg with your deflation, continuously monitoring the blood pressure and stopping to infuse fluid when a drop of 5 mmHg occurs.
6. If the patient experiences a sudden precipitous drop in blood pressure while you are deflating, stop and reinflate the garment.

Application of Antishock Trousers to a Patient Requiring a Traction Splint

1. Have your partner hold traction on the fractured leg.
2. Unfold the trousers and lay them flat on a long backboard.
3. Log-roll the patient, holding traction on the injured leg and keeping the neck stabilized.
4. Slide the backboard and the patient so that the top of the trousers is just below the lowest rib. If the patient is already on a backboard, you may simply unfold the trousers and slide them under the patient while maintaining traction on the injured leg.
5. Wrap the trousers around the injured leg and fasten the Velcro® strips.
6. Wrap the trousers around the other leg and fasten the Velcro® strips.
7. Wrap the abdominal compartment around the abdomen and fasten the Velcro® strips. Be sure that the top of the garment is below the bottom ribs.
8. Apply a traction splint (Thomas, Hare, or Sager) over the trousers. Attach the straps and apply traction.
9. Inflate the trousers in the usual sequence.

OPTIONAL SKILL 2: Esophageal Gastric Tube Airway

Objectives
Upon completion of this skill station, you should be able to:

1. Explain seven essential points about the use of this airway.
2. Correctly insert the esophageal gastric tube airway (EGTA).

Introduced in the early 1970s, blind insertion airway devices (BIADs) were designed for use by EMS personnel who were not trained to intubate the trachea. All of these devices (EOA, EGTA, PtL®, and Combitube®) are designed to be inserted into the pharynx without the need for a laryngoscope to visualize where the tube is going. All of these devices have a tube with an inflatable cuff that is designed to seal the esophagus, thus preventing vomiting and aspiration of stomach contents as well as preventing gastric distention during bag-valve mask or demand-valve mask ventilation. It was also thought that by sealing the esophagus, more air would enter the lungs and ventilation would be improved. These devices have their own dangers and require careful evaluation to be sure that they are in the correct position. None of the BIADs are equal to the endotracheal tube, which has become the invasive airway of choice for advanced EMS providers.

Esophageal obturator airways (EOA) are designed to be inserted into the esophagus at a level beyond the carina. A cuff is then inflated to reduce the likelihood of gastric distension or regurgitation during bag-valve mask or demand-valve mask ventilation. A more recent design, the esophageal gastric tube airway, has been introduced and should replace the older EOA. This design allows for the placement of a nasogastric tube through the lumen of the obturator for decompression of the stomach. In addition, ventilation occurs directly into the oropharynx rather than through the holes of the obturator.

You must remember seven essential points about the EGTA:

1. Use only in patients who are unresponsive and without protective reflexes.
2. Do *not* use in patients with upper airway or facial trauma in whom bleeding into the oropharynx is a problem. Do *not* use in any patient with injury to the esophagus (e.g., caustic ingestions) or in children who are below the age of 15 and of average height and weight.
3. You must ensure an adequate mask seal; this means appropriate lifting forward of the jaw, with every attempt to avoid movement of the head and neck.
4. Pay careful attention to proper placement. *Unrecognized intratracheal placement* is a lethal complication that produces complete airway obstruction. Such an occurrence is not always easy to detect, and the results are catastrophic. One of the great disadvantages of this airway is that you can determine correct placement only by auscultation and observation of chest movement—both may be quite unreliable in the prehospital setting.
5. You must insert gently and without force.
6. If the patient becomes conscious, you must remove the EGTA, as it will cause retching and vomiting.
7. The EGTA is only recommended when endotracheal intubation is impossible or unsuccessful.

TECHNIQUE

The airway is relatively easily inserted and must never be forced. In the supine patient the following procedure is followed:

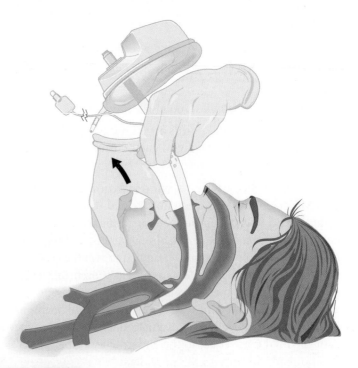

Figure A-2A Insert the esophageal airway completely assembled. Lift up and forward on the jaw as you insert.

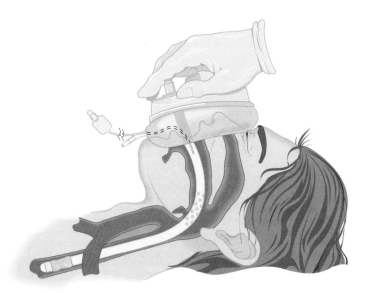

Figure A-2B Advance the tube until the face mask fits snugly over the patient's nose and mouth.

1. Ventilate with a mouth-to-mask or bag-valve mask and suction the pharynx before insertion of the airway.
2. After liberal lubrication, slide the airway, with mask attached, into the oropharynx while the tongue and jaw are pulled forward.
3. Advance the airway along the tongue and into the esophagus. Take care to observe the neck. Tenting of the skin in the area of the pyriform fossa or anterior displacement of the laryngeal prominence indicates that misplacement has occurred and indicates that you should reposition by pulling back and reinserting the airway.
4. Gently insert the airway so that the mask now rests easily on the face; then seal the mask firmly on the face as you pull the jaw forward to ensure a patent airway (see Figures A-2a and b and A-3).
5. Before inflating the cuff, attempt ventilation with a mouth-to-mask or bag-valve mask device. If you see the chest rise, hear breath sounds, and feel good compliance, inflate the cuff of the airway with 35 cc of air.

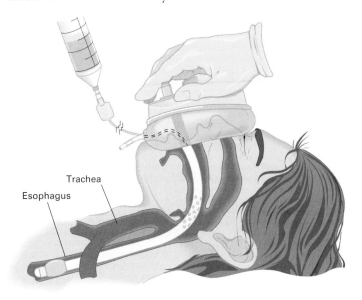

Trachea

Esophagus

Figure A-3 Final position of the esophageal airway.

6. Following inflation, auscultate the lung fields again and feel the chest wall and observe for chest wall movement. The epigastrium should not distend.

If there is any doubt about placement of the airway, remove it and reinsert. If the patient becomes conscious, you must remove the EGTA. Extubation is likely to cause vomiting; be prepared to suction the pharynx and turn the backboard.

OPTIONAL SKILL 3: Pharyngotracheal Lumen Airway

Objectives
Upon completion of this skill station, you should be able to:

1. Explain the five essential points about use of this airway.
2. Correctly insert the pharyngotracheal lumen airway (PtL®).

Introduced in the early 1970s, blind insertion airway devices (BIADs) were designed for use by EMS personnel who were not trained to intubate the trachea. All of these devices (EOA, EGTA, PtL®, and Combitube®) are designed to be inserted into the pharynx without the need for a laryngoscope to visualize where the tube is going. All of these devices have a tube with an inflatable cuff that is designed to seal the esophagus, thus preventing vomiting and aspiration of stomach contents as well as preventing gastric distention during bag-valve mask or demand-valve mask ventilation. It was also thought that by sealing the esophagus, more air would enter the lungs and ventilation would be improved. These devices have their own dangers and require careful evaluation to be sure that they are in the correct position. None of the BIADs are equal to the endotracheal tube, which has become the invasive airway of choice for advanced EMS providers.

The pharyngotracheal lumen airway is another airway developed for EMS providers who are not trained to perform endotracheal intubation. The PtL consists of a smaller-diameter long tube inside of a short large-diameter tube (see Figure A-4). The longer tube goes either into the trachea or the esophagus, while the shorter tube opens into the lower pharynx. Each tube has a cuff; the longer tube's cuff seals the esophagus or trachea, and the shorter tube's cuff seals the oropharynx so that there is no air leak when you ventilate the patient. You insert the PtL blindly into the pharynx, and then you must carefully determine whether the longer tube is in the esophagus or the trachea. If the long tube is in the trachea,

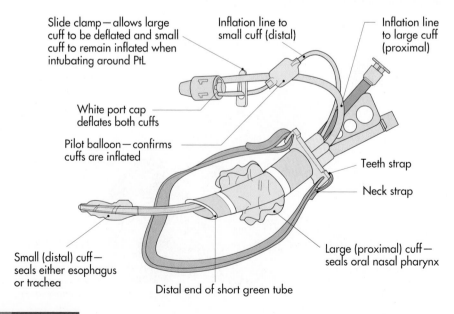

Slide clamp—allows large cuff to be deflated and small cuff to remain inflated when intubating around PtL

Inflation line to small cuff (distal)

Inflation line to large cuff (proximal)

White port cap deflates both cuffs

Pilot balloon—confirms cuffs are inflated

Teeth strap

Neck strap

Small (distal) cuff—seals either esophagus or trachea

Distal end of short green tube

Large (proximal) cuff—seals oral nasal pharynx

Figure A-4 Parts of the PtL® airway.

you ventilate through it. If the tube is in the esophagus, you ventilate through the larger tube in the pharynx. The PtL has advantages over the EGTA in that you don't require extra hands to keep a seal with a face mask; also, the cuff in the pharynx prevents blood and mucous from entering the airway from above.

You must remember five essential points about the PtL:

1. Use only in patients who are unresponsive and without protective reflexes.
2. Do *not* use in any patient with injury to the esophagus (e.g., caustic ingestions) or in children who are below the age of 15 and of average height and weight.
3. Pay careful attention to proper placement. *Unrecognized intratracheal placement* of the long tube is a lethal complication that produces complete airway obstruction. Such an occurrence is not always easy to detect, and the results are catastrophic. Like the EGTA, one of the great disadvantages of this airway is that you can determine correct placement only by auscultation and observation of chest movement—both may be quite unreliable in the prehospital setting.
4. You must insert gently and without force.
5. If the patient regains consciousness, you must remove the PtL, as it will cause retching and vomiting.

TECHNIQUE

The airway is relatively easily inserted and must never be forced. In the supine patient the following procedure is followed:

1. Ventilate with mouth-to-mask or bag-valve mask and suction the pharynx before insertion of the airway.
2. Prepare the airway by checking to be sure that both cuffs are fully deflated, that the long no. 3 tube (see Figure A-5) has a bend in the middle, and that the white cap is securely in place over the deflation port located under the no. 1 inflation valve.

A

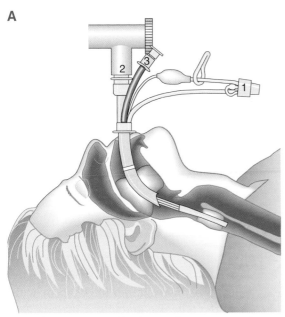

The PtL® airway inserted in the esophagus. Air and/or oxygen delivered into the short no. 2 tube passes into the lungs. An inflated cuff at the end of the long no. 3 tube seals the esophagus, while another inflated cuff seals the oropharynx and prevents air loss from the mouth and nose.

B

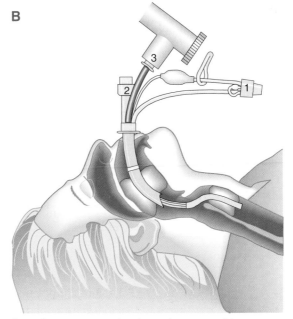

The PtL® airway inserted in the trachea. Air and/or oxygen is delivered into the long no. 3 tube after the stylet is removed. The inflated cuff at the end of the long tube keeps air from leaking from the trachea into the esophagus. The large cuff that is sealing the oropharynx serves as a secondary seal.

Figure A-5 The PtL® in place in (A) the esophagus or (B) the trachea.

3. After liberal lubrication, slide the airway into the oropharynx while the tongue and jaw are pulled forward.

4. Holding the PtL in your free hand so that it curves in the same direction as the natural curvature of the pharynx, advance the airway behind the tongue until the teeth strap contacts the lips and teeth. On very small patients you may have to withdraw the airway so that the teeth strap is up an inch from the teeth. Conversely, on very large patients you may have to insert the teeth strap into the mouth, past the teeth.

5. Immediately inflate both cuffs. Make sure that the white cap is in place over the deflation port located under the inflation valve. Deliver a sustained ventilation into the inflation valve. You can detect failure of the cuffs to inflate properly by failure of the external pilot balloon to inflate or by hearing or feeling air escape from the patient's mouth and nose. This usually means that one of the cuffs is torn and that the airway must be removed and replaced. When you determine that the cuffs are inflating, continue inflation until you get a good seal.

6. Immediately determine whether the long no. 3 tube is in the esophagus or the trachea. First ventilate through the short no. 2 tube. If you see the chest rise, hear breath sounds, feel good compliance, and hear no breath sounds over the epigastrium, the long no. 3 tube is in the esophagus, and you should continue ventilating through the no. 2 tube.

7. If you do not see the chest rise, hear breath sounds, and feel good compliance when the no. 2 tube is ventilated, the no. 3 tube is probably in the trachea. In this case, remove the stylet from the no. 3 tube and ventilate through the no. 3 tube. If you see the chest rise, hear breath sounds, feel good compliance, and hear no breath sounds over the epigastrium, the no. 3 tube is in the trachea, and you should continue ventilating through the no. 3 tube.

8. When you are sure that the patient is being adequately ventilated, carry the neck strap over the patent's head and tighten it in place. Continually monitor the appearance of the pilot balloon during ventilation. Loss of pressure in the balloon signals a loss of pressure in the cuffs. If you suspect a cuff is leaking, increase pressure by blowing into the no. 1 inflation valve or replace the airway.

Like the EGTA, if the patient becomes conscious, you must remove the PtL. Remove the white cap from the deflation port to simultaneously deflate both cuffs. Extubation is likely to cause vomiting; be prepared to suction the pharynx and turn the backboard.

OPTIONAL SKILL 4: Esophageal Tracheal Combitube

Objectives
Upon completion of this skill station, you should be able to:

1. Explain the five essential points about use of this airway.
2. Correctly insert the Combitube®.

Introduced in the early 1970s, blind insertion airway devices (BIADs) were designed for use by EMS personnel who were not trained to intubate the trachea. All of these devices (EOA, EGTA, PtL®, and Combitube®) are designed to be inserted into the pharynx without the need for a laryngoscope to visualize where the tube is going. All of these devices have a tube with an inflatable cuff that is designed to seal the esophagus, thus preventing vomiting and aspiration of stomach contents, as well as preventing gastric distention during bag-valve mask or demand-valve mask ventilation. It was also thought that by sealing the esophagus, more air would enter the lungs and ventilation would be improved. These devices have their own dangers and require careful evaluation to be sure that they are in the correct position. None of the BIADs are equal to the endotracheal tube, which has become the invasive airway of choice for advanced EMS providers.

The Combitube is like the PtL airway in that it has a double lumen. However, in the Combitube the two lumens are separated by a partition rather than one being inside of the other (see Figure A-6). One tube is sealed at the distal end, and there are perforations in the area of the tube that would be in the pharynx. When the long tube is in the esophagus, the patient is ventilated through this short tube. The long tube is open at the distal end, and it has a cuff that is blown up to seal the esophagus or the trachea, depending on which it has entered. When inserted, if the long tube goes into the esophagus, the cuff is inflated and the patient is ventilated through the short tube. If the long tube goes into the trachea, the cuff is inflated and the patient is ventilated through the long tube. Like the PtL airway, this device has a pharyngeal balloon that seals the pharynx and prevents blood and mucous from entering the airway from above. The Combitube is somewhat quicker and easier to insert than the PtL airway but, as with the other BIADs, you must be sure that you are ventilating the lungs and not the stomach.

You must remember five essential points about the Combitube:

1. Use only in patients who are unresponsive and without protective reflexes.
2. Do not use in any patient with injury to the esophagus (e.g., caustic ingestions) or in children who are below the age of 15 and of average height and weight.
3. Pay careful attention to proper placement. Unrecognized intratracheal placement of the long tube is a lethal complication that produces complete airway obstruction. Such an occurrence is not always easy to detect, and the results are catastrophic. Like the EGTA and PtL, one of the great disadvantages of this airway is the fact that you can determine correct placement only by auscultation and observation of chest movement—both may be quite unreliable in the prehospital setting.
4. You must insert gently and without force.
5. If the patient regains consciousness, you must remove the Combitube, as it will cause retching and vomiting.

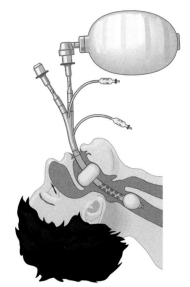

Figure A-6

Esophageal placement of the Combitube® — ventilate through tube #1.

TECHNIQUE

1. Insert the tube blindly, watching for the two black rings on the Combitube that are used for measuring the depth of insertion. These rings should be positioned between the teeth and the lips (see Figure A-6).
2. Use the large syringe to inflate the pharyngeal cuff with 100 cc of air. When inflated, the Combitube will seat itself in the posterior pharynx behind the hard palate.
3. Use the small syringe to fill the distal cuff with 10 to 15 cc of air.
4. The long tube will usually go into the esophagus. Ventilate through the esophageal connector. It is the external tube that is the longer of the two and is marked no. 1. As with the PtL airway, you must see the chest rise, hear breath sounds, feel good compliance, and hear no breath sounds over the epigastrium to be sure that the long tube is in the esophagus.
5. If you do not see the chest rise, hear breath sounds, feel good compliance, and you hear breath sounds over the epigastrium, the tube has been placed in the trachea (see Figure A-7). In this case, change the ventilator to the shorter tracheal connector, which is marked no. 2. Again you must check to see the chest rise, hear breath sounds, feel good compliance, and hear no breath sounds over the epigastrium in order to be sure that you are ventilating the lungs.

Like the EGTA and PtL, if the patient becomes conscious, you must remove the Combitube. Extubation is likely to cause vomiting; be prepared to suction the pharynx and turn the backboard.

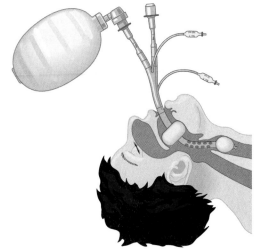

Figure A-7

Tracheal placement of the Combitube®—ventilate through tube #2.

Radio Communications

Corey M. Slovis, M.D., F.A.C.P., F.A.C.E.P.

It is imperative that you provide your hospital base station physician with an accurate, succinct, on-scene assessment. This is an essential skill to develop. In general, the physician or nurse at the other end of the radio transmission will not be able to focus on more than three to five key bits of information. Thus, before beginning your call, you should spend a few moments thinking about what specifics of the history and physical exam need to be transmitted. The purpose of radio communication is not to give all of the available findings to the physician, but to transmit only that information needed for appropriate care in the field, or to ready the emergency department (ED) for patient arrival. If you are requesting medications or procedures, then your radio report should focus on the information that justifies your request. Due to responsibilities to patients already in the ED, the physician receiving the call would like to spend a minimum of time on the radio.

When speaking over the radio, no matter how emergent the situation, you should speak clearly and avoid speaking rapidly in an emotional, high-pitched voice. However, using a slow monotone voice in reporting a cardiac arrest would be inappropriate as well. You should try to convey the urgency of the situation in a professional manner. The radio microphone should be held a few inches from your mouth to allow accurate voice transmission but not so far (more than six inches) as to allow interference from other noises at the scene.

The following format for communications is designed to maximize the efficient transfer of information (see Tables B-1 and B-2). It may also be used for calls not involving trauma.

FOUR-PHASE COMMUNICATION POLICY

The BTLS communications policy is divided into four parts. The first of these phases is devoted to the EMS unit confirming radio contact with a specific hospital or base station.

Phase 1: Contact Phase

Step 1—Identification: In attempting to establish radio contact, you should state what EMS service is calling, the unit's level of function (e.g., basic, paramedic), and the unit's identification number. For example, "This is county advanced unit 501 calling county hospital." It is important for you to identify your level of function so the physician knows which procedures and medications to consider. The EMS service should be identified, because different services operating in the same area may function with different protocols. The EMS unit's own identification number needs to be included for potential recontacting and for retrospective tape audit purposes. As different hospitals may have the same radio frequency, the specific facility being called should be stated by the caller each time contact is initiated.

Step 2—Facility Response: The base station or receiving hospital should now respond by identifying the facility, which person is on the radio, and to what EMS unit they are responding. An example might be: "This is Dr. Thomas Smith at county hospital. Go ahead county advanced unit 501." By restating the EMS unit's service and number, confusion will be minimized when multiple units are involved with a single receiving facility. It is recommended that hospital-based radio operators identify themselves. This is important because the initial response is often not by a physician. It is just as important that physicians identify themselves so that you may record who is giving you orders.

TABLE B-1	BTLS Communications Format.

Phase 1: Establishing Contact

1. Initiation of call
   EMS service
   Level of function (basic, paramedic, etc.)
   Unit number
   Medical control facility being contacted

2. Receiving facility response
   Name of facility
   Name and title of radio operator
   Renaming of calling EMS service

Phase II: In-the-Field Report

3. Reidentification
   EMS service
   Level of function (basic, paramedic, etc.)
   Unit number

4. Chief complaint/on-scene report
   One brief sentence
   Includes age, sex, complaint, and/or mechanism of injury

5. Lifesaving resuscitation
   Patient's response to lifesaving maneuvers

6. Vital signs/primary survey abnormalities
   Vital signs in stable patient
   or
   Primary Survey in unstable patient

7. ETA
   State ETA

8. Request for orders
   State what is desired
   or
   State "no orders requested"

Phase III: Base Station (Hospital)-Controlled Activity

9. Physician response
   Agree or deny or state desired orders
   Request for additional history and/or information

10. Rescuer response
    Clarification or response to requested maneuver or therapy

Phase IV: Sign-Off

11. EMS unit sign-off
12. Base station sign-off

TABLE B-2	Do's and Don'ts of Successful Radio Communications.

Do's

Think about your report before making radio contact.

Be brief and concise.

Talk clearly.

Relate only the key points of the history—don't give every single fact you've learned about the patient.

State the patient's primary problem and what you are requesting early in the call.

Ask questions if you are unsure of the base station's reply.

Ask for clarification on therapies you think are wrong or dangerous.

Call your supervisor for "unresolvable" problems.

Don'ts

Don't make a speech.

Don't ramble.

Don't use jargon, codes, or abbreviations.

Don't significantly alter how you normally talk.

Don't assume anything.

Never give a therapy you think is dangerous.

Don't make unprofessional comments that will embarrass you when the tape is replayed.

Don't argue over the radio.

Phase II: In-the-Field Report

The second phase of communications is the most important. Here you should give all-important Primary Survey information and request appropriate orders. This phase of communication is divided into the six steps that follow.

Step 3—Re-identification: Once contact has been confirmed, the in-the-field report begins by your re-identifying the EMS service, its level of function, and unit number. This information may not yet have been recorded or even heard by the physician, who has probably just arrived at the radio console.

Step 4—Chief Complaint/On-Scene Report: After you have identified your level of function and unit number, the next sentence should provide the physician with the most complete picture of the patient possible. This sentence should include the patient's approximate age, sex, complaint, and/or mechanism of injury. Having information such as the victim's approximate age and sex allows the physician to get a mental picture of the patient. Similarly, by knowing the chief complaint and/or type of injury, the physician has an idea of the type of emergency call that he will be handling. An example of this part of communication might be: "We are on the scene with a 23-year-old female restrained driver involved in a deceleration motor vehicle collision. She is complaining of chest pain," or "We are on the scene with a 23-year-old female who has a gunshot wound to the chest." The patient's medications, additional complaints, or more complete description of injuries should not be given at this time.

Step 5—Lifesaving Resuscitation: If any emergency maneuvers or lifesaving therapy has been performed during the Primary Survey, it should be reported next. Thus, if an airway maneuver has been performed or CPR started, it should be reported at this point. Examples of this include, "The patient's sucking chest wound has been sealed," or "We have begun CPR and defibrillated the patient." The result of a fingerstick glucose, if already performed on a comatose patient, should be reported during this phase.

Step 6—Vital Signs/Primary Survey Abnormalities: In the next sentence, you should give vital signs and/or Primary Survey abnormalities. In stable patients with a normal Primary Survey, a complete set of vital signs are blood pressure, pulse, respiratory rate, skin temperature (if pertinent), and oxygen saturation by pulse oximetry (if available—see Chapter 5). A typical communication might be: "The patient has a normal Primary Survey with vital signs of: blood pressure 130/90, pulse 90, respiration 16, and oxygen saturation of 98% on room air." If, however, there is an abnormal Primary Survey, a full set of vital signs does not always need to be reported. In this type of unstable patient, problems with airway, breathing, cardiovascular stability, and screening neurologic exam would be reported to the physician. In this so-called load-and-go type of call, unimportant physical findings, historical facts, or medication usage do not need to be reported at this time. A typical communication would be: "Primary Survey as follows: no palpable pulses present, respiration is 40, chest exam reveals a sucking chest wound; patient is confused and combative." Another example: "Blood pressure is 70 by palpation, pulse is 130 and weak, patient is very hot and dry. We found him in a warm, enclosed room."

Step 7—Estimated Time of Arrival: You should now state how much time it will take to get to the hospital from the present location. If you are en route, this should be reported. If, however, significant additional time is required to extricate or load the patient into the EMS vehicle, this should be specifically stated. Examples of the estimated time of arrival (ETA) phase of communication include: "We are en route to your location; our ETA is less than 4 minutes," or "We are still on-scene and will require 10 to 15 minutes before we begin transport to the hospital."

Step 8—Request for Orders: Before relinquishing radio control to the base station, you should state what orders are desired, that no orders are desired, or that the base station physician's help is needed to determine what to do for the patient. Examples of these respective situations include: "Requesting two large-bore IVs of normal saline to maintain blood pressure," or "No orders requested," or "Base station, how do you advise?"

Phase III: Base Station (Hospital)-Controlled Activity

In this phase of communication you are no longer in charge of the radio. You should now respond to the physician's approval or denial of orders. In other cases there may be talk back and forth between you and the physician.

Step 9—Physician's Response: It is now up to the physician to determine how to proceed with management of the patient. The physician may merely agree with your request by stating, "Go ahead with your requested therapy" or might completely disagree, "Orders denied, transport the patient as soon a possible." With complicated patients, the physician may need more information than you have transmitted. This is not a criticism of the rescuer's radio abilities, but merely a need for the physician to obtain additional information. For example, "Are the patient's neck veins flat or distended?" Or "Does the patient seem to improve in the Trendelenburg position?" You should be prepared to answer routine questions readily and to perform requested maneuvers.

Step 10—Your Response: You should confirm any given orders by repeating them. If the base station has given orders either that are incomplete or with which you disagree, it is now appropriate to give additional history or request an order. Examples of these problems include: "Be advised that the patient has a long history of cardiac problems and is on multiple medications," or "Base station, did you copy that the patient is hypotensive and that we are requesting an IV of Ringer's lactate?" If you cannot answer the questions, tell the physician. Examples of this type of exchange would be: "We don't have any available information on downtime," or "We are unable to attempt this, the patient is still trapped inside the vehicle."

Phase IV: Sign-Off

The final phase of EMS–base station communications is the sign-off. You should make it very clear that the unit is leaving the medical frequency and returning to dispatch frequency.

Step 11—EMS Unit Sign-Off: You should now advise the base station that you are ending communications. Although everyone seems to favor a different phrase to end with, each EMS service should agree on a common sign-off phrase. The use of a time signal at the end of a comment is recommended but optional. Acceptable closings include: "Advanced unit 501 is clear," or "Unit 501 is out at 13:59 hours." Avoid using code numbers, as many physicians do not understand them or may use similar codes for different purposes; thus "Unit 501 is 10-8 your location code 3" is not recommended, nor is "501, 10-8, 1359."

Step 12—Base Station Closing: The base station physician should similarly end communication with the same agreed-upon phrase: for example, "County hospital clear."

Keep a copy of Table B-1 by the EMS radio in the hospital. You should try to concentrate on transmitting the most information with the least amount of words.

Documentation: The Written Report

Arlo F. Weltge, M.D., F.A.C.E.P.

With the recognition of the important and increasing role of the prehospital care provider has come deserved respect. However, with this recognition comes the expectation of a standard of care and resultant liability when the care does not meet that standard.

This appendix will show how to create a document that chronicles the medical care given, communicates medical information, and provides a permanent record that can be used as evidence that the standard of care was delivered.

THE WRITTEN REPORT

The EMS system written report can vary dramatically from being primarily a billing form to an excellent narrative medical record. In most EMS systems the written report usually will provide enough space for medical documentation to be adequate for the majority of transports, since most runs do not require much more than a simple transport.

It is important to use the system written report effectively. There should be enough space for a chief complaint, simple history and assessment, and space for other comments. All written reports should be filled out completely. Even though the transport may have been "simple," failure to document vital signs, to complete checkoff boxes for the history and physical, and to enter times, events, and other simple information may reflect poorly on the care delivered if the report is ever reviewed.

If the system report does not provide adequate space for a reasonable history and assessment, or if the case is more difficult, for example, requiring intervention or long transport times, or involving potential patient complications, it may be necessary to include a continuation sheet. The continuation sheet can be a simple form. It does require some basic information, including the patient's name, date, identification of the EMS system, and the run identification number. The report should be written at or near the time of the run, and the original must be signed and kept as a regular part of the system's medical records and attached to the regular written report. A simple continuation form is shown in Figure C-1.

A simple continuation sheet can be used for almost any situation or problem. The written, or narrative, report, using the continuation sheet, requires much more effort, however, since there are not a host of fill-in-the-blank or checkoff boxes to use when writing the report. To document a complex case adequately using the continuation sheet, you need to be familiar with the general form or sequence of a written narrative report. The form is dictated by convention (or otherwise known in the medical community as a generally agreed-upon habit or standard). Effective documentation requires using this convention as well as skill and practice.

The written report should be brief, yet, like the verbal report, relevant and focused. There are times when the clinical problem is confusing and the report must be lengthier, but length does not necessarily reflect accuracy or relevancy. The report should document relevant events and discrepancies and should be written so another reader can reconstruct the events. The report should also justify the action, even if one's impression at the time was wrong. A "mistake" may have been entirely justified given the circumstances at the time, but that mistake can be justified only if the circumstances are clearly and honestly documented as part of the record.

THIS MUST BE ATTACHED TO CORRESPONDING EMS REPORT

DATE _____   HO NO: _____

NAME _____

ATTENDANT: _____

EMT REPORT:	TIME	B.P.	PULSE	RESP. RATE	TEMP.

SIGNATURE X

EMT CONTINUATION

P & S AMBULANCE TEXAS, INC.
7849 ALMEDA
HOUSTON, TEXAS 77054

WHITE - FINANCE, CANARY - HOSPITAL, PINK - SUPERVISOR

Figure C-1 Example of a continuation sheet.

The report contains the following information, but rarely will include all the information. In fact, it is more important to effectively treat the patient and document that treatment than it is to get all the information while the patient suffers because of lack of treatment or delay in transport. It is reasonable to take brief notes and to fill out the written report at the hospital before returning to service. Care of the patient is the first goal.

1. *Run Call:* Note how the call was dispatched, particularly if there is discrepancy between the dispatch description and the actual findings. It is helpful, for example, to explain delays in transport if a call came in as a sick party when actually it was a motor vehicle accident with multiple victims. Document time whenever possible. The dispatch time is important because, realistically, it may be the last documented time until arrival at the hospital.

2. *Scene Description:* Document any scene hazards that delay or affect patient treatment or transport. It is easy to forget scene hazards, but delays may affect patient outcomes and the mention of scene hazards may help jog the memory of the run when reading the report at a later time.

   The mechanisms should be noted as well. Often this is most effectively done by stick figures (see Figure C-2). You are often the only source of the mechanism of injury for subsequent treatment providers. Clear, simple drawings of mechanisms are quick and easy, useful for communicating mechanism and suspicion of occult injuries, and can help jog the memory of the event at a later time.

3. *Chief Complaint:* Record age, sex, mechanism, chief complaint or injury, and time. These identifiers focus the thought process. If previously mentioned, mechanism does not have to be documented here.

4. *History of the Present Illness/Injury or Symptoms:* Record relevant positives and negatives. Document any relevant history that you obtain from the patient. If the history does not come from the patient but from another witness, note the source and the specific information from that person, especially when it conflicts with other history.

Additional useful information includes the patient's recollection of the events immediately prior to the accident (e.g., did the patient faint first and then fall?), prior injuries to the same location (e.g., fractured the same leg last year), and any treatment given before your arrival (e.g., patient pulled from car by bystanders).

5. *Past Medical History:* Record previous illness, medications, recent surgery, allergies, and when the patient last ate. You are usually not responsible for getting a complete medical history. However, in acutely sick and injured victims, you may be the last person able to get this information before the patient loses consciousness. Again, treating the patient is the most important priority, but a little bit of useful information may save a lot of complications.

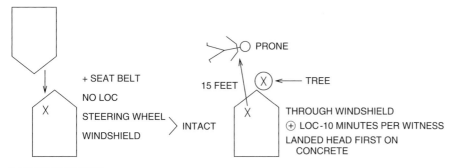

Figure C-2 Diagrams for mechanisms of injuries.

Other information that can be useful may include relevant family history (any diseases that run in the family) and social history (use of alcohol, tobacco, or other drugs). This should be documented as the SAMPLE history:

S—symptoms
A—allergies
M—medications
P—past medical history (other illnesses)
L—last meal
E—events preceding accident

6. *Physical Exam:* Record appearance, vital signs, level of consciousness, Primary Survey, and Detailed Exam. A general statement of the appearance helps focus the reader on urgencies (e.g., the patient appeared alert and in no distress or appeared in extreme pain and was ashen and short of breath). The level of consciousness should be documented with the vital signs. This is best done using stimulus and response (responds to voice/pain with moan, decerebrate posturing). The best method is to note the stimulus that provokes a response by the AVPU method:

A—alert
V—responds to verbal stimuli
P—responds to pain
U—unresponsive

Document that a complete exam was done. Simply stating the body part (back, abdomen, upper extremity) with a zero or slash afterward can indicate that the part was examined and that there were no significant findings.

One of the easiest and best ways to document the exam in a seriously injured patient is to sequentially note the findings and procedures as one does the Primary Survey and Detailed Exam. It can be helpful to write "Primary Survey," note findings, describe the resuscitation, and then start the rest of the exam with "Detailed Exam." By doing this, anyone reviewing the record can immediately recognize that you are oriented to trauma assessment, and by assumption, have performed an organized Primary Survey.

One picture is worth a thousand words and may aid the memory at a later date. Diagrams of injuries for locations or for severity (like cuts) should be simple yet contain enough detail to locate site of injury, that is, identify if it is right or left, volar (palmar) or dorsal, part of an extremity, or front or back trunk (see Figure C-3).

7. *Procedures (Indication, Procedure, Result):* Document the need, describe the procedure, and note the time and patient response when performing an invasive procedure. Any procedure potentially can have a harmful effect, sometimes delayed; all procedures should be documented (e.g., stating an IV was started in the right forearm on the second stick protects you from charges of improper technique when the

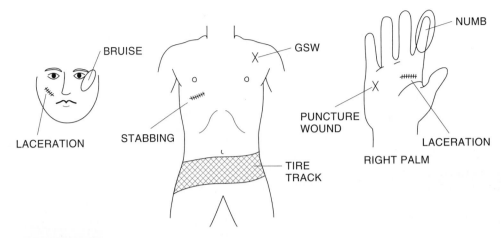

BRUISE

GSW

NUMB

LACERATION

STABBING

PUNCTURE
WOUND

RIGHT PALM

LACERATION

TIRE
TRACK

Figure C-3 Diagrams of injuries.

patient later develops a thrombophlebitis from an IV in the left arm). It may not be possible to document every IV attempt; however, when performing invasive treatment procedures such as needle decompressions and needle cricothyroidotomies, you should document the need, the confirming evidence, the procedure, and the effect—even if the effect is a negative result.

8. *Ongoing Exam (Recheck, Changes, Condition on Arrival):* Documenting the initial findings establishes a baseline, but Ongoing Exams during long transports, changes while the patient is still in your care, and condition on or just prior to arrival should be recorded as necessary to establish that decompensation did or did not occur while in your care. It is important to remember that as soon as the patient arrives, other people will perform an exam and record their findings. Any discrepancies or findings documented in their report will be presumed to have occurred while in your care unless documented by you as having existed prior to your intervention. The burden for documentation is then on you to show that complications did not occur while in transport but at the scene prior to your arrival. This is not to suggest that patients will not decompensate while in your care, but you should notice such decompensation and document that you responded to it.

9. *Impression:* Your impression may be included to summarize the significant findings. However, care must be taken not to overdiagnose. A tender forearm does not necessarily mean fracture any more than shortness of breath must mean a tension pneumothorax. Impressions should be as "generic" as possible, noting the actual finding,

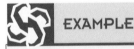 **EXAMPLE**

PROPERLY DOCUMENTED PREHOSPITAL PROCEDURE

Patient was pale, short of breath, lost the radial pulse (hypotensive), and had decreased breath sounds on right side (the suspicion). The right chest was tympanic and the trachea was deviated to the left, but neck veins were not distended (confirming findings present or absent). A 14-gauge needle was inserted over the top of the third rib in the midclavicular line with a rush of air. The patient's radial pulse returned and color improved, but respirations were still labored.

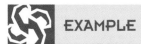 **EXAMPLE**

DOCUMENTING THE PRIORITIES (JUST THE FACTS)

Call: Single MVC.

Scene: One victim in roadway, car head-on into pole, patient through windshield supine in roadway.

Diagram: See Figure C-2.

Primary Assessment: Mid-twenties, unresponsive male, ashen, grunting respiration with contusions to face, neck, and anterior chest. Absent radial pulse, rapid, thready carotid pulse, sucking wound right chest. Abdomen distended and tender, pelvis stable, extremities appeared to have no major injuries.

Cervical spine controlled manually, no change in respiration with jaw thrust, chest wound covered with an Asherman Chest Seal®. Patient log-rolled onto long board, no obvious back injuries. Loaded and transported.

Ongoing Exam: Patient's right pupil fixed and dilated, left midposition. Respirations remained rapid and shallow. Patient given oxygen and ventilated by BVM. One 14-gauge IV RL right anticub started, arrived at city hospital in three minutes, patient still with rapid thready carotid pulse.

See Figure C-4.

---

such as pain or bruising (not the diagnosis, such as fracture or pulmonary contusion), and should include relevant information such as distal pulse. Suspicions should be noted: Shortness of breath, decreased breath sounds on right, and tender right chest. Tender right forearm, possible fracture, sensation/pulse intact.

10. *Documenting the Priorities:* The detailed description is designed for the occasion when events allow time for gathering of the information and completion of the Detailed Exam. There are times when urgent priorities limit the evaluation to treating the immediate complications and the exam never gets past the Primary Survey. Care of the patient is the first priority. Often the best way to document this is to describe the sequence as it occurs, using the Primary Survey and Detailed or Ongoing Exams.

Summary of the Narrative Report

1. Run call
2. Scene description
3. Chief complaint
4. History of the present illness/injury or symptoms
5. Past medical history
6. Physical exam
7. Procedures
8. Ongoing Exam
9. Impression
10. Documenting the priorities

IMPROVING DOCUMENTATION SKILLS

Documentation reflects on the quality of clinical practice. Like clinical care, one can improve skills by practice as well as by observing the better qualities of others. Following are suggestions to help improve the quality of documentation.

CALL: INJURED PARTY 10:15 A.M.

SCENE: AUTO-PEDESTRIAN   DIAGRAM:
          SINGLE PATIENT KNOCKED DOWN (NOT THROWN
ANY DISTANCE) AND PULLED FROM THE STREET PRIOR
TO ARRIVAL BY BYSTANDERS. PATIENT LYING ON
SIDEWALK ON ARRIVAL.

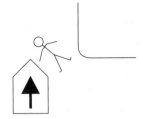

CC: MID-TEEN MALE COMPLAINING OF PAIN IN THE HEAD AND NECK.

HISTORY:
    PATIENT: DENIES LOSS OF CONSCIOUSNESS. COMPLAINS OF HEAD AND NECK AND
LEFT HIP, BUT NO OTHER INJURIES. DENIES PAIN IN ARMS, LEGS, OR BACK.

    MOTHER: BRIGHT RED HAIR AND LIPSTICK – VERY EXCITED – STATES PATIENT IS
"ALLERGIC TO EVERYTHING," DID NOT SEE ACCIDENT.

    DRIVER: STATES PATIENT STEPPED OUT AND KNOCKED DOWN – NOT THROWN –
AND NOT KNOCKED OUT.

PMH: PATIENT: NO MEDICAL PROBLEMS, NO MEDICATIONS OR SURGERY, AND NEVER
BEEN HOSPITALIZED. THINKS HE IS ALLERGIC TO PENICILLIN AND CODEINE.

EXAM: ALERT MALE, SCARED BUT NOT CONFUSED.
       BP 110/70 P 98
HEAD — HEMATOMA RIGHT OCCIPUT, FACE NONTENDER PUPILS EQUAL REACTIVE
NECK — TENDER RIGHT SIDE C-COLLAR AND PLACED ON BACKBOARD
CHEST — NONTENDER BREATH SOUNDS EQUAL
ABD — NONTENDER SOFT
BACK — 0
UP/LOW EXT—00 + DISTAL PULSE AND MOVEMENT

PATIENT TRANSPORTED CODE I TO CITY GENERAL WITH C-COLLAR AND BACKBOARD.

10:25 EN ROUTE — ALERT REPT VS: BP 118/70   P 70

10:30 ARRIVED — PATIENT ALERT, VS UNCHANGED, MOVING ALL EXTREMITIES

IMPRESSION: AUTO-PEDESTRIAN WITH INJURIES HEAD AND LEFT HIP, AND PAIN IN
NECK. NO LOSS OF CONSCIOUSNESS.

Figure C-4 Example of a completed narrative report.

Practice documentation with critique. Have somebody else try and reconstruct the events based on your narrative and evaluate what comments were useful and what comments were left out. Sometimes the most obvious events are the easiest to forget to document.

Read others' narrative reports and try to reconstruct the events.

Practice anticipating problems and criticisms. A fractured bone needs to have distal pulse and sensation checked and documented. Invasive procedures, complications, unusual events, or anticipated patient complaints can be noted and justification written. Many complications of invasive procedures, such as infections, may not be discovered for days or weeks. Anticipation of these delayed complications can be an important part of the documentation process.

Write to remind yourself. If there are specific events unique to this run or which will help you distinguish this run from other similar runs, note it in the record.

Be professional. People's lives depend on your care. Your records should reflect that you take your responsibility seriously. The medical record is not a place for humorous or derogatory comments. Use caution when describing the patient. Do not use words that could indicate your care was prejudiced by the patient's presentation. Words such as "the patient was hysterical" would be better written as "the patient was very excited and upset."

Be concise. Longer is not necessarily better. If it is of interest, write it down, but get to the point and write what is important.

Review your own records. Can you reconstruct the events and were complications anticipated? Would this record be a friend in court?

Practice quality care, including caring for the patient. A patient is a potential adversary or advocate. The excitement of the minute often results in a brusque attitude. Ask yourself if you would have been happy with the way you were treated if you had been the patient.

Important Points About the Written Report

The written report should be kept as a regular part of the patient's record and should be considered a legal document. There are some basic rules to follow:

1. Keep the report legible.
2. If there are blanks, fill them in. Empty boxes imply that the question was not asked. Open spaces imply that information might be added after the fact.
3. Never alter a medical record. If there is an error on the record, draw a single line through the error and make a note that it was an error and why.
4. The record should be written in a timely manner. Events fade and memory can be challenged. Write the chart as soon as possible after the event. If there is some delay, note the reason.
5. Always be honest on the chart. Never record observations not made. Never try to cover up actions. (We can't always be right, but we must always be honest.) The record, your primary source of support, may be discredited if any of your observations are shown not to be accurate.
6. Always make any changes or additions to the chart clearly distinguished, timed, and dated. Changes after the fact may be used against you if the appearance is that you were trying to alter the record in your favor. Such alterations give the appearance of lying.
7. What do you do if there is a complication or bad result and you did not record pertinent information on the run report? The best method is to sit down immediately and write, as accurately as possible, the sequence of events using whatever records are available and to the best of your memory. This is not as useful as a document transcribed at the time, but an accurate record even after the fact can be useful at a later date in reconstructing the events.

Appendix D
Trauma Care in the Cold

Jere F. Baldwin, M.D., F.A.C.E.P., F.A.A.F.P.

One evening during the winter of 1998 it was reported that 24 of the United States and all of the Canadian provinces had temperatures below freezing. In a multihospital study done in the United States, of 400 reported cases of frostbite, 69 came from the sunny state of Florida. Thus, for many if not most prehospital EMS providers, thought needs to be given to the application of BTLS in the cold environment. This appendix will address some of the problems encountered in applying the principles of BTLS in the cold. Although basic principles in the management of the hypothermic trauma patient (core temperature less than 95 degrees Fahrenheit or 35 degrees Celsius) are presented, this material does not pretend to be a treatise on hypothermia.

COLD WEATHER AND THE SIX STAGES OF AN AMBULANCE CALL

There are six stages of an ambulance call (see Figure D-1). The *predispatch stage* is the most important in the successful application of the principles of BTLS in the cold environment. Effective cold weather response is heavily dependent on adequate preparation before the emergency. EMS providers living in cold environments have already learned the importance of proper clothing, including hand and foot wear. Likewise, EMS systems operating in cold environments have already learned the importance of maintaining the rescue vehicle, which includes special tires and the use of engine warming blocks. EMS systems also must develop a system to keep their equipment at an appropriate temperature for immediate use. Medications can be kept in a portable box and carried to the vehicle for each run, but this is not practical for other equipment. Plastic endotracheal tubes and IV tubing must be kept warm enough so that they are malleable enough to use. Bags of IV fluid are of special concern because they could cause harm to the patient if cold IV fluids were rapidly infused into a patient. There are several methods to maintain the temperature of IV fluids. These include any type of electric warmer from electric blankets to small dog warmers on the rig. Obviously, the best solution is to keep the rescue vehicle in a heated garage.

The *travel to the scene stage* often takes on additional meaning in the winter. The shortest route, because of travel conditions, may not be the quickest or the safest. Several EMS systems have recognized that more than one mode of travel is needed. This may include any combination of helicopter, ambulance, snowmobile, or even dogsled.

The *travel to the hospital stage* may be long and arduous during winter rescue. The distances may be greater, the travel may be slower, and the vehicle more likely to break down or become stuck. Some EMS systems in North America have developed relay and backup systems for the patient. These relay systems facilitate the transfer of the patient to the nearest appropriate facility by the most appropriate mode of travel. The backup systems include a buddy system to ensure that there is someone aware of the location of the ambulance that can intervene in the event of a breakdown or a loss of communication.

Scene Size-Up

On-scene trauma assessment in the cold environment starts with the *Scene Size-up*. The hazards may not be apparent. The frozen, slippery walk or road under the snow or even the fallen power line under the snow may await the hasty rescuer. The total number of vic-

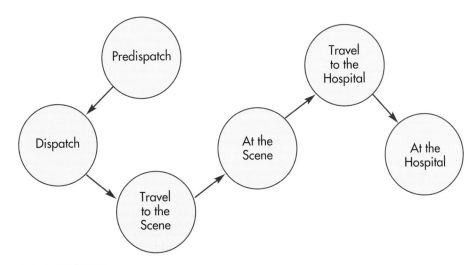

Figure D-1 Six stages of an ambulance call.

tims may not be apparent; you must look for clues to more victims. A patient left in the cold is a fatal error. It is easy to miss an unconscious, ejected patient at night or in poor visibility. The essential equipment may need to be slightly different—hydraulic equipment does not work efficiently, batteries last 25% as long, and flares last half as long. The phenomena of icy fog and the suspended vehicle exhaust from the rescue vehicles themselves cause decreased visibility. You must constantly reevaluate the safety of the scene, and you need the ability and backup equipment to react appropriately.

Determine the mechanism of injury. Look for clues to hypothermia. Even in a relatively warm 50-degree (10 degrees Celsius) environment, the patient could have hypothermia. Consider this possibility in the aged patient, the stroke victim, or the septic patient who has been lying on the bathroom floor for hours. Consider it with the intoxicated patient who has been lying at the foot of the basement stairs for hours. In the outside environment, wet clothing and wind chill can cause rapid hypothermia in the trauma patient.

Primary Trauma Survey

The BTLS Primary Trauma Survey is even more critical in the cold environment. Evaluation of the airway, cervical spine control, and documentation of initial level of consciousness is the same. However, you must consider that the decreased level of consciousness could be a result of hypothermia in addition to any trauma or shock. The evaluation of breathing is the same; however, a decreased rate and depth of respiration may be due to hypothermia in addition to head injury or intoxication from alcohol or drugs. The treatment of an inadequate respiratory effort is the same: adequate ventilation with 100% oxygen. If the patient has *isolated hypothermia*, ventilate with *warm* humidified oxygen. Do not hyperventilate.

The evaluation of the circulation has the same importance that was described in Chapter 2; however, the cold environment may make it more difficult to evaluate. Note the rate and quality of the radial pulse. Check a carotid pulse if you can't feel a radial pulse. This may take longer than usual because of the vasoconstriction caused by the exposure or because the pulse is slowed by the hypothermic state. It is important not to start chest compressions on the hypothermic patient who simply has a slow weak pulse; the compressions could induce ventricular fibrillation. The examination of the skin color and condition may be nonproductive. Because of the peripheral vasoconstriction, the skin may be pale and cool even when the patient is not hypothermic. All cold patients (except those with spinal cord injuries) will have pale, cold extremities and delayed capillary refill. Initially the best way to get an idea of the patient's temperature is to put your hand down the back of the neck and feel the skin of the back. This is quicker and easier to do than trying to feel down the front of the chest.

The patient in a cold environment, especially the patient who is thought to be hypothermic, cannot be exposed for a complete examination of the chest, abdomen, pelvis, and extremities. Assess the head and the neck. Application of the cervical immobilization device may be difficult at this time because of the patient's clothing. Palpate the patient's back with your bare hand (covered only with a latex glove) under all the layers of clothing. Palpate for tenderness, instability, and crepitation (TIC). Feel for adequate and symmetric chest wall rise. Your hand should also note the patient's temperature. If the back (or anterior chest) underneath the clothing feels in any way cool, then the patient may be hypothermic. You may at this point decide that the patient is suffering from hypothermia in addition to the other injuries you may have found. The converse is that patients who have obviously frozen hands or feet may still be warm to touch under their clothes (frostbite is more common than significant core hypothermia). *Handle the hypothermic patient very gently to prevent a lethal cardiac arrhythmia.* Even if the patient is hypothermic, you must complete the Primary Survey. Auscultate the lungs, and examine the neck, abdomen, pelvis, and extremities as best as you can. You should try to spend no more than two minutes doing this entire evaluation in the cold environment, in part to conserve body heat and to prevent further heat loss. At this point the patient can be log-rolled and put on a backboard.

Critical Interventions and Transport Decision

When the Primary Survey is complete, you have enough information to decide if the patient is critical or stable. If you find that the patient falls into the load-and-go category outlined in Chapter 2, perform critical interventions and package the patient on a wooden or plastic backboard (not metal) and immediately load into an ambulance for transport. If the patient appears stable but is in a cold environment, or if it is cool but the victim is also wet, consider this a load-and-go situation. Gently transfer the patient to the warm ambulance for the Detailed Exam, additional critical care, and the Ongoing Exams. Close the ambulance door quickly to prevent any further heat loss from the vehicle so you can remove the patient's wet clothes (if necessary). At this point the baseline vital signs and further patient history can be obtained.

Detailed Exam

When the weather is cold, you should perform the Detailed Exam in the ambulance. Remove wet and cold clothing and cover the patient with warm blankets. The patient with hypothermia must have wet, cold clothes removed in order to be rewarmed. Down clothing probably should not be cut off in the usual fashion since the heater in the ambulance will blow the feathers into the patient's wounds and the EMS equipment. Begin to rewarm the patient by both passive external rewarming with dry blankets in the warm ambulance and by core rewarming with warm (100 degrees Fahrenheit) humidified oxygen. This is usually an adequate method of rewarming for the patient with mild hypothermia (core temperature of 90 degrees Fahrenheit or greater). Do not massage or put hot compresses on the cold extremities. This may block the shivering reflex and may cause an "afterdrop" in core temperature. Rapid warming of the skin abolishes the vasoconstriction, allowing the cold blood in the extremities to return to the core causing a further lowering (afterdrop) of temperature. Patients who are still shivering have only mild hypothermia and will do fine with passive rewarming with just warm blankets. Perform the Detailed Exam as described in Chapter 2.

Critical Care and Ongoing Exam

Critical care is usually performed in the ambulance during transfer. Not only is this advantageous for the patient, but also your warm hands are better able to provide the care. Advanced airway management is easier in the ambulance than in the bitter cold outside. The endotracheal tube is more malleable and is less likely to stick to the warm mucous membranes, and your glasses do not fog up in the cold. Tube placement confirmation with the Colorimetric End-Tidal Carbon Dioxide Detection Device may prove unreliable in the cold environment. Provide the patient with warm humidified oxygen in the ambulance; the plastic humidifier bottle can be filled with saline warmed to about 45 to 55 degrees Celsius (80–100 degrees Fahrenheit). Heated saline or water in a thermos will provide some help. Any other warming unit must be carefully checked for safety to ensure that the patient is not harmed. Perform frequent Ongoing Exams during transport. Especially watch the pulse, blood pressure, and the cardiac rhythm. The mildly hypothermic patient will often have muscle artifact (sometimes from the shivering), there may be sinus bradycardia, there may be a J or Osborne wave immediately after the QRS complex, or there may be atrial fibrillation. These dysrhythmias require no treatment other than warming the patient. At 82.4 degrees Fahrenheit (28 degrees Celsius) core body temperature, there may be ventricular fibrillation that is unresponsive to defibrillation, and below 69.8 degrees (21 degrees Celsius) there may be asystole. Currently there is no medication that has proven effective for treating ventricular fibrillation in the severely hypothermic patient. The abdomen needs to be examined frequently. Your initial assessment may miss an abdominal catastrophe in the hypothermic patient. You should also frequently check and record the neurological exam.

You should decide about IV fluids during transport. If fluids are indicated, they should be at least the ambient temperature of the warm ambulance. Warmed fluids are preferable to room temperature fluids in the hypothermic patient but have very little effect in raising the core temperature. Fluid resuscitation may be necessary for hypovolemic shock or for hypothermia. Prolonged cold exposure causes prolonged peripheral vasoconstriction, resulting in more blood perfusing the kidney. This causes a "cold diuresis," an inappropriate diuresis of fluid induced by the cold. The patient will become hypovolemic. Patients with frostbite also benefit from warm fluids, which help the poor circulation in the vasoconstricted extremities. There is currently some exciting research going on about some new devices that may be used to warm the hypothermic patient in the field.

Contacting Medical Direction

If your patient is hypothermic, it is extremely important to contact Medical Direction early. Even though it may take considerable time to arrive at the nearest appropriate medical facility, the facility needs time to assemble the proper trauma team or to arrange for more expeditious transfer to another facility. Medical Direction needs to know how long the patient was exposed to the cold and the patient's core body temperature. Remember that axillary and skin temperatures are not closely correlated with core body temperature in the cold environment. The oral temperature is inaccurate at temperatures below 96 degrees. A tympanic membrane thermometer is the most practical method to take an accurate core temperature in the ambulance. Multiple temperature assessments must be performed. Medical Direction may order the use of some IV medications, but this will depend on individual circumstances.

Notes for Wilderness Rescuers

If you are required to be in the cold for long periods of time (hiking or skiing in to rescue someone in a wilderness area), there are several things to remember:

1. *Blood is heat.* Good circulation is necessary to prevent frostbite. Drink plenty of fluids and keep your canteen under your clothing so it is warm. You can force more blood (heat) to your cold, vasoconstricted hands by "windmilling" your arms (sling your arm in a circle, forcing blood into the hands).
2. *Never go into the wilderness without a partner.* You need someone to help watch you for signs of frostbite or hypothermia and who will allow you to warm your cold hands or feet in their axilla or groin under their clothing or snuggle with you in a sleeping bag (wilderness friends are close friends indeed).
3. *Good clothing and equipment are essential* so that you maintain your temperature and don't become hypothermic or develop frostbite (don't become a victim). If you have skin areas (face, scalp, hands, etc.) exposed to the cold, not only will they vasoconstrict but they will cause generalized surface vasoconstriction. Thus the saying, "If your feet are cold, put on a hat."
4. *Your perception of cold is not related to your core temperature but rather to your surface temperature.* Beware the heated hand warmer that makes you feel warm while your core temperature is dropping.

TABLE D-1	Signs and Symptoms of Hypothermia.

Neuromuscular System

Amnesia, dysarthria, poor judgment (34 degrees Celsius)

Loss of coordination, appearing "drunk" (33 degrees Celsius)

Shivering ceases (32 degrees Celsius)

Progressive decrease in level of consciousness (29 degrees Celsius)

Pupils dilated (29 degrees Celsius)

Loss of deep tendon reflexes (27 degrees Celsius)

Gastrointestinal System

Ileus

Respiratory System

Initial hyperventilation (34 degrees Celsius)

Progressive decrease in rate and depth of respiration (<34 degrees Celsius)

Noncardiac pulmonary edema (25 degrees Celsius)

Cardiovascular System

Sinus bradycardia

Atrial fibrillation (30 degrees Celsius)

Progressive decrease in blood pressure (29 degrees Celsius)

Progressive decrease in pulse (29 degrees Celsius)

Ventricular irritability (28 degrees Celsius)

Hypotension (24 degrees Celsius)

Kidneys, Blood, Electrolytes

Cold diuresis leading to hypovolemia and hemoconcentration

Lactic acidosis and hyperglycemia

SUMMARY

The application of the principles of BTLS in the cold is challenging and rewarding. You need a thorough understanding of the principles of BTLS and knowledge of the conditions and limitations imposed by the cold environment. You also must always be aware that your patient may be hypothermic. The signs and symptoms of hypothermia are listed in Table D-1. This appendix has described how the presence of a cold environment and/or the existence of hypothermia change the application of the BTLS principles.

BIBLIOGRAPHY

1. Auerback, P. S., and E. C. Geehr. *Management of Wilderness and Environmental Emergencies,* 2nd ed. St. Louis, MO: C. V. Mosby, 1989.

2. Gregory, J. S., J. M. Bergstein, and others. "Comparison of Three Methods of Rewarming from Hypothermia: Advantages of Extracorporeal Blood Warming." *Journal of Trauma,* Vol. 31 (1991), pp. 1247–1252.

3. Hector, M. G. "Treatment of Accidental Hypothermia." *American Family Physician,* Vol. 45, No. 2 (1992), pp. 785–792.

4. Ornato, J. P., J. B. Shipley, and others. "Multicenter Study of a Portable Hand-Size, Colorimetric End-Tidal Carbon Dioxide Detection Device." *Annals of Emergency Medicine,* Vol. 21 (1992), pp. 518–523.

5. Sterba, J. A. "Efficacy and Safety of Prehospital Rewarming Techniques to Treat Accidental Hypothermia." *Annals of Emergency Medicine,* Vol. 20 (1991), pp. 896–901.

Role of the Air Medical Helicopter

Russell B. Bieniek, M.D., F.A.C.E.P.

Pam Kirkpatrick, R.N.

Air medical helicopters were used extensively to transport injured servicemen during the United States military conflicts of Korea and Vietnam. On October 12, 1972, Flight for Life, the first United States hospital-based civilian air medical helicopter service, went into operation at St. Anthony Hospital in Denver, Colorado. In the years following this, similar programs were established at multiple hospitals and various other organizations across the United States and throughout the world. In 1998, according to the Association of Air Medical Services' (AAMS) database, there were over 200 air medical helicopter programs, transporting approximately 300,000 patients per year, both by their U.S. members and a limited number of international members. The structure and role of these air medical programs vary tremendously, as does their integration with the local EMS system and involvement in trauma care.

The sponsoring agency and organizational structure of an air medical service encompass a wide range of models. They may be military or other government service—federal, state, or local; they may be independent or work in cooperation with local medical care providers to provide rescue and/or transportation of injured patients. The crews may be on call and/or the helicopter may need to be reconfigured or additional equipment may need to be brought on board. The far end of the spectrum is the fully dedicated medical helicopter that flies only critically injured or ill patients and whose interior is specifically designed and configured, always medically staffed and consistently available for a medical mission.

The role may be one of primary interfacility transport (hospital to hospital), scene transport (field to hospital) or, as is most frequently the case, a combination of the two with varying percentages of each type. The involvement that an air medical service may have in the local EMS community may depend on its percentage of scene involvement.

The type of patient a service transports is usually a mixture of clinical classes, including neonatal, pediatric, cardiac, maternal, medical, and trauma. The service may transport all patients, they may limit their transports to specific types of patients, or they may have specific teams that accompany each clinical class of patients. The medical crew on board also varies with the specific program. An industry survey in 1997 revealed that 94% of medical helicopter programs utilize two medical attendants and 6% utilize one. The credentials of crewmembers vary widely, ranging from an EMT-B to a physician. The most common configuration for a two-attendant crew consists of a nurse and a paramedic. The makeup of the crew also may vary by the type of medical mission to which the helicopter is dedicated.

If an air medical service is available in your region, it is important that you become acquainted with them and know in advance the type of cases for which you will utilize them. You also will need to know how to access them and how to involve them in your system to help improve patient care.

Multiple factors influence the availability of an air medical helicopter. These include scheduled maintenance, mechanical factors, weather, and being committed on a previous mission. This resource can be very beneficial to the EMS service and the patient, but there shouldn't be dependence on it. They may not be able to respond or have to cancel en route. Contingency plans must always be in place.

Regarding safety, there needs to be prior education and training with the air medical service. This education would entail learning proper communications between ground and air, picking and describing a safe landing zone, and coordinating unloading and loading of the aircraft. In the uncommon, but possible, event of an aircraft accident, correct knowledge of the helicopter's equipment and access could be vital to crew and ground personnel. Safety must always be the first concern, as in your BTLS training: "Is the scene safe?"

THE AIR MEDICAL HELICOPTER AND THE TRAUMA PATIENT

Caring for the trauma patient can be extremely challenging; however, it is quite rewarding to you and the patient if all the components are in place and things are done properly. As an established component and resource to an EMS service, the air medical helicopter can improve patient outcome by providing assistance in two areas. The first is speed of transportation; the second is the introduction of a higher level of clinical expertise, equipment, or procedures at the scene or en route to the hospital.

Helicopters obviously are able to transport patients quicker than ground units over long distances. This involves their ability to travel at high speeds and in a straight line. They also do not have to fight road conditions, either environmental or traffic. This decreases the exposure of the general public or the caregivers themselves to the potential dangers of an ambulance rushing through busy streets with other traffic and pedestrians.

In many areas of the United States the only care available at an accident scene is BLS. An air medical helicopter would then be able to provide ALS assessment and care at the scene and en route to the hospital. Often, even in areas where ALS is available, the air medical crew may be able to provide additional critical care expertise, skills, and/or equipment. Some of these may include, but are not be limited to, needle or surgical cricothyroidotomy, needle or tube thoracostomy, intraosseous needle insertion, pericardiocentesis, and various medications for such things as sedation and chemical paralysis of the head-injured patient for control of the airway and to assist in controlling increased intracranial pressure. Additional equipment might include pulse oximetry, end-tidal CO_2 monitors, positive pressure ventilators, and Doppler-assisted blood pressure monitoring devices, to mention a few. Many services also carry packed red blood cells to use in the field. The air medical service personnel also usually handle a higher volume of critically injured trauma patients than the average provider in a rural ground system, so they may exhibit greater familiarity and comfort in working with these patients.

For interfacility transports, the patient is evaluated by the nursing and physician staffs at the referring hospital, which determine whether the patient requires additional evaluation and/or treatment at a facility with more resources available to handle the serious trauma patient. The air medical helicopter provides the vehicle, crew, and speed necessary to provide a continuum of the critical care environment en route during transport.

BTLS AND THE AIR MEDICAL HELICOPTER

BTLS provides a common language that can be used through the continuum of care for the seriously injured trauma patient. This requires coordinated education and training in a region and possibly could be an educational program offered by the air medical service. Trauma patients would then be assessed rapidly, accurately, and completely in the field by the prehospital providers, and the decision scheme that is developed for the region on utilizing the air medical service could be partly based on the results of this assessment, other specific trauma scores, types of injuries, and mechanism of injury. The air medical service would then understand the assessment and initial treatment that was done prior to their arrival, and the report could be accomplished quickly. The helicopter medical crew can then quickly do their BTLS assessment and begin transport with further treatments if necessary.

You must constantly evaluate your skills at doing a rapid assessment of the trauma patient. When you turn your patient over to another service, such as an air medical service for transport, you will not get immediate feedback on the outcome of the patient, as you do when you deliver the patient to the hospital yourself. The air medical service may serve as a link between you and the hospital to help obtain this important information. When cases are reviewed, the BTLS assessment and initial management can be used as a standard to compare with the actual care given.

SUMMARY

Air medical helicopter services are one of many special tools available to you and the hospital. As with all tools, there needs to be initial and continued education and training to ensure proper and safe usage. This will improve the utilization of resources in your service area and help achieve everyone's common goal of maximizing patient outcome.

BIBLIOGRAPHY

1. Walters, E. "Program Profile, 20 Years of Service." *Journal of Air Medical Transport,* Vol. 11, No. 9 (1992).

2. Association of Air Medical Services (AAMS) Database, 110 N. Royal St., Ste. 307, Alexandria, VA 22314 (1998).

3. "1997 Medical Crew Survey." *AirMed,* Vol. 5 (1997).

Trauma Scoring in the Prehospital Care Setting

Leah J. Heimbach, R.N., NREMT-P, J.D.

Trauma scoring systems consist of assigning a numerical rating or score to various clinical signs, such as vital signs or response to pain. They are used to assess the severity of injury and are especially valuable in assessment of the trauma patient with multiple injuries. Trauma scoring systems have important uses in trauma systems at all levels, including the hospital setting and the prehospital setting and in overall health care system analysis. There are several methods of scoring severity of injury in trauma patients, including the Glasgow Coma Score and the Revised Trauma Score (see Tables F-1 and F-2).

In the hospital setting, trauma scoring systems have several uses, including the following:

1. Standardizing triage between health care facilities (deciding when it is appropriate to transfer a patient to a trauma center).
2. Allocating medical resources.
3. Evaluating the health care facility's overall effectiveness in providing patient care.
4. Conducting audits (making sure that patients who are predicted to survive their traumatic event actually do survive).
5. Predicting morbidity and mortality of patients based on a particular trauma score.

Although prehospital care providers should never delay transport to complete a trauma score, trauma scoring systems can provide an objective and standardized way for you to triage patients appropriately (including whether a patient should go to a trauma center) and to communicate injury severity, using a common language, to other members of the health care team. Trauma scores recorded in the field are also useful in the analysis and research of EMS systems. This analysis can then be used to develop protocols for prehospital care to meet the needs of a specific EMS region. The BTLS patient assessment includes a neurological assessment, using the AVPU method (alert, responds to verbal stimulus, responds to painful stimulus, and unresponsive), and identifies parameters to determine whether the patient is a load-and-go. Communicating this information along with a list of the patient's injuries to the receiving hospital will allow the hospital personnel to gather the necessary resources to optimize care.

The use of trauma scores in the prehospital setting can be confusing at a time when patient assessment, injury management, and communication to the receiving hospital need to be concise. It is recommended that you report the following information to the receiving facility:

1. Age, sex, and chief complaint.
2. Mechanism of injury.
3. Level of consciousness.
4. What parameters led to the load-and-go decision.
5. A list of the patient's injuries.
6. What treatment was rendered.
7. The patient's response to treatment.

Many EMS regions will require the use of some type of trauma score system in the prehospital setting to facilitate patient care and/or to promote prehospital research. An

TABLE F-1	Glasgow Coma Score.

Eye Opening	Points	Verbal Response	Points	Motor Response	Points
Spontaneous	4	Oriented	5	Obeys commands	6
To voice	3	Confused	4	Localizes pain	5
To pain	2	Inappropriate words	3	Withdraws	4
None	1	Incomprehensible sounds	2	Abnormal flexion	3[*]
		Silent	1	Abnormal extension	2[**]
				No movement	1

[*]Decorticate posturing to pain
[**]Decerebrate posturing to pain

example of the Revised Trauma Score is shown in Table F-2. An example of the Pediatric Glasgow Coma Score and Pediatric Trauma Score is shown in Tables F-3 and F-4.

BIBLIOGRAPHY

1. Champion, H. R., and others. "A Revision of the Trauma Score." *Journal of Trauma,* Vol. 29 (1989), p. 623.
2. Tepas, T. A. "Pediatric Trauma Score." *Journal of Pediatric Surgery,* Vol. 22 (1987), p. 14.

TABLE F-2	Revised Trauma Score.

Score	Score	Contribution to Revised Trauma
Total Glasgow Coma Score (see Table F-1)	13–15	4
	9–12	3
	6–8	2
	4–5	1
	3	0
Systolic blood pressure (mmHg)	>89	4
	76–89	3
	50–75	2
	1–49	1
	None	0
Respirations (per minute)	10–29	4
	>29	3
	6–9	2
	1–5	1
	None	0

Note: If total score is 11 or less, the patient should be taken to a trauma center.

TABLE F-3 — Pediatric Glasgow Coma Score.

		> 1 Year	< 1 Year	
Eyes Opening	4	Spontaneously	Spontaneously	
	3	To verbal command	To shout	
	2	To pain	To pain	
	1	No response	No response	
		> 1 Year	**< 1 Year**	
Best Motor Response	6	Obeys		
	5	Localizes pain	Localizes pain	
	4	Flexion–withdrawal	Flexion–normal	
	3	Flexion–abnormal (decorticate rigidity)	Flexion–abnormal (decorticate rigidity)	
	2	Extension (decerebrate rigidity)	Extension (decerebrate rigidity)	
	1	No response	No response	
		> 5 Years	**2–5 Years**	**0–23 Months**
Best Verbal Response	5	Oriented and converses	Appropriate words and phrases	Smiles, coos, cries appropriately
	4	Disoriented and converses	Inappropriate words	Cries
	3	Inappropriate words	Cries and/or screams	Inappropriate crying and/or screaming
	2	Incomprehensible sounds	Grunts	Grunts
	1	No response	No response	No response

TABLE F-4 — Pediatric Trauma Score.

Score	+2	+1	−1
Weight	>44 lb (>20 kg)	22–44 lb (10–20 kg)	<22 lb (<10 kg)
Airway	Normal	Oral or nasal airway	Intubated Tracheostomy Invasive airway
Blood pressure	Pulse at wrist >90 mmHg	Carotid or femoral pulse palpable 50–90 mmHg	No palpable pulse <50 mmHg
Level of consciousness	Completely awake	Obtunded or any loss of consciousness	Comatose
Open wound	None	Minor	Major or penetrating
Fractures	None	Closed fracture	Open or multiple fractures

Drowning, Barotrauma, and Decompression Injury

James H. Creel Jr., M.D., F.A.C.E.P.

John E. Campbell, M.D., F.A.C.E.P.

DROWNING

Approximately 7,000 people drown annually, making drowning the third leading cause of accidental death in the United States. Freshwater drownings are more common than saltwater drownings, and there are more immersion accidents in pools than in lakes, ponds, and rivers. The peak incidence occurs in the warm months and most commonly involves teenagers and children under the age of 4.

Drowning is death from suffocation after submersion in the water. There are two basic mechanisms:

1. Breath holding, which leads to aspiration of water and wet lungs.
2. Laryngospasm with glottic closure and dry lungs.

Both these mechanisms can lead to profound hypoxia and death. Most adults who have drowned, have about 150 cc of fluid in their lungs. The amount (2.2 cc per kilogram) is enough to produce profound hypoxia. It is thought to take about 10 times this amount to get electrolyte changes, and this is rarely seen. In the prehospital phase, hypoxia is the primary concern. Survival of the victim depends on your rapid evaluation and management of the ABCs.

Initiate management as soon as possible. Be aware of surfing/diving mechanisms that indicate potential occult cervical spine injury. Protect the cervical spine during rescue of the patient. In water, CPR is generally ineffective. Remove the patient to a stable surface as soon as possible; then initiate CPR and the appropriate protocol. In cases in which hypothermia is responsible for the near-drowning, it appears to provide the brain, heart, and lungs some degree of protection (diving reflex) by slowing the metabolism. Therefore, no one is dead until warm and dead; do not stop CPR.

BAROTRAUMA

Barotrauma refers to injuries due to the mechanical effects of pressure on the body. We all live "under pressure" since the weight of the air in which we live exerts force on our bodies. At sea level the weight of air pressing on the body equals 14.7 pounds per square inch (psi). Since solids and liquids are not compressible, they are not usually affected by pressure changes. The study of barotrauma is the study of the effect of pressure on gas-filled organs of the body. Gas-filled organs are ears, sinuses, upper and lower airways, stomach, and intestines.

To understand the effects of pressure changes, you must know some properties of gases. Boyle's law states that the volume of a gas is inversely proportional to the pressure applied to it. This simply means that if you double the pressure on a gas, the volume of the gas will decrease by one-half. If you halve the pressure on a gas, the volume will double. The pressure at sea level is called one atmosphere absolute (ATA). If you go up in an airplane (or climb a mountain), you have less atmosphere above you; thus the pressure decreases and the gas inside the body expands. Most commercial airliners fly at about 35,000 feet elevation (one-fifth ATA or gas volume five times normal) but are pressurized to a cabin pressure equal to 5,000 to 8,000 feet elevation (two-thirds to three-fourths ATA), so that gas expands to only about 1.2 to 1.4 times its original volume. Airline passengers notice no change except for "popping" of the ears as the expanding gas in the middle ears vents off through the eustachian tubes into the pharynx.

Water is much heavier than air. When one descends into salt water, there is a change of one atmosphere for every 33 feet of depth (34 feet for fresh water). This means that at 33 feet of depth the body is subjected to 2 ATA, and gas in the body has been compressed to one-half of its original volume. Because of the pressures involved, divers are exposed to certain potential injuries during both descent and ascent.

Trauma of Descent: "Middle Ear Squeeze"

Since there is a large pressure change during the first few feet of a dive, skin divers and snorkelers as well as scuba divers are subject to this type of injury. Let's say that a skin diver takes a breath and rapidly descends to a depth of 33 feet: All the gas in his body will decrease in volume by one-half. This includes gas in the lungs, intestines, stomach, sinuses, and middle ears. The elastic lungs, intestines, and stomach will simply decrease in size to match the volume of gas. Problems develop with the middle ears and sinuses if the pressure cannot be equalized. The sinuses (air pockets in the bones of the face and skull) each have an opening through which air from the pharynx can enter to equalize the pressure. If the openings are blocked, the skin diver will experience pain in the sinuses and may even develop bleeding and inflammation (barosinusitis). Other than the discomfort, this causes no serious problem. Each middle ear has an opening, the eustachian tube, through which air from the pharynx can enter to equalize pressure. If the eustachian tube is blocked (mucosal congestion from allergy, infection, etc.), the pressure will push in on the eardrum and cause intense pain. This begins to be noticeable at a depth of 4 to 5 feet. If the diver cannot equalize the middle ear pressure and yet continues to descend, the pressure will eventually rupture the eardrum and flood the middle ear with cold water (even the warm waters of the Caribbean are 20 degrees below body temperature). Cold water in the middle ear causes dizziness, nausea, vomiting, and disorientation ("twirly bends"). The result can be panic and drowning or near-drowning. The diver using a self-contained underwater breathing apparatus (scuba diver) who surfaces rapidly can develop air embolism or neurologic decompression sickness. Vomiting under water can cause aspiration and drowning.

Barotitis media (middle ear squeeze) requires no prehospital treatment. The pressure is relieved when the diver returns to the surface. If there is hearing loss or continued ear pain, the diver should see a physician for treatment of ruptured eardrum or bleeding into the middle ear. The conditions that you are more likely to have to manage are the near-drowning cases caused by the disorientation from water in the middle ears.

Trauma of Ascent

Injuries from expanding gas can occur as divers ascend. These injuries are much more common in scuba divers, since such injuries usually either require some time to develop (longer than a skin diver can hold his breath) or require the breathing of compressed air.

Reverse Middle Ear Squeeze

If a eustachian tube becomes blocked during a dive, the gas in the middle ear will expand and cause pain during ascent. If there is enough expansion, the eardrum can rupture, with all the symptoms and dangers mentioned previously.

Gastrointestinal Barotrauma

If the diver swallows air while breathing compressed air or if the diver has previously eaten gas-forming foods (e.g., beans), he may accumulate a significant amount of stomach or intestinal gas during a dive. If the diver was at a depth of 66 feet, the gas will expand to three times its original volume during ascent. If he is unable to expel this gas, he will develop abdominal pain and occasionally even collapse and develop a shock-like state.

Pulmonary Overpressurization Syndromes (Burst Lung)

These occur only in divers who have been breathing compressed air. During a dive the lungs are completely filled with air, which is at a pressure equal to the depth at which the diver is swimming. If a diver panics and surfaces without exhaling, the rapidly expanding gas will overinflate the lungs and cause one of the three overpressurization syndromes listed below. Remember, the total volume of the lungs is about 6 L. An ascent from 33 feet would cause expansion to 12 L; 66 feet, 18 L; and 100 feet, 24 L. It is easy to see how delicate alveoli can be ruptured by this expansion. The expanding air will dissect into the interstitial space, pleural space, pulmonary venules, or a combination of the three.

1. *Air in the Interstitial Space:* This is the most common form of pulmonary overpressurization syndrome. As millions of tiny air bubbles escape into the interstitial tissue, they may dissect into the mediastinum and up into the subcutaneous tissue of the neck. Symptoms may develop immediately upon surfacing or may not develop for several hours. The diver may have increasing hoarseness, chest pain, subcutaneous emphysema in the neck, and difficulty breathing and swallowing. Any diver with these symptoms should get oxygen (no positive pressure ventilations unless the diver is apneic) and transport to the hospital. While interstitial air does not require treatment with a recompression chamber (hyperbaric chamber), these patients often develop air embolism or decompression sickness. They should be observed in a facility that is capable of providing recompression treatment if necessary.

2. *Air in the Pleural Space:* If the alveoli rupture into the pleural space, a pneumothorax and possibly a hemothorax will develop. The amount of pneumothorax will depend on how much air escaped into the pleural space and how far the diver surfaced after the air entered the pleural space. A 10% pneumothorax at 33 feet will be a 20% pneumothorax at the surface. A 20 to 30% pneumothorax at 33 feet may be a tension pneumothorax at the surface. The symptoms will be the same as for interstitial air except the diver will now have decreased breath sounds and hyperresonance to percussion on the affected side (may be on both sides). A tension pneumothorax will also have distended neck veins and shock (and possibly tracheal deviation—a rare sign). These patients may require a needle decompression if they have a tension pneumothorax. Otherwise, give 100% oxygen and transport immediately.

3. *Air Embolism:* The most serious syndrome of overpressurization is pulmonary air embolism. If the overdistended alveoli rupture into the pulmonary venules, the millions of tiny air bubbles can return to the left side of the heart and then up the carotid arteries to the small arterioles of the brain. These bubbles, composed mostly of nitrogen, obstruct the arterioles and produce symptoms similar to a stroke. The symptoms produced depend on which vessels are obstructed. There will usually be loss of consciousness and focal neurological signs. The symptoms almost always occur immediately when the diver surfaces. This is a very important point in differentiating air embolism from decompression sickness (which usually takes hours to develop). The patient should be placed in Trendelenburg position (30 degrees head down) on the left side, given 100% oxygen, and transported to a facility that can provide recompression treatment. The left-side, head-down position prevents further embolism of air to the brain and helps distend the vessels, thus allowing small bubbles to pass through and return to the lungs where they can be eliminated. This is one instance in which you should not hyperventilate or give positive pressure ventilations. Hyperventilation causes vasoconstriction, which will trap the bubbles. Positive pressure ventilation may force more air into the veins, worsening the injury

(if the patient is not breathing, you must give positive pressure ventilation). This patient must have immediate recompression in a recompression chamber no matter how much time has passed since the injury and no matter how far away the recompression chamber may be. In a recompression chamber, the pressure is raised to 6 ATA, which will decrease the size of the bubbles to one-sixth of their previous volume. This may allow them to pass through the capillaries back to the lungs to be expelled. Air embolism may rarely affect the coronary arteries, causing myocardial infarction, dysrhythmias, or cardiac arrest.

DECOMPRESSION ILLNESS

Decompression illness is caused by another property of gases. Henry's law states that the amount of gas dissolved in a liquid is directly proportional to the pressure applied. This means that twice as much gas would be dissolved in a liquid at a depth of 33 feet as at sea level. It also means that gas dissolved in a liquid at 33 feet will come out of solution as that liquid ascends. This is analogous to a sealed bottle of carbonated beverage that has no bubbles as long as it is sealed but bubbles the instant that the cap is removed and the pressure is released.

Nitrogen, which accounts for about 80% of the volume of inspired air, is an inert gas that dissolves in blood and fat. When a diver is under water, nitrogen dissolves in the blood and fat tissue. This nitrogen is released as he surfaces, so he must surface slowly enough to allow this nitrogen to be expelled through his lungs. The U.S. Navy has developed a set of tables of no-decompression limits that give general guidelines about how long one can stay at a certain depth without going through stage decompression during ascent. There are also standard air decompression tables for those dives that exceed the no-decompression limit. Theoretically, if one follows the recommendations of the tables, nitrogen bubbles will not form in the blood during ascent. This may not always be true because the tables were developed from a study of U.S. Navy divers, who are uniformly young, healthy, well-conditioned men who were diving in salt water. Today, there are 3 million recreational scuba divers and 300,000 new divers certified each year. Sport divers are not uniformly young, healthy, or conditioned. They are often older, poorly conditioned, and not always healthy. A special problem is obesity. Fat absorbs about five times as much nitrogen as blood or other tissue, so obese divers require longer decompression times or shorter dives. Sport divers should be very conservative when using diving tables, especially when diving in fresh water or in lakes above sea level. The greatest danger occurs when a diver who has been submerged for a significant period of time has a diving accident, panics, and surfaces rapidly. Nitrogen bubbles will form in the blood and tissue just as carbon dioxide bubbles form in champagne. This is a different injury from barotrauma or pulmonary overpressurization syndrome, and may exist along with any of the barotrauma syndromes. It is frequently seen in divers in near-drowning situations. The symptoms are almost always delayed for minutes to hours after a dive. As a general rule, symptoms that develop within 10 minutes of surfacing are caused by air embolism until proved otherwise. Symptoms developing after 10 minutes are decompression illness until proved otherwise. A special case is the vacationing diver who is asymptomatic after a deep dive and then catches a plane home the same day. This diver may develop symptoms during flight, since the cabin pressure is only two-thirds or three-fourths ATA. These symptoms may not appear until the diver has returned home far inland from the site of the dive. All emergency providers should have some knowledge of diving injuries.

Type I Decompression Illness

1. *Cutaneous ("skin bends"):* Millions of tiny nitrogen bubbles may form in the microvasculature of the skin. This causes a generalized itching rash that may be red

and inflamed or mottled with a central purple discoloration. It is called "marbleized skin." This condition requires no treatment but may be an early sign of more serious decompression sickness, so the patient must be observed. Give the patient 100% oxygen, and transport to a facility capable of recompression therapy.

2. *Musculoskeletal ("bends" or "pain-only bends"):* This is the most common presentation of decompression sickness. Over 85% of divers with decompression sickness will present with pain in the joints. The shoulders or knees are affected most commonly, but any joint may be affected. The pain is usually deep and aching, and there may be vague numbness around the affected joint. Characteristically, there are no physical findings and the pain may be eased by pressure such as inflating a blood pressure cuff. These patients require recompression therapy no matter how long it has been since the symptoms started and no matter how far the nearest recompression chamber may be.

Type II Decompression Illness

These syndromes are more serious and may be life-threatening. They are emergencies that require rapid diagnosis and treatment.

1. *Pulmonary ("chokes"):* Nitrogen bubbles forming in the vasculature of the lungs cause symptoms similar to the interstitial pulmonary overpressurization syndrome. The patient will develop cough, chest pain, difficulty breathing, and sometimes hemoptysis. These symptoms usually develop within an hour of surfacing (50%) but may be delayed for up to 6 hours and even rarely for 24 to 48 hours. Pulmonary overpressurization syndrome usually appears within a few minutes of surfacing. In either case, the patient requires oxygen and recompression therapy. Here again, be careful of positive pressure ventilation, as it may cause gas bubble emboli to the brain.

2. *Neurologic:* Nitrogen bubbles in the nervous system may present with any symptom from personality changes to specific localized neurologic changes. By far the most common symptoms involve the lower spinal cord and often produce weakness or paralysis of the legs and urinary bladder. Bladder problems are so common that historically, urinary catheters were considered essential equipment for divers. These patients must have recompression therapy or irreversible paralysis will occur.

MANAGEMENT OF DIVING INJURIES
History

1. *Type of Diving and Equipment Used:* This is very important. Remember that skin divers and snorkelers cannot get overpressurization syndrome or decompression sickness, but all divers can drown. The treatment for near-drowning is very different from that for decompression sickness or air embolism.

2. *History of the Dive:* You need to know where the dive occurred, at what depth, how many dives, how long on the bottom, and any in-water decompression. This information is also needed for dives during the preceding two days.

3. *Past Medical History:* Pulmonary problems that predispose to air trapping (asthma or obstructive lung disease) are frequently associated with overpressurization syndrome.

4. *Exactly When the Symptoms First Occurred:* This may be helpful in differentiating air embolism and decompression illness.

5. *Complications of the Dive:* Did the diver run out of air? Was there an attack by marine animals? Did a diving accident occur?

6. *Travel After the Dive:* Traveling at higher altitudes may precipitate decompression sickness.

Initial Management

1. Follow standard patient assessment protocol: Primary Survey, critical interventions and transport decision, Detailed Exam, and Ongoing Exam.
2. If there is any chance of overpressurization syndrome or decompression illness, do not hyperventilate or give positive pressure ventilation. Positive pressure ventilation is indicated only for apneic patients.
3. Check for hypothermia (see Appendix D) in all diving accident victims.
4. Patients with air embolism or neurologic decompression sickness should be placed on the left side in the head-down position.
5. All diving accident patients should get 100% oxygen.
6. Shock and other injuries are treated by routine protocols.
7. If a recompression facility is needed and you need information about the one nearest to your facility, you may obtain assistance 24 hours a day through the National Diving Alert Network at Duke University: (919) 684-8111.

SUMMARY

No matter how far you may live from a large body of water, you may be called upon to manage a patient with near-drowning or diving injuries. When treating the near-drowning patient, the performance of the ABCs is most important in the prehospital phase, but don't forget the possibility of hypothermia. When treating barotrauma, you should not only follow the basic principles of BTLS, but also remember the importance of the history, patient positioning, the possibility of hypothermia, and the dangers of positive pressure ventilation.

BIBLIOGRAPHY

1. Jeppeson, S. *Open Water Sport Diving Manual,* 4th ed., pp. 2, 25–49. Englewood, CO: Jeppeson Sanderson, 1984.
2. Kizer, K. W. "Dysbarism." In *Emergency Medicine,* ed. J. E. Tintinalli, 3rd ed., pp. 678–688. New York: McGraw-Hill, 1992.

Injury Prevention and the Role of the EMS Provider

Janet M. Williams, M.D.

Jonathan M. Rubin, M.D.

THE INJURY EPIDEMIC

Every day prehospital health care providers serve the public by delivering quality emergency care. The BTLS curriculum has been developed to convey the principles of acute prehospital care of the injured patient. Well-trained prehospital care providers with BTLS skills save many lives of injured patients each year. Unfortunately, over 50% of trauma deaths occur immediately after the injury event. As a result, you often arrive at the scene only to find a patient who has died or is dying and for whom no life-saving measures can be taken. These cases illustrate the importance of recognizing injury as a preventable disease. Your role extends far beyond the acute care of the injured patient. The entire EMS community must become active in preventing injury from occurring in the first place.

Though underrecognized, injury is a major public health problem worldwide. In the United States, injury is the single greatest killer between the ages of 1 and 44 and is responsible for more years of potential life lost than cancer and heart disease combined. In the United States alone, the cost of injury is estimated to be over $210 billion annually.

Injury has been misconceived by the public as being a result of an unavoidable "act of God," an "accident," due to "bad luck," or a result of a behavioral problem on the part of the injured individual. In reality, injuries are health problems that behave like classic infectious diseases. Injuries may be characterized by demographic distributions, seasonal variations, epidemic episodes, and risk factors. In addition, they are predictable and preventable. An analogy has been made between the cause of an injury and the cause of a disease such as malaria. Table H-1 illustrates how disease causation can be applied to both of these entities.

Traditionally, medical education programs have emphasized the treatment of acute injury and have neglected the concept of injury prevention and control. It is interesting that patients presenting with cardiac symptoms are nearly always asked if they have risk factors such as history of smoking, diabetes, hypertension, hypercholesterolemia, and family history of heart disease. In addition, these patients are counseled as to how to reduce their risk for heart disease. As health care providers, we have a responsibility to do the same for injured patients. Besides playing a vital role in the acute care of injured patients, prehospital care providers have a unique opportunity to assess risk factors for injury, to examine patients in the injury setting, to provide valuable injury information to other medical care providers, and to educate the public on injury prevention. In addition, prehospital care providers often see the "near-miss" patient who survives what could have been a fatal injury event. Such circumstances are an opportune time for prehospital care providers to give injury prevention advice.

WHAT IS AN INJURY?

Injury may be defined as any damage to the human body that results from acute exposure of physical energy or from an absence of vital entities such as heat and oxygen. There are five basic forms of injurious energy: thermal, mechanical, electrical, radiating, and chemical. Roughly three-fourths of all injuries are caused by exposure to mechanical or kinetic energy during incidents such as motor vehicle crashes, falls, and firearm discharges.

TABLE H-1	An Etiologic Comparison of Injury and a Classic Infectious Disease.			
Disease	**Host**	**Agent**	**Vector/Vehicle**	**Exposure Event**
Malaria	Human	*P. vivax*	Mosquito	Mosquito bite
Injury (i.e., head injury)	Human	Kinetic energy	Motor vehicle	Crash

Examples of injury resulting from a lack of heat or oxygen are frostbite and drowning. An individual's tolerance for injury depends on factors such as physical size, age, and presence of underlying disease.

Injury has also been defined as a disease that results from the interaction of three components of the epidemiology triangle: host, agent, and environment (see Figure H-1). The host refers to the human being or victim, the agent is the form of energy involved, and the environment provides the opportunity for the agent (energy) to be transmitted to the host.

The environment may be either protective and prevent injury or hostile and encourage injury (see Figure H-2).

The mechanism by which the agent or energy is transferred to the host is referred to as the vector. For example, during a motor vehicle crash, the automobile is the vector that may transmit physical (kinetic) energy to the host if the environment is permissive.

Injury may be classified as intentional or unintentional. Intentional injuries include those such as suicide, assault, and homicide. Unintentional injuries include those that are not deliberate or planned, such as falls, motor vehicle crashes, and burns. In some cases, it may be difficult to distinguish intentional from unintentional injury. Injury also may be categorized by the actual type of injury (such as fracture or head injury), by the mechanism or cause of injury (such as motor vehicle crash or fall), or by the population at risk (such as pediatric, black males, or the elderly).

THE INJURY PROCESS AND WHY INJURIES OCCUR

Injury results when the victim is exposed to energy in amounts that exceed the threshold of human tolerance. In most cases, energy is transmitted as the victim is attempting to perform a specific task or action. The performance of a task refers to how well the individual executes an action, and the task demand is the amount of skill that is required to successfully perform the task. Any time that an individual's performance is below the task demand for the action, there is potential for release of injurious energy (Figure H-3). For example, a drunk driver may lack the skills necessary to drive an automobile and ultimately crash. The crash results in the release of kinetic energy (motion), which may be transmitted to the driver, causing injury. In an unprotective environment, the energy is transmitted to the individual and results in an injury.

The environment may also protect the victim from injury in cases in which the road conditions are favorable, guard rails are present to prevent driving over an embankment, or the victim is restrained (Figure H-4).

Analyzing Injury Events

An injury event can be analyzed by separating it into three phases: the preinjury phase, the injury event, and the postinjury phase. Within each phase, host, vehicle, and environmental factors may contribute to the injury process. Preinjury factors either contribute to or inhibit the potential release of energy prior to the injury event. The

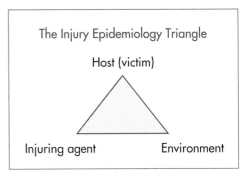

Figure H-1

The injury epidemiology triangle.

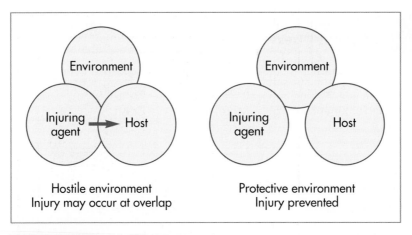

Figure H-2 The relationship of the environment, injuring agent, and host.

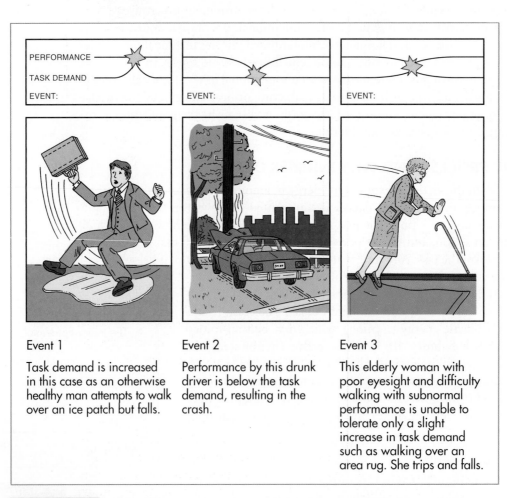

Event 1

Task demand is increased in this case as an otherwise healthy man attempts to walk over an ice patch but falls.

Event 2

Performance by this drunk driver is below the task demand, resulting in the crash.

Event 3

This elderly woman with poor eyesight and difficulty walking with subnormal performance is unable to tolerate only a slight increase in task demand such as walking over an area rug. She trips and falls.

Figure H-3 The relationship of performance and task demand in the injury process.

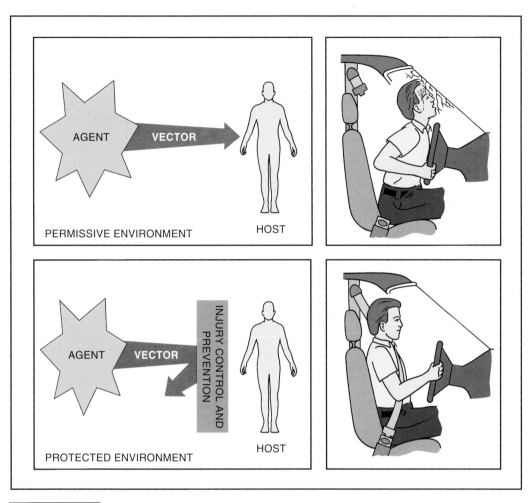

Figure H-4 The role of injury control and prevention in providing a protective environment.

injury phase has factors that may enhance or inhibit transmission of energy to the host during the injury event. Postinjury factors tend to contribute to or diminish the severity of the injury once it has occurred. Prehospital care providers play a major role in the postinjury phase by providing rapid and high-quality care to injured victims in the field.

The analysis of the three phases of an injury event with respect to host, vehicle, and environmental factors is referred to as Haddon's matrix. Table H-2 provides an example of an analysis of a motor vehicle crash using Haddon's matrix. This tool is very useful for identifying factors contributing to the outcome of an injury event, broadening the discussion for developing prevention strategies, and revealing that most injuries are the product of a large number of causal factors and are not just random happenings.

WHAT IS INJURY PREVENTION AND CONTROL?

Perhaps the most important principle of injury prevention and control is that injury is a disease that is subject to prevention by modifying transmission of energy to the individual. The goal of primary injury prevention is to prevent injury from occurring in the first place. Examples include wearing a seat belt, helmet use by motorcyclists and bicyclists, and the installation of smoke detectors. Strategies that attempt to minimize further injury or death after the initial trauma or injury event has occurred are called *secondary injury prevention.* Prehospital care providers practice secondary injury prevention, or acute care,

TABLE H-2	Haddon's Matrix.

| | | | Factors | |
Phases	Host	Vehicle	Physical Environment	Sociocultural Environment
Pre-event	Impaired capacity due to alcohol, age, poor vision, fatigue, inexperience, poor judgment	Defective parts (brakes, tires), poor maintenance, dirty windshield/windows, improper brake lights, ease of control, speed of travel	Narrow road shoulder, poor lighting, road curvature and gradient, road surface type, weather conditions, divided highway, visibility of hazards, signalization	Attitudes about alcohol, drunk driving laws, speed limits, injury prevention programs
Event	Tolerance of body to energy, injury threshold due to aging, chronic disease (osteoporosis), etc., safety belt use	Placement hardness and sharpness of contact surfaces (dash, steering wheel), automatic restraints, vehicle size	Recovery areas, guard rails, fixed objects (trees, telephone poles), median barriers, embankments	Attitudes about seat belt use, enforcement of child safety seat laws
Postevent	Extent of injury sustained, knowledge of first aid, physical condition and age	Fuel system integrity (bursting gas tank), entrapment of victim	Access to EMS, quality of EMS care, availability of extrication equipment, rehabilitation programs	Training of EMS personnel, trauma system programs
Results	Physical and mental impairment	Cost of vehicle repair	Damage to environment	Legal costs, costs to society (loss of lives and income)

by ensuring adequate airway, breathing, and circulation as well as cervical spine immobilization and rapid transportation to the closest appropriate medical facility.

Injury Surveillance

Injury surveillance data forms the foundation of injury control. Accurate and detailed data are needed to determine the incidence of specific injury events, the demographic distributions, the cause of an injury event, and injury risk factors, as well as other factors involved in injury. Prehospital data such as location of the injury site, mechanism of injury, host factors, agent factors, and environmental factors are required. Prehospital care providers are in a crucial position to document the mechanism of injury in great detail, including information such as the extent of damage to a motor vehicle (starred windshield or deformed steering wheel). Description of the location and conditions of the injury site also may be useful in identifying a dangerous section of road where motor vehicle crashes occur time and again or a hazardous area such as an unsafe playground where injuries occur frequently.

Risk Factors

Injuries are not random events. Some special populations, such as males, alcoholics, and certain age groups, are at higher risk for injury than others. A risk factor is a variable that makes an individual more likely to be injured. We can prevent injuries by reducing or eliminating risk factors. An example of a host risk factor that may predispose an individual to injury is the use of drugs or alcohol while driving a motor vehicle. A high-risk group is defined as a subset of the population that has a higher incidence of injury. This group may be exposed to hazards more frequently, may be unable to avoid a hazard, or may have a lower injury threshold. Young males are one well-known group that is at higher risk for being involved in a motor vehicle crash than the general population.

Preventive Interventions

Haddon's matrix can be used to identify the factors affecting the extent of injury during specific injury events. Some of the factors may be amenable to prevention strategies or interventions designed to reduce the incidence or severity of injury.

There are three types of interventions: educational, enforcement, and engineering. Interventions may also be classified as either active or passive. An active intervention requires a change in behavior by the individual in need of protection. Educational programs such as those that encourage seat belt use or installation of home smoke detectors are examples of active interventions that attempt to persuade individuals to alter their behavior for increased self-protection. These programs may increase public awareness but are often ignored by those who are at highest risk for injury such as the economically and educationally deprived. Laws against drunk driving and mandatory helmet use by motorcyclists are other examples of active interventions that are aimed at changing an individual's behavior. However, the introduction of a legal intervention does not necessarily imply that it will be enforced by the authorities or adhered to by the public. Unfortunately, alcohol continues to play a part in half of all fatal motor vehicle crashes despite laws against driving under the influence of alcohol. Active education and enforcement interventions are more effective when used together.

Passive interventions provide automatic protection and are generally more effective than active interventions, since they do not rely on human behavior change. Modifications in the engineering and design of vehicles and the environment have been very effective in reducing the incidence and severity of injuries. The incorporation of airbags and softer dashboards into automobiles has significantly reduced the incidence and severity of motor vehicle-related injuries. Engineering improvements in road design also have been found to be effective countermeasures in preventing motor vehicle crashes.

Designing Interventions: When developing injury prevention programs, it is critical to recognize potential pitfalls for failure as well as ingredients for success. Many intervention programs are difficult to initiate, expensive to maintain, and require the use of limited community resources. The following suggestions will be helpful in selecting injury prevention activities:

1. Target efforts toward a problem that occurs frequently or results in severe injury in your community. In some regions, this may be house fires and, for others, motor vehicle crashes.

2. Address the problem injuries that have specific countermeasures that are known to be effective. Focus on limited, concrete solutions to specific injury events and avoid diffuse, general approaches. Examples of directed specific solutions include fire-safe cigarettes, smoke detectors for house fire prevention, and helmets for bicycle-related head injury prevention.

3. Make the intervention as simple as possible to increase public acceptance and minimize the chance of misuse.

4. Develop a critical mass of community awareness through broad-based grass-roots support, legislation, enforcement, and professional action. Prehospital care providers should take advantage of their connections with local and regional community leaders to build coalitions for effective prevention programs.

5. Promote institutionalization of programs that will last beyond the initial volunteer effort or temporary grant funding. Injury prevention programs should be designed to become a permanent component of prehospital care.

Table H-3 provides examples of injury-specific interventions that have been developed and found to be successful.

ROLE OF THE EMS PROVIDER IN INJURY PREVENTION AND CONTROL

There are four areas in which prehospital personnel can make an impact and prevent injuries in their community:

1. *Acute Care/Secondary Injury Prevention of the Injured Patient:* Medically trained personnel, such as BTLS providers, are the initial and vital link in the trauma care system. By providing prompt and appropriate care, many lives are saved each year.

2. *Community Education/Primary Injury Prevention:* As respected and credible members of the community, prehospital care providers have a unique opportunity to practice primary injury prevention, since they interact directly with injured patients and their families. Less severely injured patients and their families and friends can be counseled about how the present and any future injury could be prevented. Examples include advising the public to wear helmets when riding bicycles, motorcycles, and all-terrain vehicles, as well as wearing seat belts and using child car seats in automobiles. By assessing the scene of the injury, prehospital personnel may identify specific injury prevention strategies for a given family, such as how to "childproof" a home or ways to make the home of an elderly person less risky for falls. As community spokespersons, prehospital care providers often interact with groups such as the local Parent Teachers Association and the Rotary Club. In doing so, community leaders will become more aware of the important concepts of injury prevention and work toward developing a safer community.

3. *Public Policy:* Seat belt and fire-safe cigarette legislation are two examples of regulations that have been instituted with the support of EMS personnel. Seat belt legislation has been very effective in increasing the number of people who wear seat belts and decreasing the number of highway deaths. For those states without seat belt laws, EMS personnel can be effective in encouraging the passage of such legislation.

TABLE H-3	Examples of Injury-Specific Interventions.

Injury Event	Risk Factor	Examples of Injury-Specific Intervention
Drowning	2-year-old to 5-year-old males	Install fencing around pools at least one meter high with self-locking door; water motion alarm; swimming lessons; prominent "no diving" notices near shallow water; easy access to EMS
Bicycle	5-year-old to 12-year-old males	Encourage helmet use; use of safety reflectors; bicycle traffic lanes; rider education programs
Poisoning	1-year-old to 5-year-old children	Package medicines in childproof containers; install safety latches on storage cabinets
Falls	Elderly with poor vision and/or unstable gait	Remove throw rugs; use nightlights; hand rails on stairs; access to activate EMS

Similarly, it was prehospital care providers who found that the most common cause of fatal house fires is cigarette smoking. With their support, a fire-safe cigarette has been developed. Prehospital care providers may be the first to recognize a new injury pattern or high-risk group for a specific injury. By reporting this type of information to local and state authorities, injury prevention strategies may be put into place by legislators in hopes of reducing fatal and serious injuries.

4. *Research/Injury Surveillance:* Accurate documentation of the circumstances surrounding injuries such as demographics, location, mechanism of injury, and associated risk factors is important in identifying problem injuries and designing and implementing prevention strategies. Providing reliable information to local community leaders, legislators, and physicians such as the location of the "dangerous intersection," the poorly supervised quarry, and the "unsafe" playground can lead to the development of effective injury prevention strategies and a safer community.

SUMMARY

Prehospital care providers are a vital link in the chain of the national injury control effort. Their interaction with the public is an opportunity to practice both primary and secondary injury prevention. As part of the medical community, EMS personnel provide information to emergency physicians and nurses, which is important in the acute care of injured victims as well as in injury control research. The injury epidemic can be addressed only through a concerted effort by the medical, community, and legislative organizations.

BIBLIOGRAPHY

1. American College of Emergency Physicians. *Guidelines for Trauma Care Systems.* Dallas, TX: The College, September 16, 1992.

2. Baker, S., B. O'Neill, M. J. Ginsburg, and G. Li. *The Injury Fact Book.* New York: Oxford University Press, 1992.

3. Centers for Disease Control and Prevention. *Injury Control in the 1990s: A National Plan for Action.* Atlanta, GA: The Centers, 1993.

4. Centers for Disease Control and Prevention. *Setting the National Agenda for Injury Control in the 1990s: Position Papers from the Third National Injury Control Conference.* Atlanta, GA: The Centers, 1992.

5. Committee on Trauma Research, Commission on Life Sciences, National Research Council, and the Institute of Medicine. *Injury in America: A Continuing Public Health Problem.* Washington, DC: National Academy Press, 1985.

6. Christoffel, T., and S. P. Teret. *Protecting the Public, Legal Issues in Injury Prevention.* New York: Oxford University Press, 1993.

7. Kaalbfleisch, J., and F. Rivera. "Principles in Injury Control: Lessons to Be Learned from Child Safety Seats." *Pediatric Emergency Care* (1989), pp. 131–134.

8. Martinez, R. "Injury Control: A Primer for Physicians." *Annals of Emergency Medicine,* Vol. 19 (1990), pp. 72–77.

9. The National Committee for Injury Prevention and Control. *Injury Prevention: Meeting the Challenge.* New York: Oxford University Press, 1989.

10. Wilson, M. H., and others. *Saving Children, A Guide to Injury Prevention.* New York: Oxford University Press, 1991.

Multicasualty Incidents and Triage

David Maatman, NREMT-P/IC
Roy Alson, Ph.D., M.D., F.A.C.E.P.
Jere Baldwin, M.D., F.A.C.E.P., F.A.A.F.P.
John T. Stevens, NREMT-P

Objectives

Upon completion of this appendix, you should be able to:

1. Compare and contrast the definitions of a Disaster and Multicasualty Incident.
2. Define span of control.
3. List the responsibilities of Medical Command, Triage Officer, Transport Officer, Treatment Officer, and Staging Officer.
4. Describe the Initial Assessment.
5. Identify Priority 1, 2, 3, and 4 patients.

DEFINITIONS

Disaster: An event that overwhelms the ability of the system to respond. This definition is relative and is based on the availability of resources within the system and community.

ICS: Incident Command System. An organizational structure designed to improve safety and emergency response operations of all types and complexities.

MCI: Multicasualty Incident. An incident involving a large number of persons injured in which the EMS system is unable to manage the situation utilizing day-to-day procedures. An MCI may be classified as a disaster, but not all disasters are MCIs.

Paper Plan Syndrome: Having a written MCI/Disaster Plan without training the individuals who would most likely activate and work it.

Span of Control: An effective management/supervision of subordinates. Usually limited to five subordinates per manager/supervisor.

Triage: To prioritize or sort injuries or the injured. Usually sorted into four categories: Priority 1, 2, 3, and 4 (Red, Yellow, Green, and Black).

INTRODUCTION

It is not uncommon for EMS to have more than one patient at a trauma scene; however, most day-to-day operational procedures are designed for the single patient incident. Safety, organization, and communication are paramount in all EMS activities. When faced with multiple patients, this need is even greater. It is essential that these components be effective and that all entities of the emergency system work from the same plan.

An effective and efficient way to obtain this unity is to have medical operations adopt an Incident Command System (ICS) as a template for organization. Primary functional components of a Medical Incident Command System (MICS) include Medical Command, Triage, Treatment, Transport, and Staging. Even with a single patient incident, these four components exist; however, one person usually is responsible for the functions of all components. There is a Medical Command person in charge of the patient care (team leader), injuries are triaged (prioritized assessment), treatment is provided for the patient, a transport decision is made, and deployment of on-scene vehicles is determined from a point of safety, ingress, and egress (staging).

Designing and implementing an MICS, based on an ICS, will provide EMS with dependable, reproducible results when faced with multiple patient incidents. The MICS must be simple enough for new users but expandable enough to provide the necessary structure to manage large incidents.

INCIDENT COMMAND SYSTEM

ICS was developed in southern California in the early 1970s. The typical on-scene components of an ICS are Command, Fire Suppression, Rescue/Extrication, Law Enforcement, and Medical (Figure I-1).

The structured flexibility of an ICS enables it to be adapted to all types of emergency incidents: fire, rescue, law enforcement, and multicasualty incidents. Because of its modular design, the structure of the ICS can be expanded or compressed, depending on the changing conditions of an incident. It must be staffed and operated by qualified personnel from an emergency service agency.

If an on-scene incident command system is not immediately established, other rescuers will take independent actions, which will frequently be in conflict with each other. These independent actions (freelancing) may be dangerous and disruptive in an environment that requires organization and accountability. Without organization and accountability, chaos will occur and too many people will attempt to command the incident. If you do not control the situation, the situation will control you.

MEDICAL INCIDENT COMMAND

One sector of the on-scene ICS is Medical. The medical sector is broken down into manageable components (subfunctions or branches). The five primary components of an MICS are Medical Command, Triage, Treatment, Transport, and Staging (Figure I-2). It may not be necessary to have one person in each position, but it is necessary to ensure the function of each position is executed. At a scene with multiple patients, it may be necessary to have more than one person take on the function of these components. When considering the need to expand or condense the MICS, the best indicator is current or anticipated span of control. The general rule is to have one person supervise five subordinates. Some latitude may be given due to the complexity of the situation. A highly complex or difficult situation may require a span of control of 3:1, or a simple situation may allow up to 7:1.

All participants of an ICS need to know their responsibilities. Provided below are some ideas and suggestions in determining the responsibilities of the medical sector officers of an ICS.

Medical Command
1. Establishes liaisons with on-scene Incident Command.
2. Establishes working MICS with appropriate sectors.
3. Ensures that proper rescue/extrication services are activated.

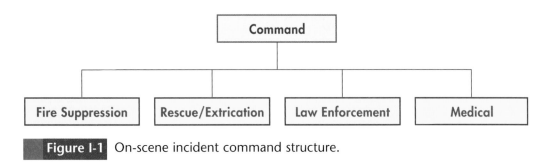

Figure I-1 On-scene incident command structure.

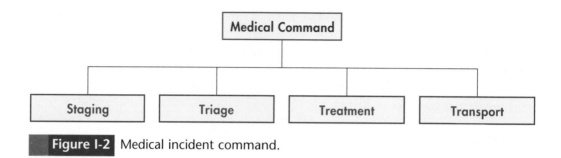

Figure I-2 Medical incident command.

4. Ensures law enforcement involvement as necessary.
5. Ensures that helicopter landing zone operations are coordinated.
6. Determines the amount and types of additional medical resources and supplies.
7. Ensures that area hospitals and Medical Direction are aware of the situation so they can prepare for casualties.
8. Designates assistance officers and their location.
9. Maintains an appropriate span of control.
10. Works as a conduit of communications between subordinates and the Incident Commander.

EMS Staging Officer

1. Maintains a log of available units and medical supplies.
2. Coordinates physical location of incoming resources (i.e., ambulances and helicopters).
3. Coordinates incoming personnel who wish to aid at the scene.
4. Provides updates to Medical Command as necessary.

Triage Officer

1. Ensures proper utilization of the Initial Assessment triage system or other local protocol.
2. Ensures that triage tags or other visual identification technique is properly completed and secured to the patient.
3. Makes requests for additional resources through Medical Command.
4. Provides updates to Medical Command as necessary.

Treatment Officer

1. Establishes suitable treatment areas.
2. Communicates resource needs to Medical Command.
3. Assigns, supervises, and coordinates treatment of patients.
4. Provides updates to Medical Command as necessary.

Transport Officer

1. Ensures the organized transport of patients off-scene.
2. Ensures an appropriate distribution of patients to all local hospitals to prevent hospital overloading.
3. Completes a transportation log.
4. Contacts receiving hospitals to advise them of the number of patients and condition (may be delegated to a communications officer).
5. Provides updates to Medical Command as necessary.

TRIAGE

As a triage officer, you are to spend less than one minute doing an Initial Assessment to determine the priority of a patient. It cannot be overemphasized that the person doing the triage does *not* render any treatment to a patient. Treatment is to be done by the treatment sector of the MICS. A triage officer who allows himself to begin treatment of victims is no longer a triage officer, and the function of triage must be reassigned. Once the medical priority of a patient has been determined, using the BTLS Triage Decision Tree (Figure I-3), the triage officer should affix an appropriately completed triage tag (Figure I-4) or other visual identification technique to the victim and move on to the next victim to be assessed.

Typically, Patients Are Prioritized into Four Categories:

Priority 1: Red tagged—Critical condition, unstable but salvageable (load-and-go)

Priority 2: Yellow tagged—Serious condition, potentially unstable

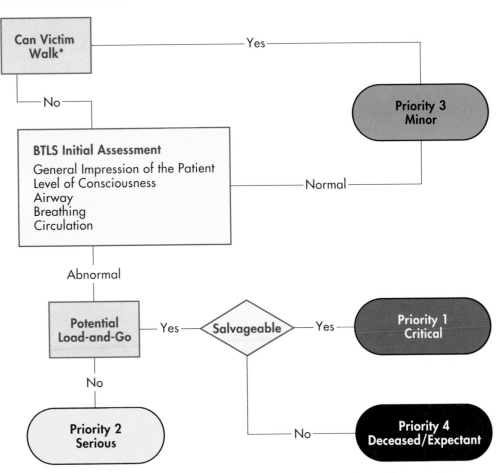

Scene Size-Up
Body Substance Isolation Precautions (PPE)
Scene Hazards
Number of Patients
Need for More Help or Equipment
Mechanism of Injury

Can Victim Walk* ──Yes──

──No──

BTLS Initial Assessment
General Impression of the Patient
Level of Consciousness
Airway
Breathing
Circulation

──Normal──

Priority 3 Minor

Abnormal

Potential Load-and-Go ──Yes── **Salvageable** ──Yes── **Priority 1 Critical**

No

Priority 2 Serious

──No── **Priority 4 Deceased/Expectant**

*In large-scale incidents with a great number of patients, have those who are able walk to a designated area to be assessed.

Figure I-3 BTLS Triage Decision Tree. This decision tree reflects the steps of initial triage. Subsequent and more detailed assessments should occur throughout patient care.

Priority 3: Green tagged—Stable condition, minor injuries, "walking wounded"

Priority 4: Black tagged—Dead or alive, but nonsalvageable*

INITIAL ASSESSMENT

Although there is a tendency to overtriage, one must refrain from this because of its impact on the resources available to the EMS system. We need to be as accurate in our triage assessment as possible.

Three basic human systems need to be quickly evaluated to determine the patient's medical priority:

1. Respiratory system.
2. Circulatory system.
3. Neurological system (LOC).

By utilizing the BTLS Initial Assessment during the triage phase and the Rapid Trauma Assessment or the Focused Assessment in the treatment phase, we will be accurate in our assessment and make the best use of resources by providing the greatest amount of good to the greatest number of patients.

General Impression (Patient Overview)

Victim's approximate age?

What position is he in?

What is his activity (aware of surroundings, anxious, in distress)?

Does he have adequate perfusion (skin color)?

Are there any major injuries or bleeding?

Level of Consciousness
Airway

Is it open and self maintained?

Is it compromised?

Breathing

Is the victim breathing?

What is the rate and quality?

Circulation

Is there a pulse?

What is the rate and quality?

Once the Initial Assessment has been completed and you have figured in a "survivability factor," you have a good idea how to prioritize the patient. An example of applying the survivability factor would be if you were presented with a geriatric patient and a pediatric patient with similar critical injuries and you only have enough resources for one. Which one do you choose, and why? The decision should be based on objective evaluations rather than emotions.

SPECIAL CONSIDERATIONS
Injured Rescuers

Many ICSs provide a separate medical component at the scene of the incident for the care and treatment of the rescuers. Structurally, this sector is part of the logistics component

---

*Some EMS systems will group the "alive but onsalvageable" patients in the Priority 1 category and work on them as long as resources are available and it does not take away from the needed resources for a salvageable patient.

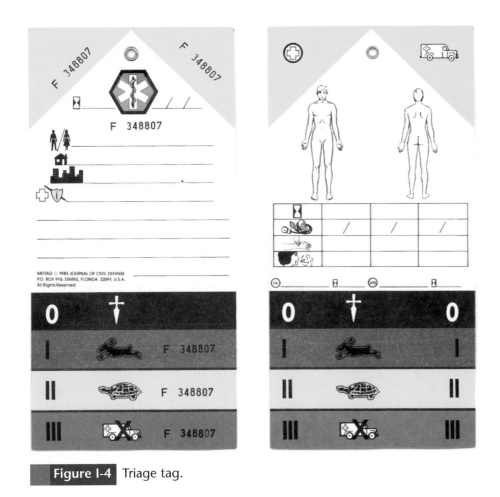

Figure I-4 Triage tag.

of a large ICS structure. In the event of illness or injury to one of our colleagues, we need to be assured that they will not fall into the triage system of the victims of the incident. We are obligated to take care of our own. This will enable our fallen colleague to return to duty quicker and help the overall operation by providing the remaining rescuers the peace of mind of knowing that their fellow rescuer has not been forgotten.

Standard of Care

When reviewing the care of a patient of an MCI, we have to consider the adverse circumstances EMS was operating under at the time of the incident. During normal day-to-day operations, standard protocols treat all patients for the worse case scenario and thus many patients are overtreated. When manpower and resources are available, it is prudent to provide such care. However, when working in an MCI or disaster environment, the inefficient use of manpower and resources may be catastrophic. The guiding principle in triage and treatment of victims of an MCI is to do the greatest good for the greatest number of patients with the least depletion of available resources.

Critique and Debriefing

The management of all MCIs and disasters should be formally critiqued. Primary focus should be on what worked and what did not. An MCI/Disaster Plan is a dynamic document, modified when there is a problem. In addition to taking time to critique the incident, time must also be taken to provide Critical Incident Stress Debriefing (CISD) for the participants of an incident. The mental health of EMS professionals is as important as their physical health.

SUMMARY

The priorities of any incident, no matter how small or large, should be safety, organization, and then patient care. To provide the most effective and efficient patient care, one must approach it in a safe and organized fashion.

To have an effective MICS requires its use in day-to-day operations, including the routine, small emergencies. The rehearsal of the MICS on smaller situations will develop proficiency and allow for a smooth transition into the larger, more complex incidents. Activating the MICS only when an incident reaches a high level can result in a lack of familiarity with its use. Routine activation of the system develops confidence in its use for all levels of command and agencies involved. To avoid the paper plan syndrome, the regular implementation and review of an MCI/Disaster Plan is paramount to having successful operations.

A MICS is not a magic wand that will save lives by itself, nor will it replace the common sense and good judgment required of experienced EMS professionals. Successful management of a situation still requires properly trained people who know what to do and how to do it. MICS properly utilized can increase the overall effectiveness of the participants by providing a proactive approach to management. If you don't manage the situation, the situation manages you. The key to effective performance in a leadership role is not necessarily rank, but the understanding of the duties of that position and the ability to properly function at that level.

For large-scale incidents an operation may last for days or even weeks and will require additional resources. As part of the disaster plan, an ICS provides the structure for the necessary administrative, planning, financial and logistical support.

MCI Case—Self-Review

SITUATION

A school bus is struck by a car. The bus rolled over with seven people on board. There is one person in the car.

Local EMS Resources

7 ground ambulances available.

1 helicopter available.

2 acute care hospitals in 30-mile radius (one designated Level I trauma center).

1 volunteer fire department with first aid training.

Response Times

Volunteer fire department and first ambulance on scene 11 minutes from time of call.

Additional ambulances on scene 15–20 minutes after first arriving ambulance.

Helicopter on-scene 25 minutes after requested.

Ground transport time to Level I trauma center 25 minutes; 20 minutes for other hospital.

TRIAGE

Review the following initial assessments of the victims. Determine what priority you would make them and discuss your decisions with others. It is not uncommon to have disagreement between EMS personnel. There may not be a single right answer.

(continued)

MCI Case—Self-Review (Continued)

TRIAGE (CONTINUED)

A. 6 y/o Female, still inside bus
   LOC—Unresponsive
   Skin—Cool/pale/moist
   Airway—Partial obstruction
   Breathing—Agonal at 6/min.
   Circulation—Radial pulses absent, carotid approximately 80/min.
   Miscellaneous—Legs pinned under a seat

B. 8 y/o Male, still inside bus
   LOC—A&O33
   Skin—Warm/pale/dry
   Airway—Open, self-maintained
   Breathing—24/min., nonlabored
   Circulation—Radial pulses approximately 80/min.
   Miscellaneous—Deformity to right femur and mangled right hand

C. 10 y/o Female, outside bus sitting against a tree
   LOC—A&O33
   Skin—Warm/normal/dry
   Airway—Open, self-maintained
   Breathing—20/min., nonlabored
   Circulation—Radial pulses approximately 130/min.
   Miscellaneous—Pain right hip, crepitus on right side of pelvis

D. 7 y/o Male, sitting up inside bus, not pinned
   LOC—A&O33 but anxious
   Skin—Warm/pale/dry
   Airway—Open, self-maintained
   Breathing—40/min. with gasping
   Circulation—Radial pulses approximately 100/min.
   Miscellaneous—Chest pain and unable to get his breath. Breath sounds clear.

E. 13 y/o Female, inside bus
   LOC—Unresponsive
   Skin—Cool/pale
   Airway—Extensive facial trauma, not self-maintained
   Breathing—Absent
   Circulation—Absent
   Miscellaneous—Open head injury

F. 9 y/o Female, sitting next to "E" hysterical
   LOC—Alert but hysterical
   Skin—Cool/pale/dry
   Airway—Open, self-maintained
   Breathing—36/min., nonlabored
   Circulation—Radial pulses approximately 120/min.
   Miscellaneous—No obvious signs of injury

(continued)

MCI Case—Self-Review (Continued)

TRIAGE (CONTINUED)

G. 55 y/o Female, restrained bus driver. She is trying to help the children
LOC—A&O33
Skin—Warm/normal/dry
Airway—Open, self-maintained
Breathing—18/min., nonlabored
Circulation—Radial pulses approximately 90/min.
Miscellaneous—3-inch laceration on forehead with slow bleeding

H. 48 y/o Male, unrestrained driver of the car, strong smell of alcohol on patient
LOC—Alert but confused
Skin—Warm/normal/moist
Airway—Open, self-maintained—slurred speech
Breathing—16/min., nonlabored
Circulation—Radial pulses approximately 100/min.
Miscellaneous—Hematoma on forehead, pupils slow to respond

Glossary

abrasion scraping or abrading away of the superficial layers of the skin; an open soft-tissue injury.

abruptio placenta early separation of the placenta from the uterus.

acidosis a condition caused by accumulation of acid or loss of base from the body.

adventitia the layer of loose connective tissue forming the outermost coating of an organ.

aerobic requiring oxygen.

air bag a passive restraint system in automobiles and other vehicles.

alkalosis a pathologic condition resulting from accumulation of base or loss of acid in the body.

anaerobic lacking oxygen.

anoxia absence of oxygen supply to the tissue.

asphyxia a condition due to lack of oxygen; suffocation.

aspirate taking foreign matter into the lungs during inhalation.

assessment to evaluate the condition of a patient.

ATV all-terrain vehicle.

AVPU a description of the level of consciousness. AVPU stands for: A—**a**lert, V—responds to **v**erbal stimuli, P—responds to **p**ain, U—**u**nresponsive.

avulsion an injury in which a piece of a structure is torn away.

axial loading compression forces applied along the long axis of the body. *Example:* a fall in which a victim lands on his feet and force is transferred up his legs to his back, causing a compression fracture of a lumbar vertebra.

bag-valve mask a system of artificial ventilation in which the oxygen inflow fills a bag that is attached to a mask by a one-way valve.

Battle's sign swelling and discoloration behind the ear caused by a fracture of the base of the skull.

beta agonists medications such as Albuterol that stimulate the beta receptors in the smooth muscles of the bronchi causing bronchodilatation. They are used to treat asthma and bronchospasm.

BIADs blind insertion airway devices, such as the esophageal tracheal Combitube®.

BLS burns, lacerations, swelling. Can also mean basic life support.

body surface area (BSA) amount of a patient's body affected by a burn.

bronchospasm contraction of the smooth muscle of the bronchi.

Broselow tape a tape used to estimate the weight of a child by measuring her length.

BSI body substance isolation. A procedure used to prevent being contaminated by a patient's body fluids. This usually entails gloves and possibly a gown and face shield.

BVM (bag-valve mask) a system of artificial ventilation in which the oxygen inflow fills a bag that is attached to a mask by a one-way valve.

caliber the diameter of a bullet expressed in hundredths of an inch (.22 caliber = 0.22 inches); the inside diameter of the barrel of a handgun or a rifle.

capillary blanch or refill test for impairment of circulation: pressure on tip of the nail will cause the bed to turn white, if it does not turn pink again by the time it takes to say "capillary refill," the circulation is impaired. The test has been found to be unreliable for early shock.

carbonaceous sputum sputum that is "sooty" or black.

carbon dioxide monitor a device used to monitor or confirm endotracheal tube placement by measuring expired carbon dioxide. These devices either measure expired carbon dioxide (capnographic) or show a color change when carbon dioxide is present (colorimetric).

carina the lowest part of the trachea, where the trachea divides to form the two mainstem bronchi.

catecholamines a group of chemicals of similar structure that act to increase heart rate and blood pressure.

C-collar (cervical collar) a device to limit movement of the neck.

central cord syndrome an injury to the spinal cord that produces more loss of sensory and motor function in the arms than in the legs.

cerebral perfusion blood flow to the brain.

cerebral perfusion pressure (CCP) the pressure moving blood through the brain.

C.N.S. central nervous system; the brain and spinal cord.

CO_2 monitor a device used to monitor or confirm endotracheal tube placement by measuring expired carbon dioxide. These devices either measure expired carbon dioxide (capnographic) or show a color change when carbon dioxide is present (colorimetric).

comminuted fracture fracture in which a bone is broken into several pieces.

compartment syndrome muscle ischemia that is caused by elevated pressure within an anatomic fascial space.

compliance the "give" or elasticity of the lungs and chest wall. This influences how easy it is for the patient to breath.

concussion a jarring injury to the brain resulting in disturbance of brain function.

contracoup an injury to the brain on the opposite side of the original blow.

contralateral situated or affecting the opposite side.

contusion bruising; the reaction of soft tissue to a direct blow.

constricted to shrink or contract.

COPD chronic obstructive pulmonary disease. The end result of asthma, chronic bronchitis, or emphysema.

copious large amount.

coup an injury to the brain on the same side as the original blow.

crepitation feeling of crackling; the sensation of fragments of broken bones rubbing together.

Cushing's reflex a reflex whereby the body reacts to increased pressure on the brain by raising the blood pressure.

DCAP deformities, contusions, abrasions, penetrations.

DCAP-BTLS deformities, contusions, abrasions, penetrations, burns, tenderness, lacerations, swelling.

DCAPP deformities, contusions, abrasions, penetrations, paradoxical movement.

deceleration to come to a sudden stop, decreasing speed.

decubent position the position assumed when lying down.

delivered volume the amount of air that you actually deliver to the lungs with each breath when you perform artificial or assisted ventilation.

denatured to destroy the usual nature of a substance.

dermis the inner layer of the skin, containing hair follicles, sweat glands, sebaceous glands, nerve endings, and blood vessels.

detailed exam a comprehensive head-to-toes exam to find additional injuries that may have been missed in the brief Primary Survey.

diaphoresis to perspire profusely.

diffuse axonal injury type of brain injury characterized by shearing, stretching, or tearing of nerve fibers with subsequent axonal damage and edema of the brain tissue.

diuretic an agent that promotes the excretion of urine.

doll's eyes oculocephalic reflex; a test of brain stem function that is never performed in the prehospital setting.

dura the tough fibrous membrane forming the outermost of the three coverings of the brain.

ecchymoses blue-black discoloration of the skin due to leakage of blood into the tissue.

EGTA esophageal gastric tube airway; an improved esophageal obturator airway.

EMS emergency medical services.

endotracheal intubation the insertion of a tube into the trachea to assist or control ventilation.

EOA esophageal obturator airway.

epidermis the outermost layer of skin.

epidural outside the dura; between the dura and the skull.

erythema general reddening of the skin due to dilation of the superficial capillaries.

ETA estimated time of arrival. An estimation of when you will arrive at the receiving hospital.

etiology the cause of a particular disease.

ET tube endotracheal tube.

evisceration the protruding of internal organs through a wound.

expeditious quick, speedy.

exsanguinate to bleed to death.

extrication removal of a patient from a dangerous position or situation.

FROPVD flow-restricted, oxygen-powered, ventilation device. An artificial ventilation device that provides 100% oxygen at a flow rate of 40 L/min at a maximum pressure of 50 ± 5 cm water.

full-thickness burn third degree burn.

gastric insufflation the filling of the stomach by air when performing positive pressure ventilation.

genioglossus muscle the muscle that pulls the tongue out of the mouth.

grunting a deep, guttural noise made in breathing; a sign of respiratory distress in small children.

GSC (Glasgow Coma Score) A method to measure the severity of injury of a head-injury patient.

Hare splint a type of traction splint.

Heimlich maneuver a method of dislodging food or other material from the throat of a choking victim.

hemiparesis partial paralysis affecting one side of the body.

hemoptysis to spit up blood or blood-stained sputum.

hemothorax the presence of blood in the chest cavity within the pleural space, outside the lung.

hypercarbia high blood carbon dioxide level.

hyperresonant giving an increased vibrant sound on percussion; tympanic.

hypertympany hyperresonant.

hyperventilation increased rate of breathing; >20 breaths per minute for an adult.

hypoventilation decreased rate of breathing, <10 breaths per minute for an adult; insufficient respiration demonstrated by an elevated blood carbon dioxide level.

hypovolemic shock hemorrhagic shock; shock caused by insufficient blood or fluid within the body.

hypoxia a deficiency of oxygen reaching the tissues of the body.

ICP intracranial pressure. The pressure inside the skull.

impaled object a penetrating object that is still in place in a patient's body.

Initial Assessment part of the Primary Survey. This is a rapid exam of airway, breathing and circulation. It is performed on all patients.

intra-abdominal within the abdomen.

intracranial within the skull.

intrathoractic within the chest.

ipsilateral situated on or affecting the same side.

JVD jugular vein distention. Distended jugular veins in the neck.

kinematics the phase of mechanics that deals with possible motions of the body.

labial angle corner of the mouth.

laryngeal mask airway (LMA) An invasive airway device to assist ventilation.

lateral decubitus position position assumed when lying on one's side.

lesion an injury or abnormal condition of a part.

LMA laryngeal mask airway. An invasive airway device to assist ventilation.

LOC level of consciousness.

MAP mean arterial blood pressure.

MAST military antishock trousers. Also called pneumatic antishock garment (PASG). A device that applies circumferential pressure to the legs and abdomen to raise the blood pressure in hypotensive patients.

MCI multiple casualty incident. An emergency situation in which there are multiple injured patients.

mean arterial blood pressure diastolic blood pressure plus 1/3 (systolic minus the diastolic blood pressure).

medial toward the middle.

minute volume the volume of air breathed in and out in 1 minute. This varies from 5 to 12 liters per minute.

mortality frequency of death or death rate.

MVC motor vehicle collision.

nasopharyngeal airway an artificial airway positioned in the nasal cavity.

necrosis the death of tissue.

neonate newborn infant.

nonrebreather mask an oxygen mask that allows the patient to breath oxygen at a concentration close to 100%

NP airway nasopharyngeal airway. An artificial airway positioned in the nasal cavity.

occult injuries injuries hidden or concealed from view.

OPIM other potentially infectious material (cerebrospinal fluid, synovial fluid, amniotic fluid, pericardial fluid, pleural fluid, or any fluid with gross visible blood).

oropharyngeal airway an artificial airway positioned in the oral cavity to keep the tongue from occluding the airway

osteomyelitis inflammation or infection of a bone or bones.

pallor paleness, absence of skin color.

palpate to examine by touch.

paradoxical motion the motion of the injured segment of a flail chest, opposite to the normal motion of the chest wall.

parenchymal the essential elements of an organ.

paresis slight or incomplete paralysis.

paresthesia abnormal sensation; a "tingling" sensation.

partial-thickness burn a burn that does not injure the full thickness of the skin. A first degree burn involves only the epidermal layer. A second degree burn involves the epidermis and part of the dermis.

PASG pneumatic antishock garment. Also called military antishock trousers (MAST). A device that applies circumferential pressure to the legs and abdomen to raise the blood pressure in hypotensive patients.

patent open.

pathophysiology the basic processes of the disease.

perfusion the passage of blood or fluid through the vessels of an organ.

personal watercraft (PWC) a small motorized watercraft that one or two persons can ride. Much like a motorcycle except it travels on water.

pia mater innermost of the three layers of tissue that envelop the brain.

placenta previa an abnormal location of the placenta, so that it covers the opening of the uterus (cervical os).

PMS pulse, motor, sensory. Description of the exam of an injured extremity

pneumothorax the presence of air within the chest cavity in the pleural space, but outside the lung (collapsed lung).

pocket mask a small face mask for performing assisted ventilation. It is made to be carried in the rescuer's pocket.

potential space a space that does not exist except under abnormal circumstances. *Example:* Normally the lungs completely fill the chest cavity so that the pleural space (between the lungs and the chest wall) is only a potential space. If the pleural space contains blood it is a hemothorax.

PPE personal protection equipment such as gloves, face shields, and impervious gowns.

primary survey a brief exam to find immediately life-threatening conditions. It is made up of the Initial Assessment and either the Rapid Trauma Survey or the Focused Exam.

pulse oximeter a noninvasive device that monitors the oxygen saturation of the blood hemoglobin.

pulse pressure the sensation given by the heart contraction to the palpating finger on an artery.

raccoon's eyes swelling and discoloration around both eyes; a late sign of basilar skull fracture.

respiratory reserve lung tissue over and above the body's need to provide oxygenation for the body.

rhabdomyolysis disintegration (lysis) or dissolution of muscle; this releases myoglobin into the blood, which can precipitate in the kidneys, causing renal failure.

RTSS radio telephone switch station; a type of radio that accesses the telephone lines.

Sager splint a type of traction splint.

SAMPLE history the least amount of information needed on a trauma patient. S—symptoms, A—allergies, M—medications, P—past medical history, L—last oral intake (last meal), E—events preceding the injury.

scaphoid shaped like a boat. When used to describe the abdomen, scaphoid means sunken in.

scuba diver a diver who is able to remain under water by breathing compressed air from a breathing apparatus needing no connection with the surface. SCUBA stands for self-contained underwater breathing apparatus.

Sellick maneuver a maneuver (posterior pressure on the cricoid cartilage) to prevent gastric insufflation and vomiting.

sheering forces forces that occur in such a direction to cause tearing of an organ.

sibling brother or sister.

skin diver a diver who holds his breath when swimming under water. He uses no artificial breathing methods.

SMR spinal motion restriction; the act of stabilizing the spinal column to prevent as much motion as possible.

snoring to breathe in a hoarse, rough noise, usually with the mouth open.

snorkeler a diver who uses a short tube (snorkel) in order to float on the surface and observe underwater life. When diving, a snorkeler must hold her breath.

spontaneous pnemothorax collapsed lung caused by the rupture of a congenitally weak area on the surface of the lung.

stridor breathing that has a high-pitched, harsh noise; a sign of impending airway obstruction.

stroke volume the amount of blood pumped by the heart in one beat.

subcutaneous emphysema the presence of air in soft tissues, giving a very characteristic crackling sensation on palpation; the Rice Krispies feeling.

tachypnea adult respiratory rate of 24 or more breaths per minute.

tamponade compression of a part of the anatomy, as the compression of heart by pericardial fluid.

TBI traumatic brain injury.

tension pneumothorax a condition in which air continuously leaks out of the lung into the pleural space, increasing pressure within the space with every breath the patient takes.

Thomas' splint a type of traction splint.

TIC Tenderness, Instability, Crepitation. An acronym for the description of the exam of a bony area.

tidal volume the amount of air that is inspired and expired during one respiratory cycle.

traction the action of drawing or pulling on an object.

trajectory the direction a missile takes in flight or after striking a body.

transected to cut transversely.

Trendelenburg position patient supine with lower body elevated about 30 degrees.

vallecula the space between the base of the tongue and the epiglottis.

vasomotor affecting the size of a blood vessel.

venous pressure pressure of the blood in the veins.

viscera any large interior organ in any one of the three great cavities of the body, especially the abdomen.

volatile a substance that evaporates rapidly at room temperature when exposed to air.

wheezing whistling sounds made in breathing; a sign of spasm or narrowing of the bronchi.

Index